Core Concepts in Renal Transplantation

Anil Chandraker • Mohamed H. Sayegh
Ajay K. Singh
Editors

Core Concepts in Renal Transplantation

Springer

Editors
Anil Chandraker, MB, FASN, FRCP
Harvard Medical School, Renal Division
Brigham and Women's Hospital
Francis Street 75
Boston, MA 02115, USA
achandraker@partners.org

Mohamed H. Sayegh, MD
Harvard Medical School, Renal Division
Brigham and Women's Hospital
Francis Street 75
Boston, MA 02115, USA
msayegh@rics.bwh.harvard.edu

Ajay K. Singh, MB, FRCP(UK)
Harvard Medical School, Renal Division
Brigham and Women's Hospital
Francis Street 75
Boston, MA 02115, USA
asingh@rics.bwh.harvard.edu

ISBN 978-1-4899-8943-7 ISBN 978-1-4614-0008-0 (eBook)
DOI 10.1007/978-1-4614-0008-0
Springer New York Dordrecht Heidelberg London

Softcover re-print of the Hardcover 1st edition 2012

Printed on acid-free paper

Springer is part of Springer Science+Business Media (www.springer.com)

This book is dedicated to my parents Khetram and Draupadi Chandraker for all the years of love and support.

Preface

Over the last few years there have been many changes in the field of transplantation. This book aims to summarize these changes and is meant for both the nephrologist and the nonspecialist with an interest in kidney transplantation. All of the chapters provide up-to-date information on the various aspects of transplantation, from basic immunobiology to medical care of the transplant recipient.

The first successful kidney transplant, conducted over 50 years ago, dramatically changed the face of medicine. It helped spur development in the areas of nephrology, immunology, drug development, and surgery. It also helped develop transplantation as a treatment for chronic diseases for other organ systems such as heart, lung, liver, and pancreas among others. Historically, the technical ability to transplant a kidney preceded the ability to suppress the immune response against foreign tissue; in fact the way in which the immune system targeted the transplanted kidney was poorly understood at the time of the first kidney transplant.

Even though kidney transplantation is now viewed as a routine procedure, the field remains very fluid, with innovations leading to continuous improvements in care. The number of living kidney donors has overtaken the number of cadaveric transplants carried out within the United States. The importance of protecting the living donor's health while allowing the benefit of transplantation to the recipient has led to greater emphasis on how we should be following our potential living donors.

Our understanding of transplant immunobiology has increased dramatically recently, with a better understanding of how the immune system is activated and responds to the allograft. This understanding has been translated into development of biologic agents, such as those targeted to block T cell co-stimulation, with the idea of suppressing the alloimmune response without the broad toxic side effects of conventional immunosuppressive medications. The introduction of new induction agents has also allowed the development of novel immunosuppression avoidance strategies, for example steroid avoidance, once thought impossible for safe transplantation in kidney recipients, to become commonplace. Key developments that have helped with immunosuppressive modulation have been in the area of tissue histocompatibility testing. This area has dramatically changed with the introduction of the solid phase antibody screening using technology such as luminex assays.

These technological advances have allowed better recognition and diagnosis of antibody-mediated rejection and shown that anti-HLA antibodies are a common cause of acute and chronic graft dysfunction. This particular field remains a very exciting area that is likely to see the development of new diagnostic and therapeutic advances over the next several years.

As we use more powerful immunosuppression, the risk of infectious complications increases; the discovery of new pathogens along with the implications for kidney transplant recipients is an expanding area, and screening for infection and use of prophylaxis antimicrobials remain an important part of posttransplant care of recipients. It is our hope that this book will be a useful resource for practicing physicians and provide relevant and timely information on care of the transplant recipient.

Boston, MA, USA Anil Chandraker

Contents

Contributors

Daniel C. Brennan, MD Department of Internal Medicine, Renal Division, Washington University in St. Louis, St. Louis, MO, USA

Mark D. Denton, MD, PhD Renal Unit, Beaumont Hospital, Beaumont Road, Dublin, Ireland

Erik R. Dubberke, MD, MSPH Department of Medicine, Washington University School of Medicine, St. Louis, MO, USA

Steven Gabardi, PharmD Department of Medicine, Renal Division, Brigham and Women's Hospital and Harvard Medical School, Boston, MA, USA

Austin Hunt, MBChB Renal Unit, Derriford Hospital, Plymouth, England, UK

Julie Lin, MD, MPH Department of Medicine, Renal Division, Brigham and Women's Hospital and Harvard Medical School, Boston, MA, USA

Colm C. Magee, MD, MPH FRCPI Beaumont Hospital, Dublin, Ireland

Sayeed K. Malek, MD Division of Transplant Surgery, Brigham and Women's Hospital, Boston, MA, USA

Martina M. McGrath, MB, BAO, BCh Renal Division, Brigham and Women's Hospital, Boston, MA, USA

Mario F. Rubin, MD Massachusetts General Hospital, Boston, MA, USA

Eric M. Tichy, PharmD Department of Pharmacy, Yale New Haven Hospital, New Haven, CT, USA

Kathryn J. Tinckam, MD, MMSc, FRCPC Department of Medicine, University Health Network, University of Toronto, Toronto, ON, Canada

Stefan G. Tullius, MD, PhD Division of Transplant Surgery, Brigham and Women's Hospital, Boston, MA, USA

John Vella, MD, FRCP, FACP, FASN Department of Medicine/Nephrology and Transplantation, Maine Medical Center, Portland, ME, USA

Melissa Yeung, MD, FRCPC Renal Division, Transplantation Research Center, Brigham and Women's Hospital, Boston, MA, USA

Chapter 1
Transplantation Immunobiology

Melissa Yeung

Abstract Our immune system has evolved into an intricate system to protect us from invading microbes while maintaining its ability to recognize self. The very nature of its design limits the success of transplantation since the recipient recognizes the transplanted organ as foreign and mounts a robust response to target it. There are two arms of the immune system: innate (or natural) immunity and adaptive immunity. The innate immune system is evolutionarily older and does not require the recognition of specific antigens. Nonspecific recruitment of macrophages, neutrophils, natural killer cells, and the complement system provides a rapidly activated first line of defense when damage or infection is encountered. In contrast, the highly sophisticated adaptive immune system involves a more efficient recognition of specific pathogens and is able to generate immunological memory. Adaptive immunity is characterized by the involvement of T cells in cell-mediated immune response and B cells in the humoral response.

Keywords Allorecognition • Major histocompatibility complex • T cells • B cells • Tolerance

Our immune system has evolved into an intricate system that protects us from invading microbes while maintaining its ability to recognize self. The very nature of its design limits the success of transplantation since the recipient recognizes the transplanted organ as foreign and mounts a robust response to target it.

There are two arms of the immune system: innate (or natural) immunity and adaptive immunity. The innate immune system is evolutionarily older and does not

M. Yeung, MD, FRCPC (✉)
Renal Division, Transplantation Research Center,
Brigham and Women's Hospital, Boston, MA, USA
e-mail: myeung@partners.org

A. Chandraker et al. (eds.), *Core Concepts in Renal Transplantation*,
DOI 10.1007/978-1-4614-0008-0_1, © Springer Science+Business Media, LLC 2012

require the recognition of specific antigens. Nonspecific recruitment of macrophages, neutrophils, natural killer cells, and the complement system provides a rapidly activated first line of defense when damage or infection is encountered. In contrast, the highly sophisticated adaptive immune system involves a more efficient recognition of specific pathogens and is able to generate immunological memory. Adaptive immunity is characterized by the involvement of T cells in cell-mediated immune response and B cells in the humoral response. The components of the immune system do not function exclusively and often work in concert with one another. For example, antigen-specific T cell activation leads to production of cytokines that recruit innate immune cells, assists B cells production of alloantibody, and generates $CD8^+$ T cell-mediated cytotoxicity.

Allorecognition

The process of how immune cells recognize transplanted grafts was first described by Snell and Gorer in a skin transplant model between strains of inbred mice [1]. When donor and recipient were of the same strain, the *syngeneic* graft was not rejected. However, when donor and recipient were of different strains, the *allogeneic* graft was rejected. These observations led to the identification of the major histocompatibility complex (MHC) as the locus of polymorphic genes encoding the key antigenic determinants of graft rejection. In humans, the MHC locus is found on the short arm of chromosome 6 and their protein products are known as human leukocyte antigens (HLA). There are two types of MHC molecules: class I and class II molecules. In humans, class I genes include HLA-A, HLA-B, and HLA-C. The class II genes are HLA-DP, HLA-DQ, and HLA-DR.

MHC class I molecules are comprised of a polymorphic α(alpha) chain and a nonpolymorphic β(beta)2-microglobulin chain, and are expressed on all nucleated cells. MHC class II molecules consist of a polymorphic α(alpha) chain and a polymorphic β(beta) chain and are constitutively expressed only on antigen-presenting cells (APCs) such as dendritic cells, B cells, and macrophages. They can, however, be upregulated on a variety of other cell types including endothelial and epithelial cells in inflammatory conditions [2]. Both classes of MHC antigens possess a peptide-binding groove. The specific amino acid sequence within this groove determines which specific peptide can bind for presentation to T cells. Class I molecules bind shorter peptides that are usually derived intracellularly, such as viral proteins, whereas class II molecules bind longer extracellular peptides that have been brought into the cell via endocytosis. They are both stably expressed on the cell surface when bound with peptide and are readily upregulated by a variety of proinflammatory cytokines. This enables constant, repeated antigen presentation in areas of inflammation. In the absence of infection or foreign allograft, MHC antigens may present self-peptides as a way of maintaining peripheral tolerance to self.

MHC molecules are polymorphic and able to express any one of hundreds of different molecules, with more than 1,600 different alleles presently documented in humans [3]. Clearly, there is evolutionary benefit to having extensive MHC polymorphism since it allows for a wide variety of microbial peptides to be bound and presented to T cells. However, in the context of transplantation, this polymorphic property becomes detrimental since matching of donor and recipient at each of the MHC loci (HLA in humans) is more difficult. The corollary is that the greater the degree of HLA matching between donor and recipient, the less likely the allograft will reject. Unfortunately, this polymorphism also increases an individual's likelihood of developing alloantibodies, which can occur with exposure to nonself HLAs through blood transfusions, pregnancy, or previous transplantation (sensitization).

Non-HLA Antigens

Although HLA mismatch is the major barrier to allogeneic transplantation, graft rejection (whether acute or chronic) can still occur despite identical HLA between donor and recipient. ABO antigens (see "ABO incompatibility" below) represent the most common non-HLA antigen, and the chance that any two individuals in the United States will be ABO incompatible is 35% [4]. However, despite ABO matching, it has been reported that 38% of deceased donor graft failures could be attributable to immunological reactions against other non-HLA factors [5]. Growing appreciation for this phenomenon has led to the identification of a plethora of non-HLA antigens including minor histocompatibility (mH) antigens, vascular endothelial receptors, and adhesion molecules.

Minor antigens are derived from various endogenous proteins that exhibit genetic polymorphisms between individuals. They are recognized as peptides bound to self-MHC and elicit a class I restricted $CD8^+$ cytolytic T cell response [6]. Over 40 mH antigen differences have been identified in mouse inbred strains and in murine models of skin and cardiac transplantation; these differences can lead to rapid rejection of the allograft [7–9]. In human hematopoietic stem cell transplantation (HSCT), HLA-matched but mH antigen-mismatched transplants show higher rates of graft rejection and graft-versus-host disease (GVHD) [10, 11]. Perhaps the most important human mH antigens are HA-1 and HY. HA-1, whose function is unknown, exists in two allelic forms. T cells recognize one HA-1 variant through its association with HLA A2, but cannot recognize the second variant because it is unable to bind with HLA A2. While mH antigens appear to be important in HSCT, their role in solid organ transplantation remains less well defined. Some have found an association of HA-1 mismatches with chronic rejection and reduced graft survival rates [12]; others have failed to demonstrate this effect [13].

MHC class I polypeptide-related sequences A (MICA) and B (MICB) have also garnered increasing attention as non-HLA target antigens in acute and chronic allograft rejection [14, 15]. MICA and MICB are highly polymorphic genes that are located near the HLA-B locus. They encode for cell-surface glycoproteins that are expressed constitutively on endothelial cells, fibroblasts, and monocytes and upregulated on lymphocytes upon stimulation [16]. In contrast to mH antigens, the effector mechanism involved in MICA/MICB-related rejection appears to be antibody mediated. Other non-HLA antigens that have been implicated in rejection include vimentin (expressed on endothelial cells), ICAM-1 (intercellular adhesion molecule-1), and AT_1R (angiotensin type 1 receptor) [16].

ABO Incompatability

ABO blood group antigens are cell surface glycosphingolipids initially identified as the targets on red blood cells leading to blood transfusion reactions. They are recognized by "hemagglutinins," natural antibodies that cause red cell agglutination. These antibodies develop in response to carbohydrate antigens expressed by bacteria that colonize our intestines. All individuals have a common core O antigen with an attached H antigen. The ability of an individual's glycosyltransferase enzyme to modify this H antigen determines their blood type. Individuals homozygous for the O allele of the enzyme produce a protein that lacks enzymatic activity while individuals who possess the A allele have an enzyme capable of glycosylating the H antigen to produce the A antigen, and those who possess the B allele form the B antigen. It turns out that ABO antigens are also expressed on other cell types such as endothelial cells, and hemagglutinins can cause hyperacute rejection via recognition of the graft vascular endothelium. In current practice, hyperacute rejection because of ABO mismatch is extremely rare because donor and recipient pairs are matched for ABO blood type. In addition, desensitization protocols have been successfully employed to allow for transplantation across ABO barriers in living donation [17, 18].

Alloimmune Response

Alloantigen Presentation

The first step in the alloimmune response involves the encounter between T cells and transplant antigens. Recipient T cells can respond to donor MHC peptides in two distinct, but not mutually exclusive, manners. The first is via direct allorecognition, where recipient T cells recognize intact MHC–peptide complexes on donor cells. These cells can be donor APCs that are transferred within the graft or graft endothelial cells. Graft endothelial cells express MHC class I, but can upregulate MHC class II expression in the context of inflammation [2]. The second pathway is through indirect allorecognition. In this case, donor MHC molecules are shed from their cell surface, taken up by recipient APCs, processed and presented as peptides on recipient MHC molecules. This second pathway is analogous to the physiologic antigen recognition that occurs with microbial exposure. In contrast, direct allorecognition is unique to transplantation and thought to be the predominant pathway in early alloimmune response.

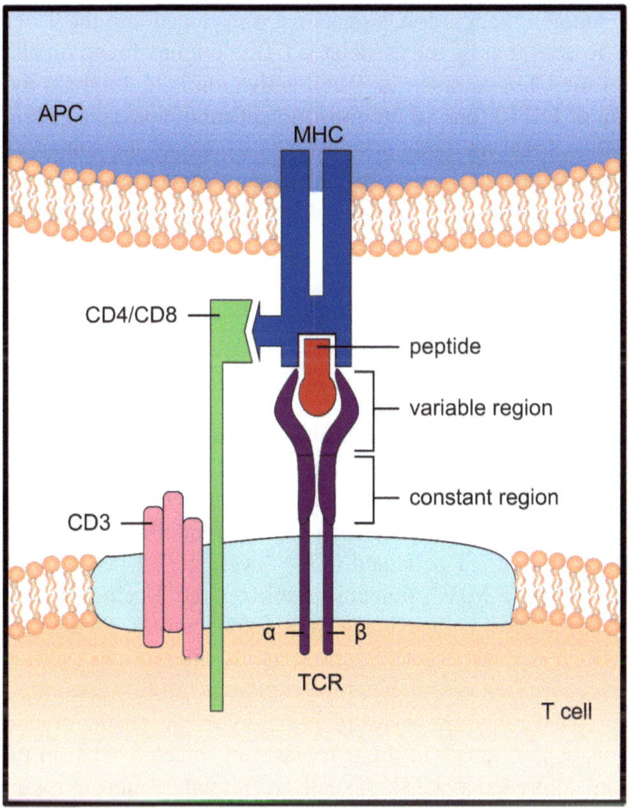

Fig. 1.1 T cell receptor (TCR). T cells recognize the MHC–peptide complex through the TCR, which is a heterodimer composed of two transmembrane polypeptide chains (α(alpha) and β(beta)). Each of these polypeptide chains has a variable and a constant region. Hypervariable regions within the variable region allow for T cells with differing TCRs to recognize a diverse set of MHC–peptide complexes. Following antigen recognition, signals are transduced into the T cell cytoplasm by the CD3 complex with the aid of the CD4/CD8 coreceptor

T-Cell Receptor

Regardless of whether it is through the direct/indirect pathway, recipient T cells recognize the MHC–peptide complex through the T cell receptor (TCR) (Fig. 1.1). The TCR is a heterodimer composed of two transmembrane polypeptide chains (α(alpha) and β(beta)) which are covalently linked by a disulfide bridge. Each of these polypeptide chains has a variable (V) and a constant (C) domain. Within the V regions of each of the α(alpha) and β(beta) chains are short stretches of amino acids where the variability between different TCRs is concentrated. These are known as the hypervariable or complementarity-determining regions (CDRs) and allow for T cells with differing TCRs to recognize a diverse set of MHC–peptide complexes.

Following antigen recognition, signals are transduced into the T cell cytoplasm not by the TCR itself, but by the associated CD3 complex found on all T cells. The importance of the CD3 complex in T cell activation is highlighted by the mechanism of action of OKT3, one of the most potent immunosuppressive medications. OKT3 is a monoclonal antibody which binds to one of the subunits of the CD3 complex, leading to destabilization and subsequent endocytosis of the TCR. Loss of the TCR from the cell surface inhibits activation and renders the T cell ineffective in generating an immune response.

CD4/CD8 Coreceptors

In addition to the CD3 complex, T cells also express other membrane receptors that aid in their response. CD4 and CD8 are transmembrane proteins that bind to non-polymorphic regions of MHC class II and class I molecules, respectively. Mature T cells express either CD4 or CD8 and their expression defines the two major subsets of T cells: $CD4^+$ "helper" T cells and $CD8^+$ "cytotoxic" T cells. Binding of CD4/CD8 to their respective MHC molecule stabilizes the T-cell/APC immunological synapse and facilitates signaling by the TCR/CD3 complex. Physiologically, $CD4^+$ "helper" T cells function in host defense against microbes that have either been ingested by macrophages or that need to be recognized by antibodies to be eradicated. $CD8^+$ cytotoxic T lymphocytes (CTLs) serve to eliminate infections by intracellular organisms that reside in the cytoplasm of infected cells. In the context of transplantation, alloreactive $CD4^+$ T cells differentiate into cytokine-producing effector cells that cause injury to the graft through reactions that resemble delayed-type hypersensitivity (DTH). $CD8^+$ T cells activated by the direct pathway differentiate into CTLs that kill nucleated cells in the graft, all of which express allogeneic class I MHC molecules. The $CD8^+$ CTLs that are generated by the indirect pathway are self MHC restricted and, as such, they cannot directly kill the foreign cells in the graft. Because of this, it has been suggested that $CD8^+$ CTLs induced by direct allorecognition are most important for acute recognition of allografts, whereas $CD4^+$ effector T cells stimulated by the indirect pathway play a greater role in chronic rejection.

Costimulatory Molecules

T cells require two distinct signals for full activation [19, 20]. The first is the aforementioned binding of the TCR with the MHC–peptide complex. The second signal occurs with engagement of "costimulatory" molecules found on the surface of T cells with their specific ligands on APCs (Fig. 1.2). Without costimulation, signaling through the TCR alone usually leads to death by apoptosis and/or a state of unresponsiveness known as anergy. It is now clear that in addition to provision of

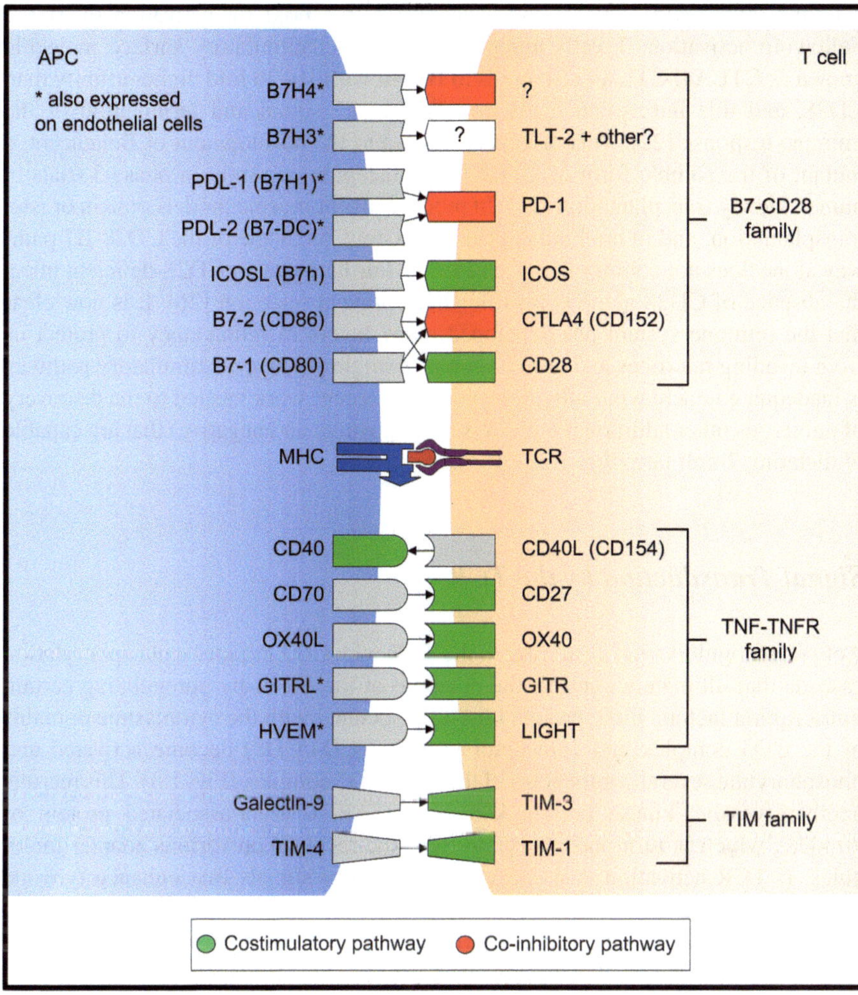

Fig. 1.2 T cell costimulatory molecules. T cells require costimulatory signals for full activation. This figure shows positive/costimulatory (*green*) and negative/coinhibitory (*red*) pathways. The receptor–ligand pairs of these pathways belong to one of three families: B7-CD28 family; tumor necrosis factor–tumor necrosis factor receptor (TNF-TNFR) family; and the T cell immunoglobulin mucin domain (TIM) family

positive signals to promote T cell activation, costimulatory pathways can also provide negative signals that terminate or attenuate immune responses [21]. The net balance of these signals determines T cell outcome and, ultimately, the fate of the allograft.

The best characterized costimulatory pathway is the CD28:B7–1/B7–2 pathway. CD28 is constitutively expressed on the surface of all $CD4^+$ and ~50% of $CD8^+$ T lymphocytes. Its interaction with B7–1 and B7–2 (also known as CD80 and CD86, respectively) on APCs leads to increased transcription of the proinflammatory cytokine interleukin-2 (IL-2) and a decreased threshold for activation of TCRs. Following activation, T cells upregulate another costimulatory surface molecule known as CTLA4. CTLA4 also binds to B7 but with 10–20 fold higher affinity than CD28, and this interaction leads to a "negative" signal and termination of the immune response [22]. This discovery has led to the development of Belatacept, a mutant of the soluble form of CTLA4. Belatacept is currently in phase 3 trials in human kidney transplantation [23]. In more stringent murine models of skin or islet transplantation, and in nonhuman primate models, blockade of the CD28-B7 pathway alone does not confer tolerance [24, 25]. Furthermore, in CD28-deficient mice, the absence of CD28 alone is insufficient to prevent rejection [26]. It is now clear that the immune system has developed many layers of redundancy to protect us from invading microbes and termination of a single positive costimulatory pathway is inadequate in achieving allograft tolerance. Recent work has led to the discovery of numerous other additional pathways (both positive and negative) that are capable of dictating T cell fate (Fig. 1.2) [20].

Signal Transduction by the TCR

Antigen recognition and clustering of the TCR with CD3 initiates a phosphorylation cascade that ultimately controls the outcome of the T cell by upregulating certain transcription factors. First, protein kinases associated with the cytoplasmic domains of the CD3 complex and coreceptor proteins (CD4/CD8) become activated and phosphorylate several components of the TCR/CD3 complex (Fig. 1.3). This recruits another tyrosine kinase protein known as ZAP-70 (zeta-associated protein of 70 kDa), which in turn phosphorylates tyrosine residues on various adapter molecules. If TCR activation is weak, or costimulatory signals that enhance tyrosine kinase activity are absent, ZAP-70 fails to achieve critical threshold and the entire phosphorylation cascade terminates. However, if the threshold is met and adapter molecules are activated, they become docking sites for cellular enzymes that initiate various downstream signaling pathways such as the calcineurin pathway, the protein kinase C (PKC) pathway, and the Ras- and Rac-mitogen activated protein kinase (MAPK) pathways. These different signaling pathways converge to generate transcription factors (such as NFAT, NFκ(kappa)B, and AP-1) that stimulate the transcription of various genes involved in cell cycle initiation, proliferation, and differentiation.

Calcineurin inhibitors work as immune modulators by interrupting one such pathway. Upon TCR engagement, phosphorylation of ZAP-70 leads to phosphorylation of PLCγ1 (phospholipase C γ(gamma)1), which hydrolyzes a membrane phospholipid PIP_2 (phosphatidylinositol 4,5-bisphosphonate) into IP3 (inositol 1,4,-triphosphate) and DAG (diacylglycerol). IP3 formation increases cytosolic calcium, and a calcium–calmodulin complex forms to activate several enzymes including calcineurin. Calcineurin is responsible for dephosphorylating NFAT (nuclear factor of activated T cells), allowing NFAT to translocate from the cytoplasm to the

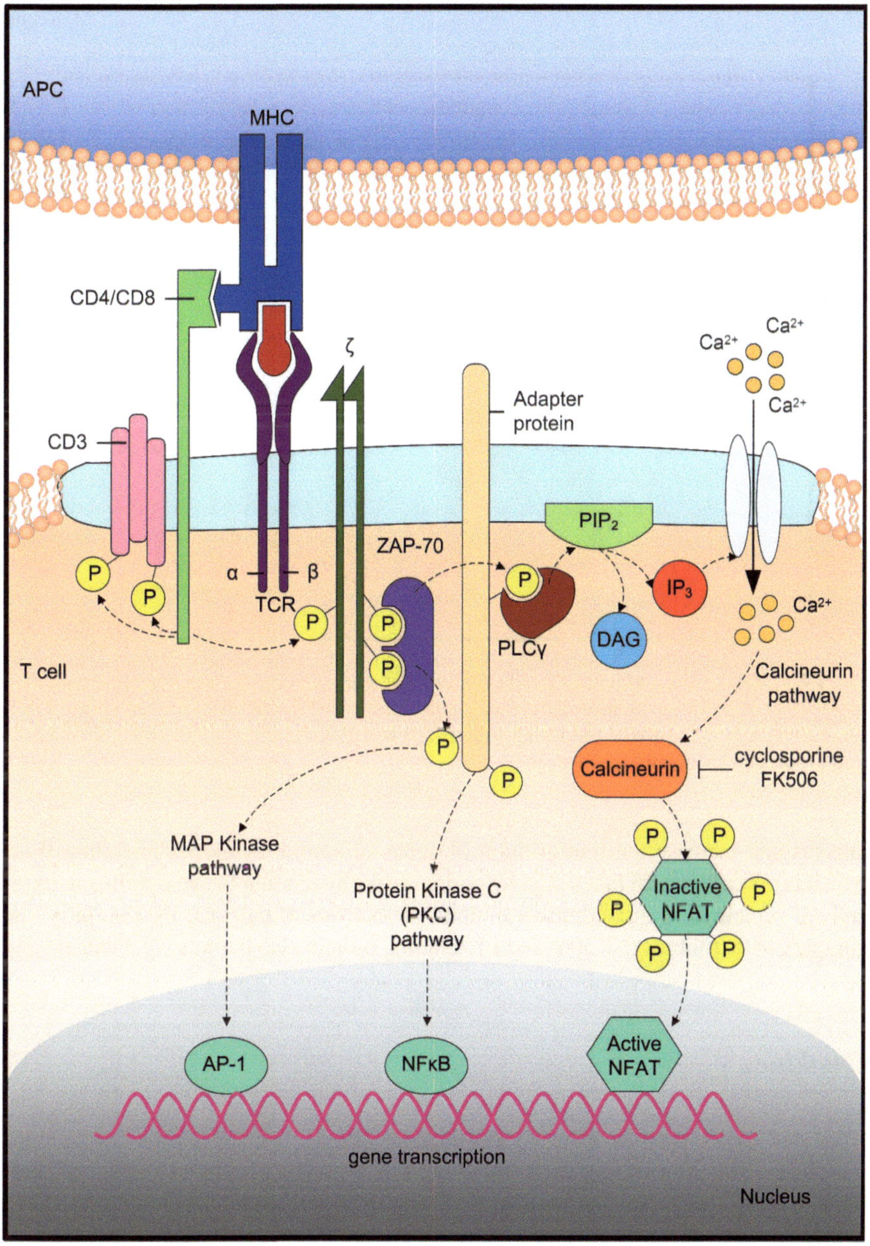

Fig. 1.3 TCR signal transduction. Antigen recognition by the TCR leads to initiation of a phosphorylation cascade. The CD4/CD8 coreceptor phosphorylates CD3 and ζ(zeta) chains. ZAP-70 binds to two phosphotyrosines of the ζ(zeta) chain and, once activated, phosphorylates various adapter molecules including PLCγ(gamma)1. These adapter proteins become docking sites for cellular enzymes that lead to activation of the mitogen-activated protein (MAP) kinase pathway, protein kinase C (PKC) pathway, and calcineurin pathway. These pathways converge to generate transcription factors AP-1 (activavtion protein-1), NFκ(kappa)B (nuclear factor κ(kappa)B), and NFAT (nuclear factor of activated T cells) which lead to gene transcription of various cytokines such as the T cell growth factor IL-2 (interleukin-2)

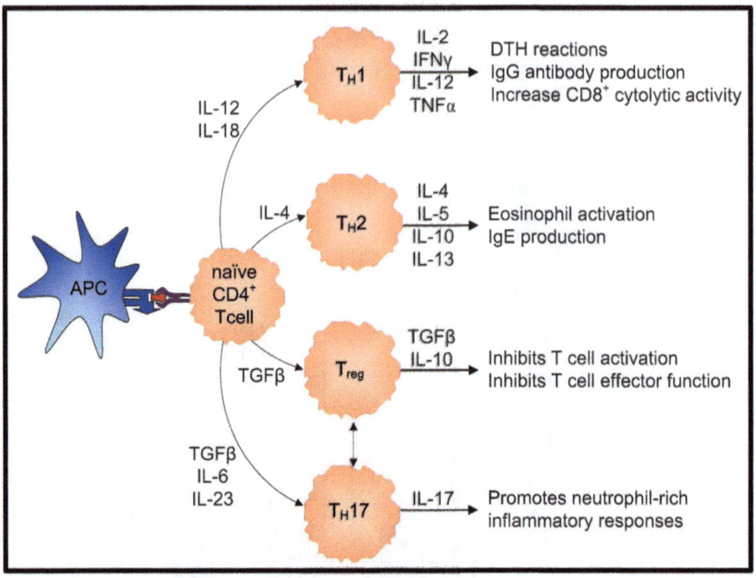

Fig. 1.4 Cytokine-induced helper T cell (T_H) differentiation. T cell activation leads to production of a variety of cytokines that promote differentiation of naïve T cells into various helper T cell subsets with distinct cytokine-producing patterns. Clonal proliferation of these differentiated cells lead to specialized effector mechanisms

nucleus and increase the transcription of genes of several cytokines including IL-2, which is a T cell growth factor. Cyclosporine works by binding to cyclophilin, an intracellular protein, and this complex inhibits the activity of calcineurin. Similarly, the complex of tacrolimus (FK506) and FK-binding protein also inhibits calcineurin.

Cytokines

Activated T cells produce a variety of cytokines (Fig. 1.4) that promote the differentiation of $CD4^+$ T cells into different subsets with distinct cytokine-producing patterns. $CD8^+$ T cells can also undergo a similar differentiation, but their significance is less well defined. Initially, two subsets were identified: Th1 $CD4^+$ T cells which secrete IL-2, IFNγ(gamma), IL-12, and tumor necrosis factor (TNF), and Th2 cells which secrete IL-4, IL-5, IL-10, and IL-13. Th1-associated cytokines stimulate DTH reactions, and promote $CD8^+$ T cell cytolytic activity and production of IgG antibodies capable of opsonization and complement fixation. Th2 cytokines activate eosinophils that stimulate the production of IgE antibody. In transplantation, rejection is thought to be mediated by the Th1 response, whereas a Th2 milieu was thought to be protective since it promoted the presence of "protective" regulatory T cells (see "Tolerance" below) [27]. However, this paradigm appears to be too simplistic.

While reduction of Th1-associated cytokines and promotion of Th2 cytokines does lead to prolonged allograft survival in murine models [27], acute rejection can occur in the absence of Th1 cytokines. For example, IL-2-knockout, IFNγ(gamma)-knockout, and STAT4-knockout mice (deficient in Th1 response) are all capable of rejecting allografts [28–30]. More recently, another subset of IL-17 producing Th17 cells have been identified as effector cells capable of mediating graft rejection [31]. To further complicate the situation, regulatory T cells can de-differentiate and become Th17 cells under certain situations [32]. This complexity and redundancy of the cytokine system, as well as the pleiotrophic effects of each cytokine, likely explains why therapeutic strategies to modulate cytokines have not been fruitful. To date, only blockade of IL-2R has translated into clinical utility, with the development of basiliximab (Simulect) and anti-CD25 monoclonal antibodies that target the IL-2/IL-2R pathway [33, 34].

Chemokines

"Chemoattractant" cytokines or "chemokines" primarily serve to recruit immune cells to sites of inflammation but have also been shown to be involved in development and differentiation of immune cells. They are produced by virtually all somatic cells. Local production creates a chemoattractant gradient to direct leukocyte trafficking through tissues and provides signals that convert the low affinity selectin-mediated leukocyte rolling into the integrin-mediated leukocyte-endothelial adhesion, bringing naïve lymphocytes into contact with antigen. To date, more than 50 chemokines have been identified and many, if not all, have been found at some stage during allograft rejection [35]. In humans, there are 20 known chemokine receptors that are differentially expressed on leukocyte populations and direct the movement or activation of these leukocytes. Each receptor often binds to more than one chemokine ligand. While certain chemokine–chemokine receptor interactions (such as the chemokines that interact with CXCR3 and CCR5 receptors) have major roles in rejection, others appear to have little to contribute [35]. Currently, molecules developed to specifically target these receptors are under investigation. Regretfully, for the most part they have not been an effective strategy in experimental models of transplantation, particularly in the case of fully mismatched allografts and in nonhuman primate models [36].

Effector Mechanisms of Allograft Rejection

Rejection of the transplanted allograft is mediated by both cellular (DTH responses and cell-mediated cytotoxicity) and humoral (antibody-mediated) components of the immune system (Fig. 1.5). In contrast to hyperacute rejection, which is the classical example of antibody-mediated rejection, both acute and chronic rejection can be caused by cellular and/or humoral components.

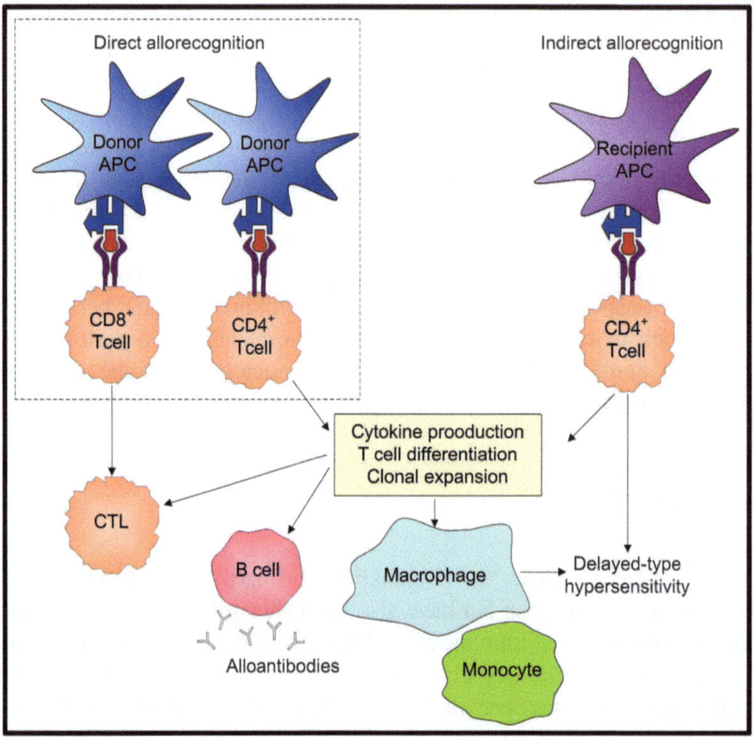

Fig. 1.5 Effector mechanisms of allograft rejection. Rejection of the allograft is mediated by both cellular (delayed-type hypersensitivity responses and cell-mediated cytotoxicity) and humoral (B cell/antibody-mediated) components. Recipient T cells respond to donor MHC peptides either by direct or indirect allorecognition. $CD8^+$ cytotoxic T lymphocytes (CTLs) are generated via the direct pathway, whereas $CD4^+$ helper T cells arise from either direct or indirect allorecognition. $CD4^+$ T cells are then able to elicit a delayed-hypersensitivity response (DTH), as well as enhance CTL activity and production of alloantibodies by B cells

T Cell-Mediated (Cellular) Rejection

T cells cause allograft rejection either by eliciting a DTH response or through cytolytic/cytotoxic activity [37]. DTH responses are primarily mediated by alloantigen-specific $CD4^+$ Th1 cells, which secrete IFNγ(gamma) and TNF-α(alpha). These proinflammatory cytokines activate monocytes and macrophages which, in turn, cause nonspecific tissue injury through the release of proteolytic enzymes, nitric oxide, and other soluble factors. These factors affect vascular tone and permeability, in addition to promoting chemotaxis and further activation and differentiation of antigen-specific T cells. While mechanisms underlying the exact nature by which DTH causes rejection are still poorly understood, it is clear that allospecific DTH response alone is sufficient to mediate experimental models of rejection, whereas graft acceptance is associated with a blunted or absent DTH response [38, 39]. Furthermore, tolerant transplant patients (i.e., patients who demonstrate long-term graft acceptance in the absence of immunosuppression) show a suppressed DTH response to donor antigens [40].

$CD8^+$ CTLs are the major players in lymphocyte-mediated cytotoxicity, and they predominate the cellular infiltrates in acutely rejecting grafts [41]. $CD8^+$ CTLs are primed and activated by recognition of donor MHC class I molecules primarily on donor APCs, but also on vascular endothelial cells [2]. Activated CTL precursors form granules containing perforins, granzymes, and other cytolytic proteins (e.g., FasL, serglycin, calreticulin, and granulysin). Once the target cell is identified via specific interactions between TCR/MHC and the CD8 coreceptor, these granules release their contents into the immunological synapse. Groups of perforins insert themselves into the target cell membrane, allowing the uptake of granzyme B into the cytoplasm, which results in apoptosis of the donor cell via a caspase-dependent mechanism [37]. This caspase-mediated cell death can also be triggered through the binding of FasL (released either via granules of direct trafficking to the synapse) to Fas on the target cell. Of these pathways, release of granzyme B to cause cell death may be the more important [42, 43]. Regardless, targeting the downstream caspase cascade may be a potential future immunomodulator: inhibitor of caspase-3 reduced apoptosis in experimental models, leading to prolonged cardiac allograft survival [44].

B Cell-Mediated (Humoral) Rejection

Alloantibody response to the graft represents the third effector mechanism contributing to graft injury. Although antibodies are produced by B cells, this arm of the immune response is dependent on help from alloreactive T cells for growth, differentiation, and immunoglobulin class switching. Naïve B cells circulate through the follicles of peripheral lymphoid organs (spleen, lymph nodes, and mucosal lymphoid tissues) until they encounter antigen that is usually presented by dendritic cells but can also exist in soluble form. Without antigenic stimulation, naïve B cells survive for a limited time, as determined by the presence of receptors for BAFF (B-cell activating factor of the TNF family or also known as BLyS, B lymphocyte stimulating factor) and APRIL (a proliferation-inducing ligand). Strategies aimed at depleting these survival factors are currently under investigation as potential targets for inducing B cell tolerance [45].

Activation occurs upon binding of antigen to membrane immunoglobulin (Ig) molecules, which together with Igα(alpha) and Igβ(beta) make up the BCR (B cell receptor) complex. Igα(alpha) and Igβ(beta) are the B cell equivalent to the CD3 and ζ(zeta) molecules that make up the TCR complex. They are required for signal transduction leading to activation of the same transcriptional factors governing T cell activation (NFAT, NFκ(kappa)B, AP-1). In addition to initiating B cell proliferation and differentiation, these events also prepare the B cells for subsequent interactions with T cells by upregulating cell surface expression of MHC and costimulatory molecules and cytokine receptors. To ensure direct interaction between T and B cells, activated T cells upregulate CXCR5, a chemokine receptor which allows it to home towards the B cell-rich primary follicles of the lymph node. Simultaneously, B cells upregulate CCR7 to respond to T cell zone chemokines CCL19 and CCL21.

T–B Cell Interaction

Although low-level B cell proliferation and antibody secretion can be induced in the absence of T cells, these functions are significantly enhanced by interaction with helper T cells. Irradiated mice (devoid of any immune cells) injected with bone marrow cells containing mature B lymphocytes, but no mature T cells, show no specific antibody production upon immunization. However, when mature T cells were also injected, antibody production is restored. Similarly, humans and mice with reduced (or deficient) numbers of $CD4^{+}$ helper T cells show defective antibody responses. These helper T lymphocytes stimulate B cell clonal expansion, isotype switching, affinity maturation, and differentiation into memory B cells.

Upon their encounter, B cells present antigen–MHC complex recognized by the TCR. Coreceptors and adhesion molecules strengthen this signal, and costimulatory molecules (particularly CD40:CD40L interactions) and cytokines released at the synapse lead to B cell proliferation, differentiation into antibody-secreting cells, and early isotype switching. With this, B cells can then make all different Ig types in addition to their constitutive expression of IgM. These initial short-lived plasma cells and memory B cells produce the first peak of specific IgM antibodies, which display low to medium affinity for antigen [46]. Days later, these B cells migrate deeper into the follicle, and rapidly proliferate to form germinal centers of antigen-specific B cell clones. With each successive cell division, numerous mutations in the variable regions of the antibodies lead to selection of long-term memory B cells and plasma cells that produce high-affinity antibody of all isotypes. Re-exposure to the same (or similar) antigen leads to an immediate robust response by these cells. A prime example of this phenomenon occurs in hyperacute rejection where preexisting antibodies against the ABO or MHC antigen on endothelial cells lead to rapid activation of the classical complement pathway.

Antibody-Mediated Damage

Antibodies exert their effector mechanism by activating the complement system through its classical pathway (Fig. 1.6). IgG or IgM recognizes alloantigen on the graft endothelium and activates C1 (made up of C1q, C1r, and C1s components). A conformational change in C1q leads to eventual cleavage of C1s, which activates C2 and C4. When C1s cleaves C4, C4a and C4b fragments are formed, exposing a

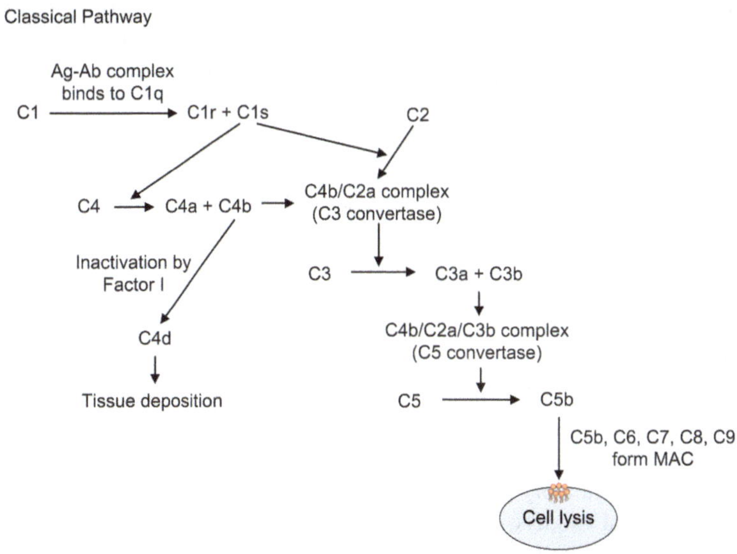

Fig. 1.6 Classical pathway of complement activation. Antibodies recognize alloantigen and activate the classical pathway by binding to C1q, a subunit of C1. This results in the formation of C3 and C5 convertases, and the eventual formation of the membrane attack complex (MAC) which mediates cell lysis. C4d, a marker of complement activation, is formed when C4b becomes inactivated by factor I

sulfhydryl group on C4b that is targeted for inactivation by factor I. The resultant inactive product, C4d remains covalently bound in tissue and its presence within the endothelium is a marker of complement activation. In clinical practice, C4d deposition detected in the allograft biopsy is a surrogate for antibody-mediated endothelial destruction. However, its presence does not denote the formation of membrane attack complexes (MAC). Without activation of MAC, graft injury may not have occurred. For graft injury to occur, C4b complexes with C2a to form C3-convertase, which then cleaves C3 into C3a and C3b. C3b then binds to the C4b/C2a complex to form C5-convertase. This cleaves C5, with C5b initiating the formation of MAC (C5b-C9), which causes lysis of endothelial cells and graft rejection. In addition, complement products have been shown to aid in T cell priming and act as chemoattractants [47].

Tolerance

The discovery of potent immunosuppressive drugs has led to reduced rates of acute rejection and greatly improved 1-year graft survival rates. However, this is often at the expense of nonspecific life-long immunosuppression (IS), which places patients at higher risk of cardiovascular disease, infections, and cancer. Allograft tolerance refers to a state of immune unresponsiveness to the transplanted graft without the deleterious effect of generalized immune suppression. In healthy individuals, immune homeostasis is maintained through a balance between effector and regulatory cells of either T or B cell lineage. Of these, $CD4^+CD25^+FoxP3^+$ regulatory T cells (Treg) have received the most attention as targets for inducing peripheral tolerance. FoxP3 (forkhead transcription factor) is a transcription factor responsible for regulating Treg development [48]. Mice and humans deficient in FoxP3 lack Tregs and develop massive T-cell hyperproliferation and severe systemic autoimmunity [49, 50]. Tregs exert their regulatory function by suppressing proliferation, differentiation, and cytokine production of effector cells via direct T cell–T cell interaction [51]. They can also cause cell death through the release of granzyme B and perforin [52, 53], as well as by inducing apoptotic pathways [54]. Additionally, Treg–APC interaction leads to an abrogated ability of these APCs to activate T cells. Finally, Tregs produce anti-inflammatory cytokines such as IL-10 and TGFβ(beta), which in turn are immunoregulatory [55–57].

In experimental models, Tregs have been shown to be important in both the induction and maintenance of allograft tolerance [58–60]. In humans, peripheral blood from operationally tolerant patients (i.e., those who have functioning grafts despite being on no IS) contain increased numbers of $CD4^+CD25^+FoxP3^+$ cells, and their presence can help predict tolerance during IS withdrawal [61, 62]. Even amongst patients on IS, the difference between stability and rejection can be attributed in part to Treg activity [63, 64]. Furthermore, during episodes of acute rejection, urinary FoxP3 mRNA levels were found to be higher in patients who successfully recovered allograft function compared with those whose rejection episodes did not reverse [65]. This is consistent with the hypothesis that during rejection, Tregs undergo expansion to try to limit alloimmunity and re-establish a tolerogenic milieu. Since the discovery of these regulatory cells in 1995, there has been an explosion of interest in harnessing them as a means to promote allograft tolerance. In fact, ex vivo expansion and infusion, as well as in vivo expansion of Tregs have been utilized successfully in experimental models of autoimmunity, graft vs. host disease, and transplantation [66, 67].

Conclusions

Our understanding of the immunobiology underlying transplantation has expanded exponentially within the last 50 years since the first successful kidney transplant. Despite this, chronic rejection and over-immunosuppression remain significant clinical problems. Our immune system has evolved into an intricate and redundant system capable of distinguishing and abolishing foreign antigens. It is unlikely therefore that a single therapy will be sufficient to achieve allograft tolerance, and a more attainable strategy will involve targeting of multiple pathways concomitantly.

References

1. Snell GD. Methods for the study of histocompatibility genes. J Genet. 1948;49:87.
2. Kreisel D, Krupnick AS, Gelman AE, et al. Non-hematopoietic allograft cells directly activate CD8+ T cells and trigger acute rejection: an alternative mechanism of allorecognition. Nat Med. 2002;8(3):233–9.
3. Sheldon S, Poulton K. HLA Typing and its influence on organ transplantation. Methods Mol Biol. 2006;333:157–74.
4. Sumitran-Holgersson S. Relevance of MICA and other non-HLA antibodies in clinical transplantation. Curr Opin Immunol. 2008;20(5):607–13.
5. Terasaki PI. Deduction of the fraction of immunologic and non-immunologic failure in cadaver donor transplants. Clin Transpl 2003:449–52.
6. Roopenian D, Choi EY, Brown A. The immunogenomics of minor histocompatibility antigens. Immunol Rev. 2002;190:86–94.
7. Derhaag JG, Duijvestijn AM, Damoiseaux JG, van Breda Vriesman PJ. Effects of antibody reactivity to major histocompatibility complex (MHC) and non-MHC alloantigens on graft endothelial cells in heart allograft rejection. Transplantation. 2000;69(9):1899–906.
8. Koulack J, McAlister VC, MacAulay MA, Bitter-Suermann H, MacDonald AS, Lee TD. Importance of minor histocompatibility antigens in the development of allograft arteriosclerosis. Clin Immunol Immunopathol. 1996;80(3 Pt 1):273–7.
9. Yang J, Jaramillo A, Liu W, et al. Chronic rejection of murine cardiac allografts discordant at the H13 minor histocompatibility antigen correlates with the generation of the H13-specific CD8+ cytotoxic T cells. Transplantation. 2003;76(1):84–91.
10. Goulmy E, Gratama JW, Blokland E, Zwaan FE, van Rood JJ. A minor transplantation antigen detected by MHC-restricted cytotoxic T lymphocytes during graft-versus-host disease. Nature. 1983;302(5904):159–61.
11. Goulmy E, Schipper R, Pool J, et al. Mismatches of minor histocompatibility antigens between HLA-identical donors and recipients and the development of graft-versus-host disease after bone marrow transplantation. N Engl J Med. 1996;334(5):281–5.
12. Krishnan NS, Higgins RM, Lam FT, et al. HA-1 mismatch has significant effect in chronic allograft nephropathy in clinical renal transplantation. Transplant Proc. 2007;39(5):1439–45.
13. Heinold A, Opelz G, Scherer S, et al. Role of minor histocompatibility antigens in renal transplantation. Am J Transplant. 2008;8(1):95–102.
14. Sumitran-Holgersson S, Wilczek HE, Holgersson J, Soderstrom K. Identification of the non-classical HLA molecules, mica, as targets for humoral immunity associated with irreversible rejection of kidney allografts. Transplantation. 2002;74(2):268–77.
15. Mizutani K, Terasaki P, Rosen A, et al. Serial ten-year follow-up of HLA and MICA antibody production prior to kidney graft failure. Am J Transplant. 2005;5(9):2265–72.
16. Dragun D. Humoral responses directed against non-human leukocyte antigens in solid-organ transplantation. Transplantation. 2008;86(8):1019–25.
17. Magee CC. Transplantation across previously incompatible immunological barriers. Transpl Int. 2006;19(2):87–97.
18. Gloor JM, Stegall MD. ABO incompatible kidney transplantation. Curr Opin Nephrol Hypertens. 2007;16(6):529–34.
19. Alegre ML, Najafian N. Costimulatory molecules as targets for the induction of transplantation tolerance. Curr Mol Med. 2006;6(8):843–57.
20. Li XC, Rothstein DM, Sayegh MH. Costimulatory pathways in transplantation: challenges and new developments. Immunol Rev. 2009;229(1):271–93.
21. Boenisch O, Sayegh MH, Najafian N. Negative T-cell costimulatory pathways: their role in regulating alloimmune responses. Curr Opin Organ Transplant. 2008;13(4):373–8.
22. Rothstein DM, Sayegh MH. T-cell costimulatory pathways in allograft rejection and tolerance. Immunol Rev. 2003;196:85–108.

23. Vincenti F, Luggen M. T cell costimulation: a rational target in the therapeutic armamentarium for autoimmune diseases and transplantation. Annu Rev Med. 2007;58:347–58.
24. Kirk AD, Harlan DM, Armstrong NN, et al. CTLA4-Ig and anti-CD40 ligand prevent renal allograft rejection in primates. Proc Natl Acad Sci USA. 1997;94(16):8789–94.
25. Levisetti MG, Padrid PA, Szot GL, et al. Immunosuppressive effects of human CTLA4Ig in a non-human primate model of allogeneic pancreatic islet transplantation. J Immunol. 1997;159(11):5187–91.
26. Yamada A, Kishimoto K, Dong VM, et al. CD28-independent costimulation of T cells in alloimmune responses. J Immunol. 2001;167(1):140–6.
27. Sayegh MH, Akalin E, Hancock WW, et al. CD28-B7 blockade after alloantigenic challenge in vivo inhibits Th1 cytokines but spares Th2. J Exp Med. 1995;181(5):1869–74.
28. Steiger J, Nickerson PW, Steurer W, Moscovitch-Lopatin M, Strom TB. IL-2 knockout recipient mice reject islet cell allografts. J Immunol. 1995;155(1):489–98.
29. Nagano H, Mitchell RN, Taylor MK, Hasegawa S, Tilney NL, Libby P. Interferon-gamma deficiency prevents coronary arteriosclerosis but not myocardial rejection in transplanted mouse hearts. J Clin Invest. 1997;100(3):550–7.
30. Zhou P, Szot GL, Guo Z, et al. Role of STAT4 and STAT6 signaling in allograft rejection and CTLA4-Ig-mediated tolerance. J Immunol. 2000;165(10):5580–7.
31. Yuan X, Paez-Cortez J, Schmitt-Knosalla I, et al. A novel role of CD4 Th17 cells in mediating cardiac allograft rejection and vasculopathy. J Exp Med. 2008;205(13):3133–44.
32. Yang XO, Nurieva R, Martinez GJ, et al. Molecular antagonism and plasticity of regulatory and inflammatory T cell programs. Immunity. 2008;29(1):44–56.
33. Nashan B, Moore R, Amlot P, Schmidt AG, Abeywickrama K, Soulillou JP. Randomised trial of basiliximab versus placebo for control of acute cellular rejection in renal allograft recipients. CHIB 201 International Study Group. Lancet. 1997;350(9086):1193–8.
34. Vincenti F, Kirkman R, Light S, et al. Interleukin-2-receptor blockade with daclizumab to prevent acute rejection in renal transplantation. Daclizumab Triple Therapy Study Group. N Engl J Med. 1998;338(3):161–5.
35. Hancock WW, Gao W, Faia KL, Csizmadia V. Chemokines and their receptors in allograft rejection. Curr Opin Immunol. 2000;12(5):511–6.
36. Fischereder M, Schroppel B. The role of chemokines in acute renal allograft rejection and chronic allograft injury. Front Biosci. 2009;14:1807–14.
37. Rocha PN, Plumb TJ, Crowley SD, Coffman TM. Effector mechanisms in transplant rejection. Immunol Rev. 2003;196:51–64.
38. Bickerstaff AA, Wang JJ, Pelletier RP, Orosz CG. Murine renal allografts: spontaneous acceptance is associated with regulated T cell-mediated immunity. J Immunol. 2001;167(9):4821–7.
39. Orosz CG, Wakely E, Sedmak DD, Bergese SD, VanBuskirk AM. Prolonged murine cardiac allograft acceptance: characteristics of persistent active alloimmunity after treatment with gallium nitrate versus anti-CD4 monoclonal antibody. Transplantation. 1997;63(8):1109–17.
40. VanBuskirk AM, Burlingham WJ, Jankowska-Gan E, et al. Human allograft acceptance is associated with immune regulation. J Clin Invest. 2000;106(1):145–55.
41. Strom TB, Tilney NL, Carpenter CB, Busch GJ. Identity and cytotoxic capacity of cells infiltrating renal allografts. N Engl J Med. 1975;292(24):1257–63.
42. Krupnick AS, Kreisel D, Popma SH, et al. Mechanism of T cell-mediated endothelial apoptosis. Transplantation. 2002;74(6):871–6.
43. Wever PC, Boonstra JG, Laterveer JC, et al. Mechanisms of lymphocyte-mediated cytotoxicity in acute renal allograft rejection. Transplantation. 1998;66(2):259–64.
44. Kown MH, Van der Steenhoven T, Blankenberg FG, et al. Zinc-mediated reduction of apoptosis in cardiac allografts. Circulation. 2000;102(19 Suppl 3):III228–32.
45. Mackay F, Schneider P. Cracking the BAFF code. Nat Rev Immunol. 2009;9(7):491–502.
46. McHeyzer-Williams MG. B cells as effectors. Curr Opin Immunol. 2003;15(3):354–61.
47. Pratt JR, Basheer SA, Sacks SH. Local synthesis of complement component C3 regulates acute renal transplant rejection. Nat Med. 2002;8(6):582–7.

48. Fontenot JD, Gavin MA, Rudensky AY. Foxp3 programs the development and function of CD4+ CD25+ regulatory T cells. Nat Immunol. 2003;4:330–6.
49. Brunkow ME. Disruption of a new forkhead/winged-helix protein, scurfin, results in the fatal lymphoproliferative disorder of the scurfy mouse. Nat Genet. 2001;27:68–73.
50. Bennett CL. The immune dysregulation, polyendocrinopathy, enteropathy, X-linked syndrome (IPEX) is caused by mutations of FOXP3. Nat Genet. 2001;27:20–1.
51. Tang Q, Bluestone JA. The Foxp3+ regulatory T cell: a jack of all trades, master of regulation. Nat Immunol. 2008;9:239–44.
52. Grossman WJ. Human T regulatory cells can use the perforin pathway to cause autologous target cell death. Immunity. 2004;21:589–601.
53. Gondek DC, Lu LF, Quezada SA, Sakaguchi S, Noelle RJ. Cutting edge: contact-mediated suppression by CD4+ CD25+ regulatory cells involves a granzyme B-dependent, perforin-independent mechanism. J Immunol. 2005;174:1783–6.
54. Nikolova M, Lelievre J-D, Carriere M, Bensussan A, Levy Y. Regulatory T cells modulate differentially the maturation and apoptosis of human CD8-T cell subsets. Blood 2009:blood-2008-04-151407.
55. Hara M. IL-10 is required for regulatory T cells to mediate tolerance to alloantigens in vivo. J Immunol. 2001;166:3789–96.
56. Maloy KJ. CD4+ CD25+ TR cells suppress innate immune pathology through cytokine-dependent mechanisms. J Exp Med. 2003;197:111–9.
57. Li MO, Wan YY, Flavell RA. T cell-produced transforming growth factor-b1 controls T cell tolerance and regulates Th1- and Th17-cell differentiation. Immunity. 2007;26:579–91.
58. Taylor P, Noelle RJ, Blazar BR. CD4+ CD25+ immune regulatory cells are required for induction of tolerance to alloantigen via costimulatory blockade. J Exp Med. 2001;193:1311–8.
59. Sanchez Fueyo A, Weber M, Domenig C, Strom T, Zheng X. Tracking immunoregulatory mechanisms during allograft tolerance. J Immunol. 2002;168:2274–81.
60. Wood KJ, Sakaguchi S. Regulatory T cells in transplantation tolerance. Nat Rev Immunol. 2003;3(3):199–210.
61. Martinez-Llordella M, Puig-Pey I, Orlando G, et al. Multiparameter immune profiling of operational tolerance in liver transplantation. Am J Transplant. 2007;7(2):309–19.
62. Pons JA, Revilla-Nuin B, Baroja-Mazo A, et al. FoxP3 in peripheral blood is associated with operational tolerance in liver transplant patients during immunosuppression withdrawal. Transplantation. 2008;86(10):1370–8.
63. Salama AD, Najafian N, Clarkson MR, Harmon WE, Sayegh MH. Regulatory CD25+ T cells in human kidney transplant recipients. J Am Soc Nephrol. 2003;14:1643–51.
64. Akl A, Jones ND, Rogers N, et al. An investigation to assess the potential of CD25highCD4+ T cells to regulate responses to donor alloantigens in clinically stable renal transplant recipients. Transpl Int. 2008;21(1):65–73.
65. Muthukumar T, Dadhania D, Ding R, et al. Messenger RNA for FOXP3 in the urine of renal-allograft recipients. N Engl J Med. 2005;353(22):2342–51.
66. Roncarolo M-G, Battaglia M. Regulatory T-cell immunotherapy for tolerance to self antigens and alloantigens in humans. Nat Rev Immunol. 2007;7(8):585–98.
67. Brusko TM, Putnam AL, Bluestone JA. Human regulatory T cells: role in autoimmune disease and therapeutic opportunities. Immunol Rev. 2008;223(1):371–90.

[illegible]

Chapter 2
Basic Histocompatibility Testing Methods

Kathryn J. Tinckam

Abstract Predicting humoral alloimmune potential in transplant recipients is the objective of histocompatibility testing and depends upon accurate donor typing and sensitive and specific testing for antibodies to human leukocyte antigen. This review for the transplant clinician will describe the evolution and current widespread practices of histocompatibility testing methods for typing, crossmatching, and antibody screening. Newer methods such as measuring T cell alloimmune potential will not be discussed as they are beyond the scope of this basic overview and are not routinely practiced in all histocompatibility laboratories at this time. Emphasis is given to the clinical applicability and limitations of each test, and the collective consideration of all tests in concert, as part of the immunologic risk assessment of the solid organ transplant recipient.

Keywords Histocompatibility • Human leukocyte antigen • Crossmatch • Panel reactive antibody (PRA) • Antibodies

Introduction

The fundamental goal of histocompatibility testing, despite a myriad of advances in technologies in the last 4 decades, remains to provide a reliable measure of the humoral immunologic risk of a transplant recipient in the context of their potential donor(s). The nature of this measurement has evolved with advances in techniques for human leukocyte antigen (HLA) typing, revealing thousands of new alleles and sources of alloimmune stimuli, as well as the improved sensitivity and specificity of

K.J. Tinckam, MD, MMSc, FRCPC (✉)
Department of Medicine, University Health Network, University of Toronto, Toronto, ON, Canada
e-mail: kathryn.tinckham@uhn.on.ca

A. Chandraker et al. (eds.), *Core Concepts in Renal Transplantation*,
DOI 10.1007/978-1-4614-0008-0_2, © Springer Science+Business Media, LLC 2012

detection methods for antibodies to HLA antigens, and more recently identification of non-HLA alloimmune targets also. This testing interrogates the risk that the recipient immune system will recognize a potential allograft as foreign to self, and thereby initiate inflammatory events resulting in allograft damage. HLA laboratory testing should be seen as the immunologic component of the clinical pretransplant risk assessment. Furthermore, HLA testing methods are no longer limited to the pretransplant period. Indeed antibody analysis is increasingly studied posttransplant, as noninvasive predictors of acute and chronic alloimmune complications. It is imperative for the clinician to understand the complex and interactive nature of these available histocompatibility testing methods in order to fully identify the immunologic risk status of a potential recipient or transplant patient.

This chapter, directed to the transplant clinician, will discuss most commonly utilized methods of HLA typing in transplant centers, HLA typing, antibody screening, and crossmatching, with an emphasis on their evolution over the last 4 decades, their current clinical utility and applicability, and the various factors that must be considered in their interpretation. In providing a practical reference of histocompatibility testing methods for the clinician, such that the basic principles are understood in the context of clinical outcomes, improved communication between the clinical service and laboratory may facilitate improved immunological understanding of the transplant patient.

HLA Typing

All nucleated cells in the body express HLA Class I molecules (A, B, and Cw), whereas HLA Class II (DR, DP and DQ) molecule expression is limited to B cells, antigen-presenting cells, and activated microvascular endothelial cells [1, 2]. A major initiator of the alloimmune response in solid organ transplantation is recognition of nonself HLA by recipient T cells. In response, T cell activation releases proinflammatory mediators with subsequent recruitment of the effector cells of the immune system [3–7]. Indeed, many HLA laboratories were initially called "Tissue Typing Labs" as their prime role was to identify the degree of mismatch between donor and recipient tissues rendering HLA typing as one of the most important risk assessment tools for predicting nonself HLA recognition by quantifying the number of HLA antigen mismatches between donors and recipients. Currently, both serologic and molecular typing methods are routinely used in a majority of HLA laboratories.

Serologic Typing

As suggested by the name, serologic typing utilizes various sera (frequently obtained from multiparous females), containing well-characterized antibodies to a wide range of HLA specificities. Although in the past laboratories often kept large banks of sera from which to make their own typing reagents, today commercially prepared trays which contain sera with antibodies to all common, and many rare HLA alleles, are the norm. Lymphocytes (expressing the HLA antigens of the patient to be typed) are mixed with the various sera in the tray wells of and incubated with complement and a vital dye.

If the cell has antigens on its surface to which antibody in a particular well is able to bind, then complement is activated in those well(s), the membrane attack complex forms and inserts into the cell membrane, cell death occurs, and the vital dye is taken up into the cell [8]. Significant cell death occurs in any well in which the cell surface antigen and serum antibody bind, which can be identified under phase contrast microscopy. Comparing and eliminating the serologic specificities of the positive wells assigns the HLA type. For example, if two wells with sera known to bind (a) B46,57,62,63,75 and (b) B57,75 are found to have significant cell death, negative wells containing antibodies binding B46,57,62,63 (in combination) therefore will assign the typing as B75.

Advantages of serologic typing include obtaining rapid results, which is of particular importance in deceased donor typing, in order to reduce cold ischemia times, and also the ability to discriminate "null" HLA alleles which have detectable DNA sequences in molecular typing, but no antigen expression on cell surfaces, and therefore may be of less immunologic relevance. A major limitation, however, is finding high quality sera with sufficient antibody specificities to reliably identify the ever-increasing number of HLA alleles [9, 10]. There is increasing clinical interest in HLA-Cw, DQ, and DP antigen contributions to allograft outcomes and the availability of serologic assays is limited for these loci. Additionally, small amino acid differences in HLA proteins are not easily detected by serologic methods yet may have potent immunologic consequences [11, 12]. For example, B44 antigen has a number of alleles including B*4402 and B*4403 which differ by a single amino acid at position 156 [10]. Serologic typing would classify a B*4402 donor and B*4403 recipient as B44 (i.e., identical) and yet the recipient could form an antibody to the epitope with the amino acid difference that would not be expected based upon serologic typing alone.

Molecular Typing

HLA proteins are encoded by DNA regions on the short arm of chromosome 6. With their sequences well described [10] molecular typing methods are increasingly used including sequence specific primer polymerase chain reaction (SSP-PCR), sequence specific oligonucleotide probes (SSOP), and direct DNA sequencing. In SSP-PCR, DNA is isolated from the subject to be typed, and amplified in multiple wells, each containing specific primers complementary to particular HLA alleles. An amplification product in a given well is formed only if the DNA probes are complementary to the sequence of the HLA molecule. The contents of the wells are then run by electrophoresis through an agarose gel with the amplification product appearing as a band on the gel; the HLA typing is assigned by matching the primers of resulting amplification products to the DNA sequences of the various candidate alleles. In SSOP, oligonucleotide probes that are complementary to the unique segments of the DNA of different alleles are mixed with amplified DNA. Unique fluorescent tags distinguish those probes that are complementary to the DNA, such that the unique HLA alleles may be identified. Sequencing determines the exact order of nucleotides in the gene of interest and the HLA type is assigned by comparison to published HLA allele sequences [10]. Regardless of the specific method, molecular typing more precisely identifies the differences in HLA antigen between donor and recipient, frequently with resolution to the amino acid level which may provide better quantification of the risk associated with mismatched donor–recipient antigens, amino acids, and epitopes [12, 13].

Crossreactive Groups, Nomenclature, and Mismatches

HLA nomenclature differs depending on the typing method used; a basic understanding of the differences is required to "translate" between techniques. Historically, as HLA antigens were (serologically) discovered, they were named in order of that discovery by gene locus, e.g., A1, A2, etc., and B7, B8, etc. Refinement of serologic methods identified even more antigens, previously thought to represent single allotypes, which in fact were serologically and genetically unique. For example, B60 and B61, which were identified as unique antigens (with therefore unique private epitopes), were earlier thought to be just one antigen, B40, based on sera binding to a shared public epitope between the two. Both B60 and B61 are considered part of the B40 crossreactive group or CREG, which itself is part of the B7 CREG. Public epitopes are those common to all the members of a CREG whereas private epitopes delineate the individual serologically defined antigens.

Serological antigen nomenclature does not represent the true heterogeneity of the HLA system. Indeed, early studies with mixed lymphocyte cultures detected this heterogeneity in HLA antigen recognition that could not be discerned by serology alone; for example, HLA A2 was found to consist of several subtypes stimulating different lymphocyte reactivity. DNA sequencing subsequently confirmed that indeed multiple alleles of each HLA antigen are known to exist, despite the fact that they may react to a single common typing serum at the antigen level. A new molecular typing nomenclature was introduced in 1987 where the locus is followed by an asterisk, then the first two digits describe the type, and then the next two digits represent a unique allele differing by at least one amino acid difference. Beginning April 1, 2010, this system was modified further, adding a colon between each two digit designation, thus allowing for greater than 99 unique alleles within each allele family. For example, HLA-A*020101 becomes HLA-A*02:01:01. Some more significant changes occur where >99 alleles have already been documented, e.g., A*0299 was followed by A*9201 in the older molecular nomenclature but will now be called A*02:101.

Table 2.1 Common HLA serologic equivalents that differ numerically from the molecular nomenclature

Molecular typing	Serologic equivalents
HLA-B*15xx	B62,63,71,72,75,76,77
HLA-B*14xx	B64,65
HLA-B*40xx	B60,61
HLA-C*03xx	Cw9,10
DQB1*03xx	DQ7,8,9
DRB1*03xx	DR17,18
DRB3*yy	DR52
DRB4*yy	DR53
DRB5*yy	DR51

xx various alleles in the allele group; *yy* allele group

Frequently, the serological and molecular nomenclature correspond (e.g., HLA-A*0201 has the serological equivalent of HLA-A2) but incongruencies do occur. For the purposes of solid organ transplantation, it is important for the clinician to recognize which system is used by their laboratory in the assignment of HLA type as well as in the assignment of antibody specificities. For example, if a donor is assigned a typing of B*1501 and the donor has an antibody defined to B62, the donor specificity of this antibody may not be immediately apparent, even though B62 is the serological equivalent of B*1501. Failure to appreciate that different nomenclature is used may result in missed recognition of a donor specific antibody (DSA). Such concerns may be easily addressed through communication with the HLA laboratory, and in addition several references are readily available [9, 10, 14]. A table is provided here as a reference for the clinician listing the most common HLA serologic antigen names where the molecular typing may not be congruent or obviously related (Table 2.1.) In addition, for Class II molecules, that are at the protein level, composed of unique alpha and beta chains, the serologic equivalent name reflects the beta chain polymorphism only. Communication with the laboratory is required to discuss if the alpha chain typng is clinically relevant (for example, if a DSA is present to the alpha chain) as the serologic nomenclature will not reflect differences in the alpha chain, and the molecular alpha chain typing may need to be specified.

When describing the typing of a donor and recipient, their dissimilarity should reflect the "alloimmune burden" that a donor presents to a recipient as it is more immunologically informative. For example, if a donor is A1,- B8,39 DR1,3 and the recipient is A1,24 B39,44 DR1,11, then this is a 0-A, 2-B,1-DR mismatch or 3 HLA mismatch transplant. However, if the donor and recipient typings were reversed then the recipient immune system would see 4 HLA antigens (1-A, 2-B, 1-DR) as nonself. The number of affirmative matches should not routinely be used. Note also that typing at HLA-A, B, C, DRB1, DRB3/4/5, DQB1, DQA1, DPA1 and DPB1 are all possible and performed in many centers. These represent up to 18 unique protein products in donors and recipients where mismatch may occur, in contrast to the commonly utilized 6 antigen mismatch approach of HLA-A, B, DRB1. Programs differ widely as to what extent these typing are used in their clinical decision making, however it is important for the clinician to be aware of all of these typing possibilities.

HLA Antibody Screening

Up to one third of waitlisted patients may have some HLA antibodies detected when the most sensitive screening methods are used. Sensitization to HLA antigens occurs with previous exposure to nonself HLA during pregnancy or after blood transfusion or prior transplant. A major consequence of preformed antibodies is decreased access to transplantation; antibodies to a greater number of HLA antigens will result in higher rates of positive crossmatches and exclusion of these donors. Indeed, even if the crossmatch is negative, permitting transplant to proceed with short-term safety, low titers of antibody directed to donor HLA are associated with higher rates of early [15] and late [16] antibody mediated outcomes (including rejection and graft loss). Therefore, both sensitive and specific identification of HLA antibodies is necessary to identify the risks faced by sensitized recipients and also to permit novel strategies for successfully transplanting these patients, such as desensitization [17], acceptable mismatching, and paired exchange [13, 18]. Repeated pretransplant antibody screening for waitlisted patients comprises a majority of solid organ transplant work in most HLA laboratories.

Cytotoxic (Cell Based) Antibody Screening

"Cell donors" (usually 20–40 in number) are randomly selected from a population to have variable HLA types and their lymphocytes form panels of cells. While these "cell donors" are not organ donors per se, their HLA typings are intended to be representative of the HLA antigen distribution in a similar population from whom deceased donors may be (also randomly) selected. In this way, the percentage of the "cell donors" panel to which a given recipient has antibodies approximates the percentage of potential organ donors drawn from that same population to whom the recipient would be expected to have a positive crossmatch. The basic method is similar to that of serologic typing except that it is now the recipient serum that is mixed with "cell donor" lymphocytes in individual wells along with complement and the vital dye. If the serum contains antibodies that bind to the cell surface with sufficient density, complement will be activated, and the vital dye uptake allows the dead cells to be easily identified (Fig. 2.1a). If in a panel of 40 cells, 30 of the reaction wells had significant cell death, the panel reactive antibody (PRA) would be reported as 75%.

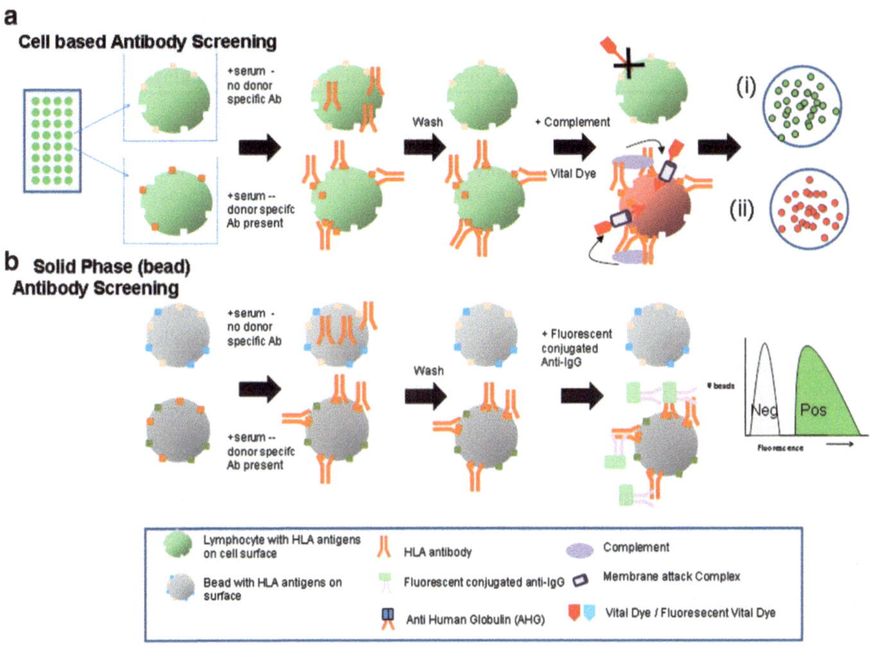

Fig. 2.1 Schematic diagram of cell based and solid phase (bead based) antibody screening. (**a**) Two representative wells are illustrated from the panel of cells that is used. Serum is added to each well in the panel. On the *top*, the antibody in the serum does not bind to the cells, on the *bottom*, donor specific antibody (DSA) does bind. Bound DSA remain after wash steps, so that when complement is added, it forms the membrane attack complex, killing the cell and allowing the vital dye is taken up by and visualized. No donor specific antibody leaves live cells (i), and when DSA are present, the vital dye identifies the dead cells (ii). (**b**) Serum is added to beads coated with purified or recombinant HLA antigen. In this case, the antibody in the serum is only specific to the bead on the *bottom*. Only beads with DSA already bound will bind the secondary fluorescent anti-IgG marker. Increased fluorescence defines positive beads with DSA bound to them

Limitations of Cytotoxic Antibody Screening

An obvious limitation of this method is that the PRA percent may numerically change (without a change in amount or type of antibody) depending on the cell panel that was used in the screening. The interpreting clinician must not overinterpret small changes in PRA as a significant change in alloimmune potential. Frequently, commercially made cell panels are used, however they may not accurately represent the HLA distribution of a particular donor region depending on the racial differences in that region, which can alter HLA antigen frequencies. Furthermore, substantial false positive results may occur due to non-HLA antibodies and autoantibodies or nonspecific IgM antibodies, as well as false negative results from low sensitivity (dependence on complement activation which requires higher titer antibodies). Complement activation requires that antibody must be of sufficient density to link complement between Fc receptors; with lower titer antibody,

Table 2.2 Antibody detection parameters of cytotoxic vs. solid phase antibody screening tests

	Cytotoxic antibody screening	Solid phase antibody screening
Detects class I HLA Ab	Yes	Yes
Detects class II HLA Ab	If B cells are used	Yes
Detects non-HLA Ab	Yes – to any target on lymphocyte	Only with antigen-specific assays (e.g., MICA)
Detects IgM Ab	Yes (DTT treatment of serum would prevent this)	No
Detects low titer Ab	No	Yes
Able to identify HLA Ab to specific antigens	Rarely	Yes (using single antigen beads)
Detects noncomplement binding Ab	No	Yes – all IgG subtypes detected

the absence of complement activation allows a true antibody to "hide" [19]. Finally, accurate and complete lists of antibody specificities and unacceptable antigens are almost impossible to obtain with this methodology as there are multiple antigens per reaction well (Table 2.2).

Cellular or *cytotoxic* PRA testing may therefore be best thought of as estimating the risk of a given recipient of having a positive *cytotoxic* crossmatch to a potential organ donor drawn from a comparable population as the cell panel donors.

Solid Phase Antibody Screening

Antibody-mediated damage has been reported in the absence of detectable antibody by cytotoxic screening methods as described earlier; the development of more sensitive assays was needed. The desire to discriminate HLA antibody from non-HLA antibody, as well as to clearly differentiate Class I and Class II antibodies stimulated the development of the currently available solid phase methodologies. These methods utilize only soluble or recombinant HLA molecules rather than lymphocyte targets which present both HLA and non-HLA molecules. Purified HLA molecules are applied to solid phase media (enzyme-linked immunosorbent assay [ELISA] [20, 21] platforms or microbeads [22]), and therefore will bind only HLA antibody when recipient serum is added. Antibodies to human IgG that are enzyme conjugated (in the case of ELISA) or fluorescent dye conjugated (microbead) are then added and detect any HLA antibody in the serum that is bound to antigen via an optical density reading (ELISA) or fluorescence detection (microbead). Microbeads may be run on a traditional flow cytometer (Flow PRA ®) or may be multiplexed in a suspension array on the Luminex® platform allowing for high throughput detection of multiple analytes in a single reaction chamber (Fig. 2.1b). Both of the microbead-based assays are up to 10% more sensitive for lower titer antibody than the ELISA which in turn is up to 10% more sensitive than antihuman globulin (AHG) enhanced cytotoxicity-based assays for the detection of HLA antibody [19]. By virtue of controlling the antigens placed on the beads, these assays are specific for HLA antibody only, Class I and Class II HLA antibody may be easily distinguished by utilizing class-specific beads, and isotype detection can be limited to IgG. Finally, precise specificities may be determined by utilizing beads that each binds only one unique HLA antigen (Table 2.2).

Limitations of Solid Phase Antibody Testing

Although the use of these platforms has addressed many of the problems associated with cellular assays, they too have their limitations including detection of both non-complement and complement binding antibody simultaneously (which may have different clinical implications), and detection of antibody well below the level associated with a positive crossmatch. The detectable antibody may not always be associated with a meaningful clinical outcome, yet if this information is used to exclude potential donors, it could limit transplants with negligible net benefit. The role of non-HLA antibodies in certain clinical outcomes is increasingly recognized, so it is important that we do not view solid phase HLA test results in isolation. As the number of HLA alleles identified continues to grow into the thousands, it is clear the full spectrum of unique HLA antigens cannot be practically represented on solid phase assays. Clear examination of donor and recipient typing must also be considered in the interpretation of any solid phase PRA result.

The outputs of solid phase assays are fluorescence or optical density readouts; these are continuous variables and considerable controversy exists as to what thresholds should be considered positive. As a result, there can be substantial interlaboratory variability; it is recommended that the clinician review how antibodies are called and how they are correlated to crossmatch results in their own HLA laboratory [23].

Crossmatching

In a 1969 landmark paper, Patel and Terasaki [24] demonstrated for the first time that recipients with DSA in their serum at transplant had substantially higher rates of hyperacute rejection and primary nonfunction. The test described in the paper was the cytotoxic assay described in the previous sections of serologic typing and cytotoxic PRA testing. Thus, the T cell cytotoxic crossmatch was implemented almost universally as the requisite immune assay before transplant [25] and resulted in a significant reduction in hyperacute rejection. Detection of donor-specific cytotoxic antibodies (a positive crossmatch) was a contraindication to transplant. In contrast to a PRA, which identifies all antibodies to a potential pool of donors, the crossmatch identifies whether a recipient has antibodies to a particular single donor of interest. Although a vast improvement over the absence of testing, the T cell cytotoxic crossmatch had a 4% false negative rate and a 20% false positive rate

Table 2.3 Differences between commonly used crossmatch methods

	CDC	AHG-CDC	Flow cytometry	Cytotoxicity with flow cytometry
Detects HLA Ab	Yes	Yes	Yes	Yes
Detects non-HLA Ab	Yes	Yes	Yes	Yes
Detects IgM	Yes	Yes	No	No
Detects low titer Ab	No	Yes but less sensitive than flow cytometry	Yes	Yes
Ab titer detected	Moderate to high	Low to moderate	Low to very low	Low to very low
Detects noncomplement binding Ab	No	No	Yes	Yes

demonstrating it was insufficient to define all relevant antibodies and may be unnecessarily excluding patients from transplant. Over time, assays have been developed to address these limitations [26–29], and the improved sensitivity has lead to a critical examination of which antibodies identified by more sophisticated techniques are predictive of significant clinical outcomes (Table 2.3). The solid phase antibody screening data should always be used in conjunction with crossmatch results to help classify them as immunologically irrelevant or relevant (high risk of rejection or graft loss, or transplant contraindicated) [30].

Complement-Dependent Cytotoxicity Crossmatch Methods

The T cell expresses Class I HLA as well as non-HLA antigens and therefore acts as an in vitro "surrogate" allograft, with the actual allograft expected to express the same cell surface proteins on its endothelium. The B cell additionally expresses Class II HLA antigens, which may be additionally expressed on the endothelium of an allograft. Similar to the method used in cytotoxic antibody screening, the cytotoxic crossmatch result is considered positive if a significant proportion of the T lymphocytes are killed after the addition of complement, inferring that substantial DSA had been bound to the cell surface (Fig. 2.2a). However, as with cytotoxic PRA screening, similar concerns of low titer but nonetheless relevant antibody potentially not detected has lead to improvements to this technique of increasing sensitivity, including longer incubation times, additional wash steps [26] and most commonly, the AHG-enhanced method [27]. AHG, a complement fixing antibody to human immunoglobulin, is added as a second step, and binds any DSA already on the lymphocyte (both complement binding as well as noncomplement binding DSA) thereby increasing the antibody density, the likelihood of activating complement, and thereby increasing sensitivity (Fig. 2.2b). Moreover, the lower titer antibodies detected by this method are found to be clinically significant; they were associated with 36% 1 year allograft loss compared with 18% loss in those with a negative test [28]. All these methods may also be applied to B cells which may identify Class I and II as well as non-HLA DSA.

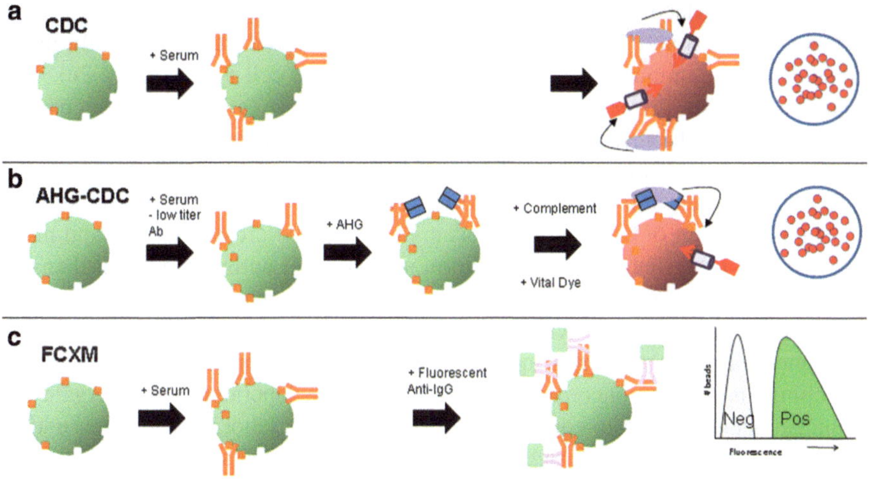

Fig. 2.2 Evolution of basic crossmatching techniques (see Fig. 2.1). (**a**) In an unenhanced complement dependent cytotoxicity crossmatch (CD), when high titer DSA is bound to the cell in sufficient density, complement is activated, the cell is killed and the vital dye is taken up identifying the dead cells. (**b**) With the AHG enhancement, lower titer antibody is less dense on the cell surface and would not naturally activate complement. Adding AHG increases the overall density of complement activating antibodies on a cell that already has some DSA bound, thereby allowing complement activation with subsequent cell death as with CDC alone. (**c**) In FCXM, donor-specific antibody binds the cell and a second fluorescent antibody to human IgG is used to detect even small amounts of bound antibody. When run through a flow cytometer, the DSA (which may be complement or noncomplement binding) is measured as fluorescence on the cells

Limitations of Cytotoxic Crossmatch

As with cytotoxic PRA, the cytotoxic crossmatch may miss low titer antibody giving false negatives, or detect non-HLA IgG antibody, autoantibody, or IgM HLA/non-HLA antibody resulting in false positives, the latter of which can be mitigated to an extent by treating serum with dithiothriotol to break the disulfide bonds in the IgM pentamer, resulting in a more immunologically relevant test result.

Flow Cytometry Crossmatch Methods

Basic Flow cytometry crossmatch (FCXM) differs from cytotoxic crossmatching in that it detects DSA regardless of the ability for complement fixation. Rather it detects only the presence or absence of IgG DSA on the donor lymphocyte. Recipient serum is incubated with donor lymphocytes, and then secondarily stained with a fluorochrome conjugated anti-IgG antibody that remains bound only if DSA from the recipient serum is initially bound to the cell surface. Additional antibodies with different fluorochromes that are specific to unique B and T lymphocyte surface proteins can be added such that when run through a flow cytometer, the B and T cells may be easily distinguished and individually interrogated for the unique DSAs corresponding to those cell types (Fig. 2.2c). The output of the flow crossmatch is at least semiquantitative (e.g., number of channel shifts of mean fluorescence above the baseline or standardized against MESF [molecules of equivalent soluble fluorescence] beads) but thresholds for positivity can vary between individual laboratories. Nonetheless, it is less subjective than visual assessment of cell death that occurs in cytotoxic crossmatching, and more biologically representative of the continuous nature of antibody amount than the dichotomous positive/negative result of cytotoxic crossmatches.

Once again, as for flow cytometric-based antibody screening, there is considerable interlaboratory variability in methods routinely used for flow cytometric crossmatching and in the concordance of results between laboratories [31]. Again the clinician is encouraged to communicate with their own laboratory to better understand the methods of crossmatch performance and reporting at their center.

A variant of flow crossmatching permits concomitant definition of the proportion of complement/noncomplement binding donor DSAs in a sample. Simultaneous measurement of complement binding cytotoxic antibodies (by various cell death markers) over a denominator of total antibody (both complement and noncomplement binding) can be determined by appropriate staining techniques in flow cytometry [32]. Whereas this test has greater sensitivity for complement binding antibody than standard complement dependent cytotoxicity assays, their role in refining a patient's immunological risk assessment has yet to be demonstrated and such tests may not be available in all labs. One cardiac transplant study of complement fixation by antibody on solid phase beads showed an incremental increase in allograft loss over noncomplement fixing antibody [33].

Non-HLA Antibodies

With the appreciation that HLA antibodies have a substantial impact on both short- and long-term allograft outcomes, it has also become clear that in some cases, antibody-mediated outcomes are clinically or pathologically suspected, but no circulating HLA antibodies are detected. There is increasing awareness that in some of these cases, immunologically relevant non-HLA antibodies may be contributing. Whereas this was first postulated over 3 decades ago [34], recent data from the Collaborative Transplant Study highlighted that even amongst HLA identical sibling transplants, high PRA recipients had worse graft outcomes, suggesting that non-HLA antibodies may be at least partly responsible for this finding [35]. In some cases, it may be seen with newer antibody technologies that HLA antibodies to Cw, DQ, and DP antigens (which only recently were able to be reliably detected on a large scale) may be responsible for some of these discrepancies, in siblings identical at HLA-A, B and DR. But in other cases it appears that exploration of non-HLA antibodies is relevant.

The etiology of these antibodies may be quite different than that of HLA antibodies. In addition to exposure to polymorphic alloantigen – which is thought to be causative in MICA (major histocompatibility complex [MHC] class I-related chain A) antibody development – other pathways may include the exposure of otherwise hidden antigens during injury which stimulate autoimmunity, molecular mimicry with antibodies to viruses crossreacting with antigenic epitopes, and nonadherence to immunosuppressive protocols.

It is very important to remember that the target antigens for these antibodies are not expressed on lymphocytes, and therefore not detected on traditional lymphocyte (cytotoxic or flow) crossmatching. As such, the assertion that non-HLA antibodies detected in lymphocyte crossmatches are not immunologically relevant remains valid. The relevance of non-HLA antibodies detected an assays specific for their detection, remains a large area of investigation.

Applications of HLA Testing in Solid Organ Transplantation

Applications of HLA Typing

Prior to modern era immunosuppression, the impact of HLA mismatch on transplant was clinically very significant [36]. With current immunosuppressive regimens we now have a majority of first allografts with HLA mismatches and still acceptable graft survival. However, large registries still show a statistically significant (though less clinically dramatic) impact of HLA mismatches on deceased donor transplants [37]. Results from the Collaborative Transplant Study indicate that shortening of cold ischemia time does not eliminate the effect of HLA matching and argue for consideration of HLA type in deceased donor allocation.

In the setting of regrafts, repeat Class I and/or Class II antigens with a prior donor may have an independent deleterious effect on graft survival, underscoring the need for accurate donor typing such that risk assessment may be properly estimated [38, 39]. Furthermore, even matching of HLA antigens within a given CREG group may be associated with better long-term allograft survival [40, 41]. The development of late antibody-mediated outcomes may require a diagnosis of DSA, which necessitates knowledge of donor typing.

Additionally, for the third of waitlisted patients who have preformed antibody to HLA antigens (see below), accurate donor typing is paramount in the identification of lower risk donors to whom the recipients do not have alloantibody, as in acceptable mismatch [11] or paired exchange programs [18, 42]. Occasionally, patients may form antibody to only certain alleles at a given locus, for example antibody to B*4402 but not B*4401. Molecular typing may be used to ensure only those donors with the allele of interest are potentially excluded, rather than all B44 donors [30, 43].

Ongoing work is examining whether incompatibilities at HLA-Cw, DP, DQ and MICA [44, 45], MICB (MHC class I-related chain B), and KIR (killer cell immunoglobulin-like receptor) [46] influence graft outcome. Molecular technologies may be easily adapted for typing at these loci as the evidence surrounding their importance is emerging.

Applications of Antibody Screening/PRA Testing

The presence of PRA/HLA antibodies has been repeatedly associated with poor transplant outcomes [35]. There has been considerable debate as to what threshold of PRA percent should be considered "high risk"; now that specificities of HLA antibodies may be more precisely defined, it is clear that it is the specificity and not the percent PRA per se that defines the clinical risk. With PRA testing output demonstrable as a continuous variable, the dichotomous approach of high vs. low risk is clearly not biologically reflective of risk which is also a continuum. The amount of antibody as well as the specificities contributes to the assessment of risk. Higher amounts of antibodies can be associated with more short-term clinical adverse outcomes (e.g., acute antibody-mediated rejection) whereas lower titers of antibodies may be associated with chronic pathologies or may take some time to develop into higher titers with a later presentation of acute pathology. Even a PRA of 5% may confer significant risk if the antibody it represents binds to donor antigens. A low titer antibody may become high titer antibody if stimulated by the appropriate antigen from a donor organ and may explain why pretransplant low titer DSA is associated with subsequent posttransplant adverse outcomes [47]. Conversely, by defining precise antibody specificities, unsuitable donors can be avoided in high PRA patients and with the selection of an acceptably mismatched donor (one to whom no antibodies are directed), they can now expect comparable long-term outcomes as nonsensitized patients [11, 48]. Therefore, the detection of any HLA antibody must be followed by the interrogation of comprehensive specificities for it is those specificities, rather than a particular PRA percent, which determines the risk assessment when considered along with the potential donor typing.

PRA percent is relevant, but should be interpreted instead as an estimate of the fraction of potential donors to whom a patient has donor-directed antibody and therefore it represents the "risk" of donor specificity occurring, but not the risk of an immunologic event in and of itself. Calculated PRA (cPRA) is a standardized approach to determining the likelihood that a recipient will have DSAs by comparing the antibody specificities (determined on solid phase assay locally) to the defined frequencies of HLA alleles in the population of interest nationally. A U.S. cPRA calculator may be found on the OPTN website for public access.

Antibody to a donor may be detected on a solid phase assay even when a crossmatch is negative, owing to the high sensitivity of these tests. The significance of these findings in studies ranges from no clinical relevance [49] to an increase in short- and long-term outcomes [15, 16, 50].

A major utilization of solid phase antibody testing is to assist in the interpretation of which crossmatches may be of immunologic relevance (see below).

Regardless of assay type, all no antibody screening test can fully evaluate the potential for memory responses. The ability to predict a future immunologic event is based only upon the serum available after patient identification and referral and cannot therefore measure antibodies that may have occurred in the past with historical sensitizing events that have subsequently waned. It does happen that when a serum appears to be free of antibodies, shortly after a repeat stimulus with a transplant, a memory response may still occur and new antibodies develop much more quickly than the 4–6 weeks required for a de novo response. As such, although largely reassuring, negative antibody screening history alone can completely exclude a potential memory response; clinical history of sensitizing events must always be considered even in an unsensitized recipient.

Virtual Crossmatching

The virtual crossmatch (VXM), despite its name, is not a true crossmatch in the sense of mixing cells and serum in a test tube, but rather an application of both solid phase antibody screening and donor HLA typing together. In essence it "mixes" the known antibody specificities of a recipient serum with the donor HLA antigens, as a prediction of the actual crossmatch results when the true in vitro test is done. The limitations of the virtual crossmatch must be carefully considered by the clinician. Antibody specificities, titers, and presence or absence can vary significantly over time. Therefore, using antibody specificities from a serum that is, for example, 6 months old cannot with certainty predict a crossmatch that is performed on current serum 6 months later. Blood transfusions, transplants, and pregnancies that occur after antibody specificities are defined may substantially change those antibody specificities that are then detected. As such, the virtual crossmatch should be performed considering all available serum results for a patient including at least one recent (<3–6 months old) serum.

The VXM may also be false positive in the case of very low titer/noncomplement binding antibody or where the crossmatch is less sensitive than the antibody detection method, and this may unnecessarily exclude donors if used for the purposes of allocation. Similarly, patients may demonstrate allele specific antibodies (e.g., antibody to DRB1*0401 but not other DRB1*04 alleles) [30] which may unnecessarily exclude other DR4 donors. Also, DNA typing may identify null alleles that are not expressed as antigens on the cell surface but would be excluded by VXM based on typing alone.

Alternatively the VXM may be falsely negative, as the ever-expanding list of all potential HLA antigens in the population cannot be completely represented on solid phase tests [9, 14]. Care must be taken to ensure that the donor alleles are completely represented on the solid phase panel in order to report a negative VXM. Correlation between VXM and actual crossmatch is highly variable depending on the methods used and the operating range must be clarified within each transplant center laboratory until better standardization is achieved. As it is not 100% predictive of positive or negative results, the currently acceptable approach is that an actual crossmatch must also be performed, either prospectively or retrospectively depending on program policies [48].

Crossmatch Interpretation and Limitations

T lymphocytes express Class I HLA and non-HLA antigens and B lymphocytes express both Class I and Class II as well as non-HLA antigens. Therefore, in general, a positive crossmatch due to HLA Class I antibody will be positive on T and B cells, and that due to HLA Class II antibody will be T cell negative and B cell positive. However, antibody to irrelevant non-HLA targets may confound these results and must be considered to clarify whether a crossmatch result is accurately identifying risk. Table 2.4 outlines a general approach to the interpretation of crossmatches in the context of other testing parameters. Individual cases of positive crossmatches that appear to be immunologically irrelevant should always be reviewed with your own HLA laboratory.

Non-HLA/Autoantibodies

Historically, a positive crossmatch was considered a contraindication to transplantation on the assumption that HLA antibody was the causative factor. We now know that false positives (i.e., not due to HLA antibodies) may be due to cytotoxic antibodies to non-HLA antigens on both T and B cells, or autoreactive IgM or IgG, which are generally considered immunologically insignificant [51, 52]. One potential exception to this is one reported association of complement fixing IgM

Table 2.4 Causes of positive crossmatches – sorted by immunologic relevance

Crossmatch type	Caused by	Supportive testing results
Immunologically RELEVANT positive crossmatches		
T and B cell	IgG class I HLA antibody	Solid phase testing will be positive for class I antibody
B cell	Low titer class I HLA antibody	Solid phase testing positive for class I antibody
B cell	IgG class II HLA antibody	Solid phase testing positive for class II antibody
T and B cell or B cell alone	IgG class I and class II HLA antibody	Solid phase testing positive for both class I and class II antibody
Immunologically IRRELEVANT positive crossmatches		
T and/or B cell	Autoantibody	Autocrossmatch positive
T and/or B cell	IgG non-HLA antibody	Solid phase testing negative for class I or II HLA Ab
T and/or B cell (CDC or AHG CDC only)	IgM non-HLA antibody	Negative after DTT treatment of serum
T and/or B cell (CDC or AHG CDC only)	IgM class I or class II HLA antibody	Negative after DTT treatment of serum
T and B cell	Thymoglobulin/ Alemtuzumab	Clinical history of drug given
B cell	Rituximab	Clinical history of drug given

non-HLA antibodies correlating with early cardiac allograft failure [53]. The autocrossmatch is performed by mixing recipient serum with recipient own cells by the same method as the allocrossmatch. If the autocrossmatch is positive, the allocrossmatch against the donor cannot be interpreted without further testing. Other non-HLA antibodies may be immunologically significant, [45, 54] but are not expressed on the lymphocyte surface and must be detected in specially designed assays.

Allo-IgM

Solid phase antibody tests when run in parallel to crossmatches allow for easy determination if a crossmatch is due to IgG HLA antibody, and is therefore relevant [20, 21, 55]. This is particularly important in the interpretation of B cell crossmatches which have a high false positive rate from non-HLA antibody [56]. By design, alloreactive IgM antibodies are detected by the solid phase manufacturer methods and appear to have no impact in studies of cytotoxic crossmatch outcomes [57]. Treating serum with dithiothriotol (DTT) or heat inactivation will break up any pentameric IgM molecule; a crossmatch that is negative with DTT or heat treatment should be considered negative in terms of immunological risk assessment in general practice.

Low Titer Antibody Detected Only by FCXM

FCXM frequently detects low titer and/or noncomplement binding antibodies not detected by cytotoxic methods. It is recognized that these antibodies still do predict risk for posttransplant rejection and graft loss. Up to 15% of primary transplants and 30% of second transplants may have positive FCXM with negative CDC/AHG-CDC crossmatches; higher rates of early graft loss (<3 months), rejection and worse 1-year allograft survival for both primary [58–60] and second transplants [59, 61] is seen in these cohorts. With FCXM in particular, it is important to confirm HLA antibodies on a solid phase assay [47, 55, 58, 59], as if none are detected, a positive FCXM has no impact on graft survival [55]. Conversely, a negative flow crossmatch in the sensitized patient predicts the similar graft survival as a nonsensitized recipient, [48] further underscoring the importance of donor specificity, rather than PRA as the main determinant of posttransplant risk.

B Cell Crossmatches

B cell cytotoxic crossmatching became common in the 1980s to ascertain the presence of Class II antibody; however, early studies of isolated positive B cell crossmatches had few associations with outcomes [62, 63]. Later studies challenge this finding [64] and solid phase testing explains it further: up to 75% of isolated B cell crossmatches are due to non-HLA or autoantibodies, [56] and in those cases, having comparably good outcomes to negative crossmatch recipients [58]. Autocrossmatching to exclude positive B cell crossmatch from autoantibody, with solid phase confirming Class II antibody presence or absence, is imperative to interpret the B cell crossmatch as relevant (due to Class I or II HLA antibody) or irrelevant.

A positive B cell crossmatch with negative T cell crossmatch may also be due to low titer Class I antibody as Class I antigen may be expressed with increased density on B cells compared with T cells [65]. When confirmed with solid phase antibody testing to be due to HLA antibody, it is associated with higher rejection rates and graft losses [64, 66].

Historic Crossmatches

The historical serum stored in the HLA lab may be viewed as a window into immunologic history and memory of the patient, for as far back as the serum was collected. Patients with a negative crossmatch to a donor using current serum, but a positive crossmatch using a historical serum (with different antibody specificities and titers), have higher rates of early graft loss and diminished graft survival [58, 67]. While not an absolute contraindication to transplant per se, a positive historical crossmatch clearly identifies increased posttransplant risk of the potential for memory response.

Posttransplant Testing

All of the above testing methodologies are routinely and systematically applied pretransplant; however, a major immune activating event is the transplant itself with subsequent alloimmune responses that, with these new technologies, can now be easily measured posttransplant. Recently, there has been increased interest in the posttransplant measurement of alloantibody in particular with strong associations between the presence of posttransplant antibodies and acute and chronic pathology and graft loss in heart [68], lung [69], and kidney transplantation [70, 71].

When studied in smaller, well-defined patient groups, it becomes clear that the application and predictive ability of these tests may vary depending on the pretransplant risk of the recipient–donor pairs. One recent study of low immunologic risk patients demonstrated little predictive ability of first year antibody testing on acute humoral rejection outcomes [72] whereas in a high risk cohort, early changes in antibody levels were strongly predictive of acute rejection [73]. Ongoing studies are required to better define these relationships and implement posttransplant standardized testing protocols analogous to those currently practiced pretransplant.

Summary

In summary, basic HLA laboratory testing in the current era results in accurate donor and recipient typing, sensitive and specific screening for HLA and non-HLA antibodies, and precise crossmatching methodologies in order to more closely describe humoral immunologic risk. DSAs to HLA and non-HLA antigens may be semiquantitatively ranked by strength such that risk may be more accurately viewed as a biological continuum rather than a dichotomous feature. Higher level antibodies may confer immediate risk requiring aggressive therapies or acceptable mismatch strategies to permit safe transplant. Lower level antibodies may identify patients who require altered immunosuppression or closer follow-up. Solid phase testing determines the immunologic relevance of cell-based assays in clinical practice. Risk continues to evolve posttransplant and the utilization of HLA testing in this time period must be systematically evaluated.

Each method outlined in the categories above has inherent strengths and limitations; no one test is intended to function in isolation as the single predictor of transplant immunologic risk. HLA typing identifies potentially appropriate donors for highly sensitized patients, who in turn must have complete and clear antibody specificities determined. Antibody screening for HLA antibody alone may miss clinically relevant non-HLA antibodies, therefore cellular-based assays continue to have a role, as do novel solid phase methods. Crossmatch results do identify DSAs but their correct interpretation for immunologic risk estimate is most predictive of relevant outcomes solid phase antibody when testing is concurrently considered. The complete risk estimate of any donor–recipient pair must therefore consider HLA typing and potentially multiple methods of antibody detection. The reader is encouraged to further examine the newer literature on T cell assays of alloreactivity including ELISpot (measuring T cell cytokine release after stimulation with specific donor antigens or peptides), Cylex ™ Immuknow (an antigen-independent measurement of T cell ATP production after stimulation), and soluble CD30 measurement in the plasma for additional newer developments.

The HLA laboratory is no longer just a "tissue typing lab" but rather one that provides sophisticated humoral risk assessment consultation in the context of the clinical patient assessment. Understanding HLA laboratory methods and their interpretive parameters is paramount for the clinician to correctly stratify patient risk for appropriate therapeutic interventions.

References

1. Arnold ML et al. Anti-HLA class II antibodies in kidney retransplant patients. Tissue Antigens. 2005;65(4):370–8.
2. Muczynski KA et al. Normal human kidney HLA-DR-expressing renal microvascular endothelial cells: characterization, isolation, and regulation of MHC class II expression. J Am Soc Nephrol. 2003;14(5):1336–48.

3. von Andrian UH, Mempel TR. Homing and cellular traffic in lymph nodes. Nat Rev Immunol. 2003;3(11):867–78.
4. Ono SJ, et al. Chemokines: roles in leukocyte development, trafficking, and effector function. J Allergy Clin Immunol. 2003;111(6):1185–99; quiz 1200.
5. Cyster JG. Homing of antibody secreting cells. Immunol Rev. 2003;194:48–60.
6. Jacobelli J et al. New views of the immunological synapse: variations in assembly and function. Curr Opin Immunol. 2004;16(3):345–52.
7. von Andrian UH, Mackay CR. T-cell function and migration. Two sides of the same coin. N Engl J Med. 2000;343(14):1020–34.
8. Prodinger WM et al. Complement. In: Paul WE, editor. Fundamentals in immunology. Philadelphia: Lippincott Williams & Wilkins; 2003. p. 1077–103.
9. Schreuder GM et al. HLA dictionary 2004: summary of HLA-A, -B, -C, -DRB1/3/4/5, -DQB1 alleles and their association with serologically defined HLA-A, -B, -C, -DR, and -DQ antigens. Hum Immunol. 2005;66(2):170–210.
10. Robinson J et al. IMGT/HLA and IMGT/MHC: sequence databases for the study of the major histocompatibility complex. Nucleic Acids Res. 2003;31(1):311–4.
11. Claas FH et al. The acceptable mismatch program as a fast tool for highly sensitized patients awaiting a cadaveric kidney transplantation: short waiting time and excellent graft outcome. Transplantation. 2004;78(2):190–3.
12. Duquesnoy RJ, Claas FH. Is the application of HLAMatchmaker relevant in kidney transplantation? Transplantation. 2005;79(2):250–1.
13. Claas FH et al. Future HLA matching strategies in clinical transplantation. Dev Ophthalmol. 2003;36:62–73.
14. Marsh SG. Nomenclature for factors of the HLA system Monthly Updates 2006–2008. http://www.anthonynolan.com/HIG/nomen/updates/updates.html. 2008. Accessed Date 14 June 2010.
15. van den Berg-Loonen EM et al. Clinical relevance of pretransplant donor-directed antibodies detected by single antigen beads in highly sensitized renal transplant patients. Transplantation. 2008;85(8):1086–90.
16. Gupta A et al. Pretransplant donor-specific antibodies in cytotoxic negative crossmatch kidney transplants: are they relevant? Transplantation. 2008;85(8):1200–4.
17. Stegall MD et al. A comparison of plasmapheresis versus high-dose IVIG desensitization in renal allograft recipients with high levels of donor specific alloantibody. Am J Transplant. 2006;6(2):346–51.
18. Gentry SE et al. Expanding kidney paired donation through participation by compatible pairs. Am J Transplant. 2007;7(10):2361–70.
19. Gebel HM, Bray RA. Sensitization and sensitivity: defining the unsensitized patient. Transplantation. 2000;69(7):1370–4.
20. Zachary AA et al. Characterization of HLA class I specific antibodies by ELISA using solubilized antigen targets: I. Evaluation of the GTI QuikID assay and analysis of antibody patterns. Hum Immunol. 2001;62(3):228–35.
21. Zachary AA et al. Characterization of HLA class I specific antibodies by ELISA using solubilized antigen targets: II. Clinical relevance. Hum Immunol. 2001;62(3):236–46.
22. Pei R et al. Single human leukocyte antigen flow cytometry beads for accurate identification of human leukocyte antigen antibody specificities. Transplantation. 2003;75(1):43–9.
23. Campbell P et al. Standardization of HLA antibody identification across multiple laboratories. Is is feasible? Hum Immunol. 2007;68(s1):s117.
24. Patel R, Terasaki PI. Significance of the positive crossmatch test in kidney transplantation. N Engl J Med. 1969;280(14):735–9.
25. Stiller CR et al. Lymphocyte-dependent antibody and renal graft rejection. Lancet. 1975;1(7913):953–4.
26. Amos DB, Cohen I, Klein Jr WJ. Mechanisms of immunologic enhancement. Transplant Proc. 1970;2(1):68–75.
27. Fuller TC et al. HLA alloantibodies and the mechanism of the antiglobulin-augmented lymphocytotoxicity procedure. Hum Immunol. 1997;56(1–2):94–105.

28. Kerman RH et al. AHG and DTE/AHG procedure identification of crossmatch-appropriate donor-recipient pairings that result in improved graft survival. Transplantation. 1991;51(2): 316–20.
29. Scornik JC et al. Outcome of kidney transplants in patients known to be flow cytometry crossmatch positive. Transplantation. 2001;71(8):1098–102.
30. Gebel HM, Bray RA, Nickerson P. Pre-transplant assessment of donor-reactive, HLA-specific antibodies in renal transplantation: contraindication vs. risk. Am J Transplant. 2003;3(12):1488–500.
31. Scornik JC et al. Multicenter evaluation of the flow cytometry T-cell crossmatch: results from the American Society of Histocompatibility and Immunogenetics-College of American Pathologists proficiency testing program. Transplantation. 1997;63(10):1440–5.
32. Saw CL, Bray RA, Gebel HM. Cytotoxicity and antibody binding by flow cytometry: a single assay to simultaneously assess two parameters. Cytometry B Clin Cytom. 2008;74:287–94.
33. Smith JD et al. C4d fixing, luminex binding antibodies – a new tool for prediction of graft failure after heart transplantation. Am J Transplant. 2007;7(12):2809–15.
34. Ahern AT et al. Hyperacute rejection of HLA-AB-identical renal allografts associated with B lymphocyte and endothelial reactive antibodies. Transplantation. 1982;33(1):103–6.
35. Opelz G. Non-HLA transplantation immunity revealed by lymphocytotoxic antibodies. Lancet. 2005;365(9470):1570–6.
36. Takemoto S et al. Survival of nationally shared, HLA-matched kidney transplants from cadaveric donors. The UNOS Scientific Renal Transplant Registry. N Engl J Med. 1992;327(12):834–9.
37. Wissing KM et al. HLA mismatches remain risk factors for acute kidney allograft rejection in patients receiving quadruple immunosuppression with anti-interleukin-2 receptor antibodies. Transplantation. 2008;85(3):411–6.
38. House AA et al. Re-exposure to mismatched HLA class I is a significant risk factor for graft loss: multivariable analysis of 259 kidney retransplants. Transplantation. 2007;84(6):722–8.
39. Lair D et al. The effect of a first kidney transplant on a subsequent transplant outcome: an experimental and clinical study. Kidney Int. 2005;67(6):2368–75.
40. Crowe DO. The effect of cross-reactive epitope group matching on allocation and sensitization. Clin Transplant. 2003;17 Suppl 9:13–6.
41. Thompson JS, Thacker 2nd LR, Takemoto S. The influence of conventional and cross-reactive group HLA matching on cardiac transplant outcome: an analysis from the United Network of Organ Sharing Scientific Registry. Transplantation. 2000;69(10):2178–86.
42. Segev DL et al. Kidney paired donation and optimizing the use of live donor organs. JAMA. 2005;293(15):1883–90.
43. Bray RA, Gebel HM. Allele specific HLA alloantibodies. Implication for organ allocation. Am J Transplant. 2005;5(s11):488.
44. Mizutani K et al. Serial ten-year follow-up of HLA and MICA antibody production prior to kidney graft failure. Am J Transplant. 2005;5(9):2265–72.
45. Zou Y et al. Antibodies against MICA antigens and kidney-transplant rejection. N Engl J Med. 2007;357(13):1293–300.
46. Tran TH et al. Analysis of KIR ligand incompatibility in human renal transplantation. Transplantation. 2005;80(8):1121–3.
47. Gebel HM et al. Flow PRA to detect clinically relevant HLA antibodies. Transplant Proc. 2001;33(1–2):477.
48. Bray RA et al. Transplanting the highly sensitized patient: the emory algorithm. Am J Transplant. 2006;6(10):2307–15.
49. Bryan CF et al. Successful renal transplantation despite low levels of donor-specific HLA class I antibody without IVIg or plasmapheresis. Clin Transplant. 2006;20(5):563–70.
50. Patel AM et al. Renal transplantation in patients with pre-transplant donor-specific antibodies and negative flow cytometry crossmatches. Am J Transplant. 2007;7(10):2371–7.
51. Cross DE, Greiner R, Whittier FC. Importance of the autocontrol crossmatch in human renal transplantation. Transplantation. 1976;21(4):307–11.
52. Taylor CJ et al. Characterization of lymphocytotoxic antibodies causing a positive crossmatch in renal transplantation. Relationship to primary and regraft outcome. Transplantation. 1989;48(6):953–8.

53. Rose ML, Smith JD. Clinical relevance of complement-fixing antibodies in cardiac transplantation. Hum Immunol. 2009;70(8):605–9.
54. Sumitran-Holgersson S et al. Identification of the nonclassical HLA molecules, mica, as targets for humoral immunity associated with irreversible rejection of kidney allografts. Transplantation. 2002;74(2):268–77.
55. Bray RA et al. Evolution of HLA antibody detection: technology emulating biology. Immunol Res. 2004;29(1–3):41–54.
56. Le Bas-Bernardet S et al. Identification of the antibodies involved in B-cell crossmatch positivity in renal transplantation. Transplantation. 2003;75(4):477–82.
57. Roelen DL et al. IgG antibodies against an HLA antigen are associated with activated cytotoxic T cells against this antigen, IgM are not. Transplantation. 1994;57(9):1388–92.
58. Karpinski M et al. Flow cytometric crossmatching in primary renal transplant recipients with a negative anti-human globulin enhanced cytotoxicity crossmatch. J Am Soc Nephrol. 2001;12(12):2807–14.
59. Kerman RH et al. Improved graft survival for flow cytometry and antihuman globulin crossmatch-negative retransplant recipients. Transplantation. 1990;49(1):52–6.
60. Mahoney RJ et al. The flow cytometric crossmatch and early renal transplant loss. Transplantation. 1990;49(3):527–35.
61. Bryan CF et al. Long-term graft survival is improved in cadaveric renal retransplantation by flow cytometric crossmatching. Transplantation. 1998;66(12):1827–32.
62. Ettinger RB et al. Successful renal allografts across a positive cross-match for donor B-lymphocyte alloantigens. Lancet. 1976;2(7976):56–8.
63. Jeannet M, Benzonana G, Arni I. Donor-specific B and T lymphocyte antibodies and kidney graft survival. Transplantation. 1981;31(3):160–3.
64. Phelan DL et al. Positive B cell crossmatches: specificity of antibody and graft outcome. Transplant Proc. 1989;21(1 Pt 1):687–8.
65. Pellegrino MA et al. B peripheral lymphocytes express more HLA antigens than T peripheral lymphocytes. Transplantation. 1978;25(2):93–5.
66. Mahoney RJ, Taranto S, Edwards E. B-Cell crossmatching and kidney allograft outcome in 9031 United States transplant recipients. Hum Immunol. 2002;63(4):324–35.
67. Turka LA et al. Presensitization and the renal allograft recipient. Transplantation. 1989;47(2):234–40.
68. Xydas S et al. Utility of post-transplant anti-HLA antibody measurements in pediatric cardiac transplant recipients. J Heart Lung Transplant. 2005;24(9):1289–96.
69. Girnita AL et al. HLA-specific antibodies are risk factors for lymphocytic bronchiolitis and chronic lung allograft dysfunction. Am J Transplant. 2005;5(1):131–8.
70. Pelletier RP et al. Clinical significance of MHC-reactive alloantibodies that develop after kidney or kidney-pancreas transplantation. Am J Transplant. 2002;2(2):134–41.
71. Piazza A et al. Impact of donor-specific antibodies on chronic rejection occurrence and graft loss in renal transplantation: posttransplant analysis using flow cytometric techniques. Transplantation. 2001;71(8):1106–12.
72. Gill JS et al. Screening for de novo anti-human leukocyte antigen antibodies in nonsensitized kidney transplant recipients does not predict acute rejection. Transplantation. 2010;89(2):178–84.
73. Burns JM et al. Alloantibody levels and acute humoral rejection early after positive crossmatch kidney transplantation. Am J Transplant. 2008;8(12):2684–94.

Chapter 3
Medical Evaluation of the Living Kidney Donor

Julie Lin

Abstract Living kidney donors have voluntarily assumed the immediate risks of elective surgery, as well as the less well-defined medium and longer term risks to their future health, in gifting half their kidney function to another person. Yet despite this considerable responsibility placed on the living kidney donor, physician advocate, and transplant team members, protocols for the evaluation of potential donors may differ substantially between centers. While a number of published expert recommendations serve as a basis for most living donor protocols, including one for living donors in the United States, the United Kingdom guidelines, and the Amsterdam Living Kidney donor guidelines, variability in guidance regarding donors of older age, with hypertension, and evaluation of diabetes risk, baseline kidney function, and anatomical imaging requirements, persist due in part to the relative lack of detailed longitudinal outcomes data. This chapter seeks to provide a comprehensive approach to the counseling and medical evaluation of potential living donor based on a critical review of the available scientific literature on potentially adverse risk factors.

Keywords Kidney donation • Screening • Hypertension • Obesity • Glucose intolerance

Introduction

Primum non nocere (Latin for "First, do no harm") has been widely attributed to the Hippocratic oath and is an exceptionally appropriate guiding principle in the medical evaluation of potential living kidney donors. Living kidney donors have voluntarily

J. Lin, MD, MPH (✉)
Department of Medicine, Renal Division, Brigham and Women's Hospital and Harvard Medical School, Boston, MA, USA
e-mail: jlin11@partners.org

A. Chandraker et al. (eds.), *Core Concepts in Renal Transplantation*,
DOI 10.1007/978-1-4614-0008-0_3, © Springer Science+Business Media, LLC 2012

assumed the immediate risks of elective surgery, as well as the less well-defined medium and longer term risks to their future health, in gifting half their kidney function to another person.

Yet despite this considerable responsibility placed on the living kidney donor, physician advocate, and transplant team members, protocols for the evaluation of potential donors may differ substantially between centers. While a number of published expert recommendations serve as a basis for most living donor protocols, including one for U.S. living donors [1], the United Kingdom guidelines [2], and the Amsterdam living kidney donor guidelines [3], variability in guidance regarding donors of older age, with hypertension, and evaluation of diabetes risk, baseline kidney function, and anatomical imaging requirements, persist due in part due to the relative lack of detailed longitudinal outcomes data.

Living kidney donation has gained wider popularity in recent years with approximately 6,000 donor nephrectomies currently performed each year in the United States. Superior renal allograft outcomes have been noted: one analysis of 14,162 living compared with 31,720 cadaveric allografts in the United Network for Organ Sharing (UNOS) database reported that 10-year graft survival for living transplants was 68% compared to 51% for cadaveric transplants [4].

This chapter seeks to provide a comprehensive approach to the counseling and medical evaluation of potential living donor based on a critical review of the available scientific literature on potentially adverse risk factors.

Overview of Living Kidney Donor Screening and Evaluation

At Brigham and Women's Hospital, we have synthesized a protocol for living kidney donor screening upon review of published guidelines above; our process is summarized in Table 3.1 and Fig. 3.1. We require that living donors have an average creatinine clearance of >90 mL/min. Because of potential errors in timed urine collections, donors with borderline creatinine clearance often undergo direct measurement of glomerular filtration rate (GFR) by ^{99}Tm-DTPA. Microalbumin and total urinary protein excretion should be in the reference ranges of <30 mg/24 h and <150 mg/24 h, respectively. It should be noted, however, that even low levels of albuminuria in the traditional "normal range" have been consistently shown to confer significantly increased risk for cardiovascular disease and all-cause mortality in large population studies [5, 6]. Whether this risk of low levels of albuminuria is directly applicable to generally very healthy living donors is not known, however, but it does raise the considerations of cardiovascular morbidity and mortality in addition to risk for progressive kidney disease after donation.

Abnormalities on urinalysis and urine microscopy are also scrutinized; in particular, the presence of microscopic hematuria receives a thorough evaluation for urinary tract as well as intrarenal abnormalities as appropriate. The indications and details for evaluation of cardiovascular risk are summarized in Fig. 3.2. Any abnormal

Table 3.1 Blood, urine, and radiology screening tests for potential living kidney donors

Blood tests
Chem 7 panel
Calcium, phosphorus, uric acid
Liver function tests
Fasting lipids
Fasting glucose, hemoglobin a1c%[a]
Complete blood count (CBC)
PT/PTT/INR
HIV
Hepatitis B and C serologies
RPR (syphilis)
Cytomegalovirus IgG
PSA for men >50 years (for African Americans >40 years)
HCG pregnancy test for women of childbearing potential
Sickle cell screening for African Americans
Tissue typing
Urine tests
Urinalysis (urine dipstick) and microscopy on two separate days
Timed 24-h urine collections on two separate days for urinary creatinine, creatinine clearance, microalbumin, total protein[b]
Urine culture
Other tests
Chest X-ray (PA and lateral)
Electrocardiogram
PAP smear within 1 year for women
Mammogram for women >40 years old
Colonoscopy recommended within past 10 years if >50 years old
Renal USG or CT if family history of PCKD[c]
Pulmonary function tests for active smokers
Cardiac stress testing (only as indicated – see Fig. 3.2)
CT angiography of kidneys

Brief directions given to patients for 24-h urine collection: (a) discard first morning urine on first day, (b) wake up at same time on second day, (c) collect all urine voids until AFTER first morning urine on second day

[a]Patients with history of diabetes mellitus in a first-degree relative should have oral glucose tolerance testing

[b]Blood creatinine needs to also be drawn on days when 24-h urines are completed to allow calculation of creatinine clearances

[c]If donor <30 years, two cysts establishes PCKD, either unilateral or bilateral by CT or MRI. If donor is 30–59 years old, two cysts in each kidney establishes PCKD, and if donors >60 years, four cysts in each kidney establishes PCKD. No donor candidates are accepted below age 30 unless genetic testing is normal

laboratory results receive repeated testing and further evaluation, including referrals to subspecialists as needed.

The extent and type of radiologic imaging for kidney donors varies between centers. At our institution, a contrast tomography (CT) angiography study with

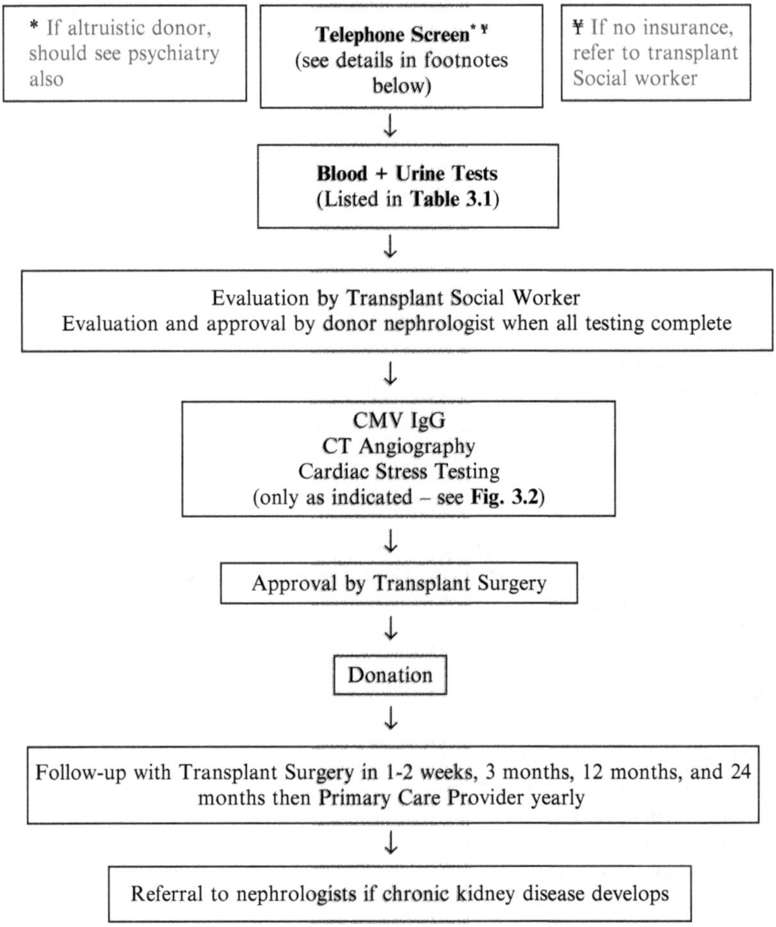

Fig. 3.1 Algorithm for evaluation of potential living kidney donors. Notes: initial telephone questions to potential donors; cancel further evaluation if any of following is present: (1) History of diabetes or diabetes during any pregnancy. (2) Symptomatic multiple kidney stones or first stone within past 1 year. (3) Any history of hypertension and age <50. (4) Hypertension, age ≥50 and on >2 antihypertensive medications (if on ≤2 BP meds, first exclude hypertension retinopathy by eye exam and LVH by ECHO, then confirm that 24-h ambulatory BP monitoring shows 24 h average BP ≤ 130/80 before proceeding with further workup.). (5) Cancer in last 5 years (do not include carcinoma-in-situ of uterine cervix or carcinoma-in-situ of breast cervix or nonmelanoma skin cancer.). (6) BMI ≥ 30 (calculated from height and weight); do advise weight loss and reassess when weight goal is reached. (7) Financial incentive. Check with nephrologists donor MD before further evaluation if any of: (1) age 18–24.9 years. (2) Kidney disease (please specify)

intravenous contrast, which includes an evaluation of the number and caliber of renal vessels, is performed when medical clearance is obtained. We emphasize to the donors that findings on the CT may provide new data, such as asymptomatic bilateral kidney stones or renal tumors, which may exclude the patient from donation.

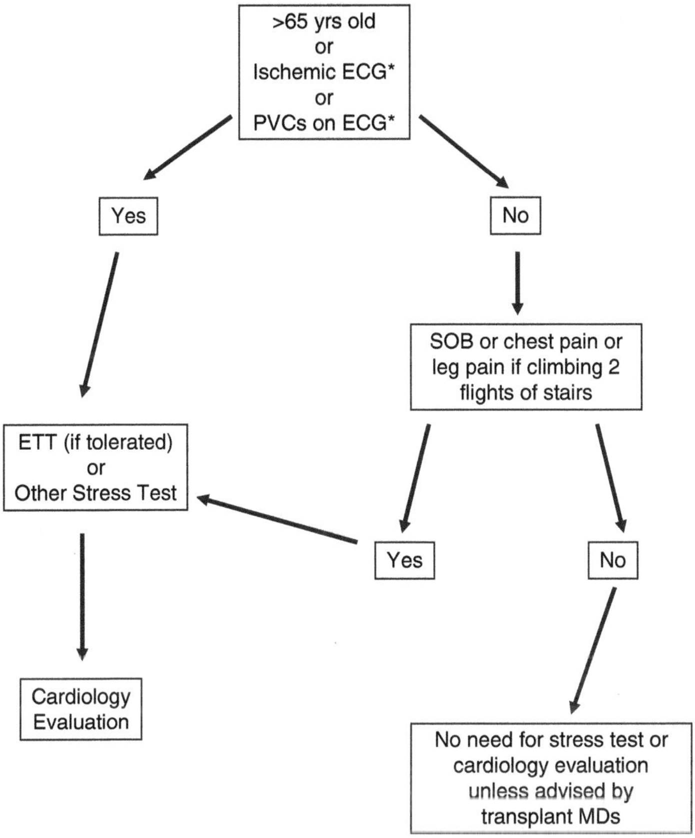

Fig. 3.2 Algorithm for cardiac testing of potential living kidney donor (patients with known cardiovascular disease will almost always be already excluded from donation). Review ECGs with donor physicians as needed. *PVCs* premature ventricular contractions (ectopy); *ETT* exercise treadmill test; *SOB* shortness of breath

Discussion of Risks, Benefits, and Expectations with Potential Living Kidney Donors

The primary role of the living kidney donor advocate is to advise and inform the potential donors about the potential risks, benefits, and alternatives (including dialysis and cadaveric transplantation for the recipient) to living donation. This includes potential psychosocial and financial, in addition to medical, considerations. Living donors are educated about the improved quality of life and decreased mortality risks in kidney transplant recipients compared to patients who do not receive transplants. The superior allograft survival noted in preemptive kidney transplants (i.e., before dialysis is needed) from living donors is also mentioned [7].

Ascertainment that the desire to donate is free of coercion (especially family pressure) and financial incentive is also important. The physician's goal is to empower the patient to make an informed and autonomous decision about whether to proceed with the donation evaluation and process. The discussion of the potential donor's decision making should be kept confidential and free of conflict of interest relative to the potential recipient. The shorter recovery time with laparoscopic donor nephrectomy, the primary approach at our institution, is also addressed. We also recommend a 4–6 week postsurgery recovery period for most patients and up to 3 months for donors who may have physically demanding and active jobs.

Our transplant center provides a folder with living donor education materials as well as access to informational videos by the American Society of Transplant Surgeons and UNOS as part of the patient education process. Additional independent research and reading by potential living donors of internet-based resources such as those provided by the National Kidney Foundation (www.kidney.org/transplantation/livingDonors/index.cfm) are also strongly encouraged.

Independent Donor Advocate and the Informed Consent Process

Each kidney transplantation center in the United States is required by the Center for Medicare Services (CMS) to have a designated living donor advocate. Ideally, in order to minimize potential issues with conflict of interest, this should be a formally trained nephrologist who is not involved with the kidney recipient evaluation or posttransplant care. The donor advocate should place the interests and well-being of the potential living donor at the forefront of the evaluation, as well as work cooperatively with the other members of the transplant team (surgeons, coordinators, social workers, psychologists, etc.) to provide detailed education about the risks and benefits of living kidney donation so that the donor can make an autonomous, informed decision about whether to proceed with the donation evaluation.

Our center also places consistent and strong emphasis on the idea that any significant lack of desire to donate a kidney constitutes a contraindication and that the potential donor may signify this at any point during the evaluation process. Moreover, in the not uncommon situation where a potential donor finds it very difficult to communicate the wish to withdraw from donating to the potential recipient (especially noted when the pair are close family members), we stress that the transplant team will tell the recipient that a reason has been found that precludes living kidney donation.

Considerations in Living Donor Age

The majority of U.S. kidney transplant centers will not consider living donors who are younger than 18 years [8]. Because the majority of living donors are close relatives of the recipients with kidney failure (and therefore may have a genetic predisposition for subsequent renal failure themselves), our center favors a more conservative lower age limit of 25 years, although we will consider living donors as young as 18 years if there are no other donors and the donor–recipient pair are parent and child,

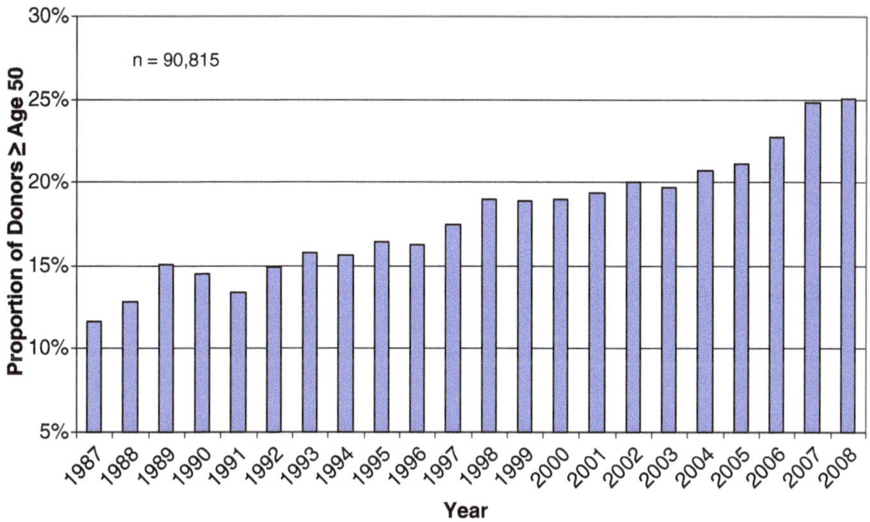

Fig. 3.3 Proportion of living kidney donors ≥50 years old at time of donation (data from the United Network for Organ Sharing (UNOS)/Organ Procurement and Transplantation Network (OPTN) dataset of living kidney donors and transplant recipients; November 2009)

for example. In potential donors with a family history of polycystic kidney disease, however, we require a minimum age of 30 years and no evidence of cystic kidney disease by radiology screening (Table 3.1).

In the medical literature, living donors aged >50 years are typically considered to be "older donors." The proportion of these older donors has been increasing over the past 20+ years in the United States, as documented in the UNOS database (Fig. 3.3) to the point where they comprise approximately one-quarter of living donors in recent years. We do not apply an absolute upper age limit that precludes kidney donation; instead we rely on clinical assessment of a potential older donor's medical history and physical findings, as well as activity and lifestyle, while recognizing that the residual kidney function after donor nephrectomy in older donors is of concern. A recent study of 178 consecutive living kidney donors who underwent predonation and postdonation renal functional reserve assessment (as measured by percent increase in iothalamate GFR with low-dose dopamine infusion) reported that older age was associated with greater loss in renal reserve after donor nephrectomy [9]. Furthermore, as blood pressure tends to increase over time in living donors with aging [10] (as in the general population), the risk of subsequent chronic kidney and cardiovascular disease in older living donors from hypertension is of additional concern.

Older donor age also has been associated with higher rates of acute rejection and graft loss in the transplanted kidney although the effect appears most significant in donors >65 years of age [11]. Therefore, as part of the informed consent process for living kidney donor nephrectomy, a discussion of how older age at time of donation may result in decreased ability of the remaining kidney to compensate for GFR should be included.

Hypertension in Living Donors

The risk conferred by hypertension in the potential living kidney donor represents an important area of concern where significant further research is needed. Because hypertension is present in the majority of progressive chronic kidney diseases and is itself a strong independent risk factor for chronic kidney disease [12] as well as cardiovascular disease, this is a chronic condition that deserves careful scrutiny in potential donors. This caution is reflected nationally as in 2007, 47% of U.S. programs exclude donors on any hypertension medications and an additional 41% exclude donors on more than one hypertension medication [8].

We acknowledge, however, that a potential living donor's short- and long-term well-being may be so closely linked to the health of the potential recipient (who is likely a relative or close friend), that after considerable discussion, we have decided to be relatively generous in our screening criteria and allow donors age 50 or greater who taking < two antihypertensive medications to be screened; however, acceptance as a donor is not assured. This is based in part on the Amsterdam criteria, which recommended that patients with "easily controlled hypertension" who are >50 years age, have a GFR > 80 mL/min, and have urinary albumin excretion ratio (AER) <30 mg/day, may "represent a low-risk group for development of kidney disease after donation and may be acceptable as kidney donors" [3].

In particular, our center evaluates the duration, severity (including how many medications), and control of hypertension (Fig. 3.1). Presence of end organ damage (such as hypertensive retinopathy or left ventricular hypertrophy) is considered an absolute contraindication to donation. Potential donors taking two or fewer hypertension medications are required to undergo 24-h ambulatory blood pressure monitoring to assess adequacy of blood pressure control. In the situation where hypertension is newly diagnosed at the time of donor evaluation, patients younger than 50 years are excluded from donating at that time and patients 50 years or older are placed on a single blood pressure agent and re-evaluated in 6 months with 24-h blood pressure monitoring.

This cautious and conservative approach is supported by original published data. In a study of Korean living donors, hypertension (defined as >140/90 mmHg that was well controlled by at most one blood pressure agent) in absence of end organ damage and other work up, in presence of GFR > 80/mL/min had an ~8 fold increased risk of GFR < 60 endpoint after >50 months of follow-up (mean 77 months) [13]. While a study by Textor et al. of 24 hypertensive (mean 24-h ambulatory blood pressure monitor values of >135/85 mmHg or on medications [$n = 3$]) compared with 124 normotensive donors reported no significant differences in the two groups, a major limitation was the short 1-year follow up [14]. Of note, there was a small 7 mL/min lower GFR directly measured by iothalamate in hypertensive donors at 1 year that was statistically significant and attributable to the lower baseline GFR seen in this group [14].

Obesity in Living Donors

Our center requires that living donors achieve a BMI of 30 kg/m^2 or better before undergoing donor nephrectomy; this is largely due to the increased difficulties and complications for laparascopic nephrectomy in patients who are obese. We often note, however, that obese or overweight patients have several risk factors for developing subsequent kidney and cardiovascular complications including higher blood pressure, borderline or overt glucose intolerance, and dyslipidemia, all of which often improve with weight loss. Therefore, we favor that potential living donors who have BMI > 30 kg/m^2 defer detailed testing until they can lose weight to achieve a BMI of 30 kg/m^2 or better.

Being overweight or obese have been identified as independent risk factors for development of chronic kidney disease [12] and progression to end-stage renal disease [15] and it is possible that transplanted kidneys from overweight donors have a greater degree of early focal segmental sclerosis as previously reported in obese adults [16]. A study of 73 kidney donors has reported those with BMI > 30 kg/m^2 had significantly greater risk for developing overt proteinuria or renal insufficiency (92 vs. 12%, $p<0.001$) [17]. Obesity in living donors has also been identified as a risk factor for longer surgical times [18] and more perioperative complications [19].

Using the UNOS database, our research group observed that median donor BMI between 2004 and 2008 was 26.4 kg/m^2 and did not vary by year. (No living donor data on weight and height from before 2004 are available.) Almost two-thirds of the living donors had BMI >25 kg/m^2; similarly, approximately 60% of their recipients had BMI > 25 kg/m^2. We have also identified extreme BMI mismatch where the living donor is heavier as conferring a significantly elevated risk for death-censored allograft loss after adjustment for known potential confounders including donor and recipient BMI and clinical characteristics [20]. By definition, these donors were all in the morbidly obese category (BMI > 35 kg/m^2) however, so there may also be an effect of donor obesity although donor BMI was not associated with allograft loss in the multivariable adjusted model.

Evaluation of Glucose Tolerance and Future Diabetes Risk

As diabetes mellitus is considered the leading cause of ESRD, current glucose tolerance and future diabetes risk is also an important consideration in living donors. We assess fasting glucose and Hgb A1c% in all living donors; patients with a family history of diabetes mellitus also undergo oral glucose tolerance testing (Table 3.1). Because women with a history of diabetes during pregnancy have a significantly higher likelihood of developing clinical diabetes later in life, we consider this an exclusion criterion although other transplant centers may consider these candidates.

A pertinent example case, which includes medical and nonmedical considerations in the living kidney donor evaluation as related to diabetes risk is illustrated below:

A 36-year-old woman originally from India who wishes to be considered as a living donor for her husband who has ESRD, on dialysis for ~6 months. She has a documented elevated fasting glucose in the 106–120 range about 3 years ago as well as elevated Hgb A1c% to 6.3%. There is a strong family history of type 2 diabetes on her father's side. She is very motivated and had already lost 25 lbs over 6 months after hiring a professional trainer.

The patient and her husband are anxious to proceed so he can return to work as they have a difficult financial situation as her father-in-law was providing some financial support for the family by report. On physical examination, her BP is 109/54 and her BMI is 29.7 (weight 173 lbs and height 64 in.); no other significant findings noted. The plasma creatinine is 0.7 mg/dL, one fasting glucose 98 mg/dL but the repeat test was 102 mg/dL, the Hgb A1c% 6.0% where the upper limit of normal for the lab was 6.1%, and no proteinuria or albuminuria are detected on multiple timed and spot urine tests.

In evaluating this patient's future risk for diabetes, we applied a number of published risk calculators for incident diabetes, most of which include sex, current fasting glucose, family history, and some measure of obesity. These revealed a 18% [21] to 33% [22] risk for incident diabetes in ~8 years even if she could improve her BMI to 25 kg/m^2 and achieve a fasting glucose of 90 mg/dL. Another prediction rule put her at 100% risk for developing clinical diabetes mellitus in 10 years with 80% sensitivity and specificity score [23]. An important caveat in using these diabetes prediction scores is that most of these cohorts used for risk development are comprised primarily of Caucasians, which may not be appropriate for this woman of South Asian descent. In fact, investigators have reported that South Asians and Chinese adults have levels impaired glucose, dyslipidemia, and hypertension comparable to Caucasians at much lower BMI levels (24 vs. 30 kg/m^2) [24], so her incident diabetes risk is likely even higher. Another caveat is that these prediction rules use only baseline clinical and laboratory characteristics; therefore, the influence of weight loss on diabetes risk is not known, per se.

Even if a highly accurate assessment of her future diabetes risk could be achieved, however, other considerations include the undefined additional risk (if any) conferred by living donor nephrectomy on her risk for kidney and cardiovascular morbidity and mortality as well as the complicated interplay of how the ability to donate may benefit the donor's overall well-being as related to benefits to her husband and family balanced with the potential medical risks.

Kidney "Swaps" and Altruistic or Undirected Living Kidney Donation

The living kidney donation process is sometimes further complicated when the living donor is not donating to a specific recipient. In situations of ABO-incompatibility, the donor–recipient pair may seek to have (1) a kidney donation to the cadaveric list in return for the recipient being moved to the top of the cadaveric list or (2) a kidney "swap" where matching with one or more ABO-incompatible donor–recipient pairs for transplants is performed. ABO-incompatible living donors should be informed, however, about the superior allograft outcomes a living compared to a deceased donor as part of the informed consent process.

A recent phenomenon is the growing popularity of undirected or "altruistic" kidney donation where a living donor indicates the desire to donate a kidney to anyone in need. A variation on this is the situation where a donor and recipient find each other using internet websites. Careful and comprehensive screening of potential altruistic donors, especially with regard to requests for monetary or other reimbursement as this is denounced by the Declaration of Istanbul on Organ Trafficking and Transplant Tourism [25].

Medical Complications After Donation

In women of childbearing age, the recent data concerning pregnancy complications after donor nephrectomy should be addressed. The Norwegian Registry Study published in 2008 analyzed 326 donors with 726 pregnancies (106 after donation) and used a random sample of nondonors and pregnancies prior to donation used as controls. The investigators reported an increased rate of preeclampsia after donation (5.7 vs. 2.6%, $p=0.026$) but not in other adverse pregnancy outcomes [26]. Second, a study from the University of Minnesota published a series of 1,085 women with 3,213 self-reported pregnancies (490 postdonation). Compared with predonation pregnancies, postdonation pregnancies were associated with lower likelihood of full-term deliveries (73.7 vs. 84.6%, $p=0.0004$), higher likelihood of fetal loss (19.2 vs. 11.3%, $p<0.0001$), higher risk of gestational diabetes (2.7 vs. 0.7%, $p=0.0001$), higher risk of gestational hypertension (5.7 vs. 0.6%, $p<0.0001$), higher risk of proteinuria (4.3 vs. 1.1%, $p<0.0001$), and higher risk of preeclampsia (5.5 vs. 0.8%, $p<0.0001$) [27]. Therefore, there appears to be a relatively small absolute but statistically significant risk for pregnancy complications after donor nephrectomy.

The literature on risk for ESRD after donor nephrectomy remains very limited. A single center study from Sweden reported that only 6 out of 1,112 (0.5%) who donated between 1965 and 2005 reached ESRD between 2001 and 2006. These donors were assessed 36–41 years after living donation with a median age 77 years [28]. Another study using the UNOS database from the United States raised the possibility that African Americans may be at increased risk after donor nephrectomy. Of the 102 previous kidney donors listed for kidney transplant between 1993 and 2005 (0.2% of 51,308 in the total donor cohort), 44% were black despite the fact that blacks comprised only 14.3% of donors during this period. The authors suggested that this may represent indirect evidence for increased ESRD risk in blacks [29].

In 2010, a study in the New England Journal of Medicine also reported that U.S. black and Hispanic living kidney donors are at higher risk for developing hypertension, diabetes, and cardiovascular disease after donation compared to white donors (as is the case with non-donors) although the additional risk directly conferred from donation was compared with a sample with prevalent rather than an incident chronic medical diseases [30].

In any study of clinically significant kidney disease in living donors, however, a number of considerations need to be acknowledged. First, although the living donors study from University of Minnesota did perform assessments of GFR at a mean follow-up of 12.2 years after donation in a subset of 255 kidney donors, the matched control group from the NHANES cohort had only baseline plasma creatinine and no follow creatinine nor direct GFR measurements [31]. Issues of survival bias (i.e., donors who are deceased may have worse kidney function as this is an established risk factor for mortality) and competing risk (i.e., death prior to ESRD) in assessing kidney function change in living donors also remain important limitations. A rigorous evaluation of kidney function change after living kidney donation would require prospective recruitment of incident donors who would be followed longitudinally with high participant retainment and ascertainment of outcomes, which has not yet been accomplished.

Long-Term Quality of Life and Mortality Outcomes in Living Kidney Donors

Few studies are currently available on long-term quality of life and medical outcomes in donors, and the available investigations may include donors who were overall younger and had lower BMI than current living donors at the time of donation. For example, one study of 339 Egyptian living donors published in 2007 reported excellent outcomes after a mean 10.7 years of follow-up, but the mean age at donation was 37.8 years and mean BMI was 23.7 [32]. A recent investigation from the University of Minnesota reported preserved renal function and excellent quality of life among a subset of 255 of their center's living donors followed for a mean of 12.2 years. Although this study appeared to have a substantial representation of donors with BMI>30 kg/m^2 (~30%), these values were measured at the time of follow up and likely do not reflect patients' BMI at donation. The mean age of this cohort at time of donation was 41.1 years, which is similar to that seen among the 2006–2008 cohorts in this study; the proportion of donors over the age of 50 was not reported [31].

Most recently, a study of the UNOS database published in 2010 examined surgical mortality and long-term survival in over 80,000 living kidney donors who had nephrectomies between 1994 and 2009. The investigators reported that "long-term risk of death" was equivalent or lower to that in age and comorbidity-matched controls from NHANES III participants including stratification by age, sex, and race [33]. It should be noted, however, that the median follow-up for living donors was relatively short at 6.3 years.

Summary and Concluding Thoughts

Comprehensive living kidney donor evaluation and education is a complex and time-consuming process if carried out in a thoughtful manner and necessitates extensive detailed communication between all members of the transplant team. The joint donor–recipient pair benefits and risks should be considered together for this elective procedure. One notable challenge is that characteristics of living donors have been changing over time with older, more overweight, and more unrelated donors over time. This makes it difficult to accurately counsel potential donors on their projected future risks.

For example, although a single factor, such as isolated hyperlipidemia, may not be an absolute contraindication to living kidney donation, when a constellation of factors coexist (i.e., hyperlipidemia plus hgb a1c% suggestive of high risk for diabetes plus borderline hypertension) in a potential living donor, recommendation to not proceed with donor nephrectomy may be warranted. The majority of factors that confer high risk for adverse medical and surgical outcomes after kidney donation are often addressed by a single intervention: *weight loss* in the overweight or obese patient. The success of living donors in keeping in the normal BMI range with a healthy and active lifestyle after nephrectomy and the long-term implications of this are not known, however.

In conclusion, the changing characteristics of living kidney donors and their recipients over time emphasize the need for new studies of donor and recipient outcomes following living kidney transplantation among a contemporary cohort, because previous longitudinal studies often included donors with ages and BMI substantially lower than those seen presently. Specific questions for future study include the incidence and risk factors for the development of hypertension, diabetes, and cardiovascular disease in living kidney donors. Prospective longitudinal studies of contemporary cohorts of living kidney donors recruited soon after donation with matched longitudinal population data from comparable healthy subcohorts are needed to compare overall mortality, incident hypertension, cardiovascular disease, and chronic kidney disease. Because the volume and popularity of both living related and unrelated kidney donation have increased dramatically in recent years, better defining the risks and outcomes for this elective procedure represents an important public health issue.

References

1. Davis CL, Delmonico FL. Living-donor kidney transplantation: a review of the current practices for the live donor. J Am Soc Nephrol. 2005;16(7):2098–110.
2. United Kingdom Guidelines for Living Donor Transplantation, Third Editionl, compiled by a Joint Working Party of The British Transplantation Society and The Renal Association, Editor. London: Triangle; May 2011.
3. Delmonico F. A report of the Amsterdam forum on the care of the live kidney donor: data and medical guidelines. Transplantation. 2005;79(6 Suppl):S53–66.
4. Cecka JM. The UNOS renal transplant registry. Clin Transpl. 2002:1–20.

5. Hillege HL et al. Urinary albumin excretion predicts cardiovascular and noncardiovascular mortality in general population. Circulation. 2002;106(14):1777–82.
6. Arnlov J et al. Low-grade albuminuria and incidence of cardiovascular disease events in nonhypertensive and nondiabetic individuals: the Framingham Heart Study. Circulation. 2005;112(7):969–75.
7. Mange KC, Joffe MM, Feldman HI. Effect of the use or nonuse of long-term dialysis on the subsequent survival of renal transplants from living donors. N Engl J Med. 2001;344(10):726–31.
8. Mandelbrot DA et al. The medical evaluation of living kidney donors: a survey of US transplant centers. Am J Transplant. 2007;7(10):2333–43.
9. Rook M et al. Nephrectomy elicits impact of age and BMI on renal hemodynamics: lower postdonation reserve capacity in older or overweight kidney donors. Am J Transplant. 2008;8(10):2077–85.
10. Gossmann J et al. Long-term consequences of live kidney donation follow-up in 93% of living kidney donors in a single transplant center. Am J Transplant. 2005;5(10):2417–24.
11. Oien CM et al. Living donor kidney transplantation: the effects of donor age and gender on short- and long-term outcomes. Transplantation. 2007;83(5):600–6.
12. Fox CS et al. Predictors of new-onset kidney disease in a community-based population. JAMA. 2004;291(7):844–50.
13. Lee JH et al. Risk factors for MDRD-GFR of less than 60 mL/min per 1.73 m^2 in former kidney donors. Nephrology (Carlton). 2007;12(6):600–6.
14. Textor SC et al. Blood pressure evaluation among older living kidney donors. J Am Soc Nephrol. 2003;14(8):2159–67.
15. Hsu CY et al. Risk factors for end-stage renal disease: 25-year follow-up. Arch Intern Med. 2009;169(4):342–50.
16. Kambham N et al. Obesity-related glomerulopathy: an emerging epidemic. Kidney Int. 2001;59(4):1498–509.
17. Praga M et al. Influence of obesity on the appearance of proteinuria and renal insufficiency after unilateral nephrectomy. Kidney Int. 2000;58(5):2111–8.
18. Heimbach JK et al. Obesity in living kidney donors: clinical characteristics and outcomes in the era of laparoscopic donor nephrectomy. Am J Transplant. 2005;5(5):1057–64.
19. Pesavento TE et al. Obese living kidney donors: short-term results and possible implications. Transplantation. 1999;68(10):1491–6.
20. Lin J et al. Longitudinal trends and influence of BMI mismatch in living kidney donors and their recipients. Int Urol Nephrol. 2011;43(3):891–7.
21. Wilson PW et al. Prediction of incident diabetes mellitus in middle-aged adults: the Framingham Offspring Study. Arch Intern Med. 2007;167(10):1068–74.
22. Stern MP, Williams K, Haffner SM. Identification of persons at high risk for type 2 diabetes mellitus: do we need the oral glucose tolerance test? Ann Intern Med. 2002;136(8):575–81.
23. Lindstrom J, Tuomilehto J. The diabetes risk score: a practical tool to predict type 2 diabetes risk. Diabetes Care. 2003;26(3):725–31.
24. Razak F et al. Defining obesity cut points in a multiethnic population. Circulation. 2007;115(16):2111–8.
25. International Summit on Transplant Tourism and Organ Trafficking. The declaration of istanbul on organ trafficking and transplant tourism. Clin J Am Soc Nephrol. 2008;3(5):1227–31.
26. Reisaeter AV et al. Pregnancy and birth after kidney donation: the Norwegian experience. Am J Transplant. 2009;9(4):820–4.
27. Ibrahim HN et al. Pregnancy outcomes after kidney donation. Am J Transplant. 2009;9(4):825–34.
28. Fehrman-Ekholm I et al. Incidence of end-stage renal disease among live kidney donors. Transplantation. 2006;82(12):1646–8.
29. Gibney EM et al. Living kidney donors requiring transplantation: focus on African Americans. Transplantation. 2007;84(5):647–9.

30. Lentine KL et al., Racial variation in medical outcomes among living kidney donors. New Engl J Med. 2010;363(8):724–32.
31. Ibrahim HN et al. Long-term consequences of kidney donation. N Engl J Med. 2009;360(5):459–69.
32. El-Agroudy AE et al. Long-term follow-up of living kidney donors: a longitudinal study. BJU Int. 2007;100(6):1351–5.
33. Segev DL et al. Perioperative mortality and long-term survival following live kidney donation. JAMA. 2010;303(10):959–66.

Chapter 4
Evaluation of Renal Transplant Candidates

Martina M. McGrath and Mario F. Rubin

Abstract The pretransplant evaluation of kidney transplant candidates is a complex process which is best carried out in the context of a multidisciplinary approach. A given patient's candidacy is determined not only by a careful assessment of the medical/surgical risks but also by a thorough determination of each individual's psychosocial aspects. What follows is our attempt to provide the reader with a series of simple facts which we hope will, in turn, facilitate an understanding of this delicate process.

Kidney transplantation is the treatment of choice for most patients with end stage kidney disease (ESKD). There is ample evidence that transplantation is associated with a superior quality and length of life at a lower economic cost. Therefore, appropriate selection of transplant candidates is one of the most important goals of a transplant team. There have been several sets of guidelines produced by experts in the transplantation field to guide the appropriate and timely evaluation of these patients. The goal pretransplant evaluation is to determine that the necessary medical, surgical, and psychosocial conditions are met to derive a maximal benefit from transplantation.

Keywords Age • Malignancy • Infections • Waiting list • Psychosocial issues

M.M. McGrath, MB, BAO, BCh
Renal Division, Brigham and Women's Hospital, Boston, MA, USA

M.F. Rubin, MD (✉)
Massachusetts General Hospital, 165 Cambridge St., Suite 302, Boston, MA 02114, USA
e-mail: mfrubin@partners.org

A. Chandraker et al. (eds.), *Core Concepts in Renal Transplantation*,
DOI 10.1007/978-1-4614-0008-0_4, © Springer Science+Business Media, LLC 2012

Introduction

Kidney transplantation is the treatment of choice for most patients with end stage kidney disease (ESKD). There is ample evidence that transplantation is associated with a superior quality and length of life at a lower economic cost [1]. Therefore, appropriate selection of transplant candidates is one of the most important goals of a transplant team. There have been several sets of guidelines produced by experts in the transplantation field to guide the appropriate and timely evaluation of these patients [2–5].

The goal of pretransplant evaluation is to determine that the necessary medical, surgical, and psychosocial conditions are met to derive a maximal benefit from transplantation. This, in turn, should lead to an increase in the longevity and quality of life of the patient.

In addition, the evaluation process should identify unsuitable candidates in a timely fashion, thereby ensuring the appropriate use of resources and the avoidance of unnecessary invasive procedures. Finally, an overriding principle is to ensure the best use of the donated kidney, fulfilling the debt to society by equitable sharing of this limited and precious resource.

Timing of Referral

Ideally, preparation for ESKD and transplantation should begin as soon as progressive chronic kidney disease (CKD) is recognized. Unfortunately, a significant proportion of patients present with advanced disease and therefore accrue time on dialysis prior to being referred for transplant evaluation.

Nephrologists need not wait for ESKD to develop in order to refer their patients for kidney transplant evaluation. Preemptive kidney transplantation (i.e., preceding the initiation of dialysis) is well known to offer improved patient and allograft outcomes. Five- to ten-year graft survival is over 20% higher in those patients who received either no dialysis or less than 6 months dialysis as compared with those on dialysis for over 2 years [6].

Within the United States the rules for listing patients with ESKD for transplantation vary from region to region and many regions only allow patients to be tested after initiation of dialysis.

Referral for kidney transplant evaluation should be considered once it is evident that the underlying renal failure is progressive. Within the United States, all Medicare patients are legally entitled to kidney transplantation education and referral. The current Center for Medicare Services (CMS) guidelines do not allow the enrollment of patients in the United Network Organization Services's transplant waiting list when estimated glomerular filtration rates are >20 mL/min/1.73m^2. Therefore, the timing of the evaluation process (which may take several months to complete) is critical.

Barriers to Referral

All patients with ESKD should be offered equal access to renal transplantation. However, there are a wide variety of factors that prevent certain patients from achieving this access. These include patient-related, educational, socioeconomic, and logistic issues as outlined in Table 4.1.

Unfortunately, candidates from more disadvantaged backgrounds, particularly lower educational achievement and minority race, appear less likely to be referred for transplantation [7].

In a Canadian study of transplant referral patterns, 42% of incident dialysis patients were referred for transplant evaluation. Forty-two percent of the remaining had a defined contraindication to transplantation. However, a further 23% had no defined contraindication and were not referred. The average age of this group was older with a greater overall burden of comorbidity [8].

Table 4.1 Documented variables that may inhibit timely referral for transplantation

- Lower level of educational attainment
- Lower socioeconomic status
- Non-English-speaking background
- Minority race
- Female gender
- Inadequate health literacy
- Certain medical diagnoses such as diabetes mellitus
- Obesity
- Dialysis in for-profit or isolated units

Contraindications to Transplantation

It is important to identify patients who have a contraindication to transplantation early on in the process (see Tables 4.2 and 4.3). Such an identification not only avoids unnecessary further investigation but also allows referral of these patients for appropriate management, as many of these conditions are treatable and it is possible that some may be suitable candidates at a later point. Nevertheless, it is essential to give patients realistic expectations, as some will remain truly unsuitable.

Table 4.2 Absolute contraindications for renal transplantation

- Active or metastatic malignancy
- Severe chronic illness with predicted survival <2 years
- Untreated current infection
- Uncontrolled psychiatric illness impairing compliance or consent
- Recalcitrant treatment noncompliance
- Active substance or alcohol abuse

Table 4.3 Relative contraindications for renal transplantation

• Active infection
• Coronary artery disease
• HIV infection (see text)
• Active peptic ulcer disease
• Advanced cerebrovascular disease
• Repeated graft loss from recurrent disease

Evaluation of Specific Risk Factors

Cardiovascular Disease

The association between CKD and arteriosclerotic vascular disease has been validated by multiple studies.

Cardiovascular disease is the most common cause of mortality following kidney transplantation with the majority of the events taking place early after transplantation. Fifty percent of the deaths that occur within the first 30 days following transplant are due to acute myocardial infarction [9–12]. Current demographics of the kidney transplant waiting list (i.e., marked increases in the number of patients older than 65 years) strengthens the need for a thorough cardiovascular evaluation.

The prevalence of angiography proven coronary artery disease (CAD) in patients undergoing transplant evaluation varies widely (42–81%) [13–18]. A good correlation has been found between angiographically defined coronary stenosis and subsequent clinical events [13–15].

Therefore, all patients referred for kidney transplant evaluation should undergo a thorough assessment of their cardiovascular disease risk factors and be screened for ischemic heart disease.

The extent of the evaluation depends upon multiple components such as the presence or absence of symptoms; previous history of cardiovascular disease; and risk factors such as smoking, hypertension, hyperlipidemia, and diabetes.

The optimal noninvasive screening test (myocardial perfusion studies, stress testing, computed tomography [CT]) has not yet been identified [19, 20]. The ideal test should have a high positive and negative predictive value for angiographically demonstrable significant CAD. Nuclear (i.e., myocardial perfusion studies) and stress echocardiography (DSE) have been evaluated in potential kidney transplant recipients and correlated with angiography demonstrable lesions and posttransplant clinical events. In the general population, they both correlate well with the presence of CAD with a sensitivity of 86–88% and a specificity of 74–81% [21, 22]. Unfortunately, their sensitivity (37–90%) and specificity (40–90%) in end-stage renal disease (ESRD) patients are quite variable [13, 23–29].

As a general rule, both studies have a good negative predictive value (i.e., identifying patients that will not have a posttransplant clinical event) but a poor positive predictive value. As a result, a significant number of asymptomatic patients with significant ischemic heart disease will be erroneously labeled as "acceptable for kidney transplantation." Therefore, high-risk patients such as those with diabetes and/or with multiple risk factors should undergo additional testing.

The detection and quantification of coronary artery calcification via the use of cardiac CT and the recent introduction of 64–320 slice CT coronary angiography have improved cardiovascular risk prediction (compared to the Framingham score) in asymptomatic patients without kidney disease [30]. On the other hand, their role in ESKD patients has not been validated and remains to be defined [31].

No consensus has been reached as to the optimal treatment (surgical, bare vs. drug eluting stents) of coronary stenosis prior to transplantation in stable asymptomatic patients although the need for anticoagulation with stents potentially complicates transplant surgery [32].

Recent large prospective studies have shown no benefit of coronary surgical revascularization over medical management in patients with stable cardiac symptoms awaiting major vascular surgery although whether these studies are equally applicable to patients with CKD/ESKD with concomitantly higher cardiovascular risk factor remains to be determined [33, 34]. To date, only a small single center study has shown an advantage of coronary surgical revascularization over medical management in stable type 1 diabetic patients [35].

There has been great variability amongst transplant centers in the pretransplant cardiac evaluation approach and the frequency of re-evaluation of patients on the waiting list. The validity and cost effectiveness of the current approach has been questioned mainly as a result of the low use of coronary interventions (2.9–9.5%) after cardiac evaluation [18, 36–38]. Therefore, consensus-based guidelines have been developed by several national organizations in an effort to standardize pretransplant evaluation practices [4, 20, 39].

Another issue which also lacks consensus is the frequency of cardiovascular re-evaluation of kidney transplant patients on a waiting list. While a prospective observational study discounted the need for periodic cardiac surveillance [40], there is a general agreement that such surveillance should occur annually for high-risk patients (i.e., diabetics and patients with a previous cardiovascular history) or whenever they become symptomatic. The aggressive treatment of risk factors (hypertension, hyperlipidemia, volume excess, smoking, etc.) of patients on a waiting list remains undisputed.

The evaluation of left ventricular function is another important aspect of the cardiac evaluation process. Many studies clearly show that the pretransplant presence of left ventricular systolic dysfunction and/or its development following transplantation are associated with poor prognosis [41, 42]. Data on the outcomes of those with diastolic dysfunction are currently not available. It must be understood that patients with uremic nonischemic cardiomyopathy should not be excluded as they tend to improve posttransplantation [43]. Consideration for a combined heart–kidney transplant should always be entertained in patients with combined ESKD and advanced or end-stage heart disease.

Another important aspect of the evaluation is the assessment of the peripheral arterial circulation [5, 44, 45]. The presence of pretransplant peripheral arterial disease (PAD) is not an absolute contraindication for kidney transplantation, but its extent and severity must be carefully evaluated. Noninvasive testing (ankle-brachial index, toe-brachial index and pulse volume recordings, noncontrast abdominal-pelvic CT) and angiography are tools frequently utilized in the evaluation process. PAD is associated with an increased risk of amputation (particularly in diabetic patients), significant morbidity, and poor patient survival. Patients with large uncorrectable abdominal aneurysms, severe occlusive common iliac disease, active gangrene, or recent atheroembolic events are not candidates for kidney transplantation. In general, the vascular anastomosis of a renal allograft to previously placed vascular prosthetic materials is not associated with good outcomes.

Cerebrovascular Disease

Traditional risk factors for cerebrovascular disease such as hypertension, dyslipidemia, and diabetes are highly prevalent in the ESKD population. Observational studies report that up to 8% of renal transplant recipients will suffer a stroke by 10 years of follow-up care [46]. Despite this data, there is no evidence that screening asymptomatic transplant candidates for the presence of cerebrovascular disease is beneficial. Criteria for consideration of carotid endarterectomy are the same as those adopted for the general population.

Those with known cerebrovascular disease should be symptom free for a minimum of 6 months prior to being considered for renal transplantation.

Autosomal dominant polycystic kidney disease (ADPKD) is associated with an incidence of cerebral aneurysms that is 5 times higher than that of the general population. Aneurysms are found in 6% of those without a family history and 16% of those with a positive family history. The consensus appears to be that patients with a positive family history, a prior ruptured aneurysm, or suggestive symptoms should be screened and followed over a long-term period. The yield of screening other ADPKD patients appears to be low and it is not currently recommended [47]. The effect of renal transplantation on preexisting cerebral aneurysms is unclear and, therefore, there are no specific recommendations for patients in this setting.

Pulmonary Disease

Intrinsic lung disease may increase the perioperative transplant risks by impairing the ventilatory response to anesthesia and by increasing the risk of infection. In addition to the standard chest x-ray (CXR) and physical examination, pulmonary function studies may be required to ascertain the degree of lung dysfunction.

The 2005 Canadian Transplantation guidelines suggest that patients with the following clinical features should not be candidates for kidney transplantation: those needing home oxygen therapy, those with uncontrolled asthma, severe Cor Pulmonale, severe chronic obstructive pulmonary disease, pulmonary fibrosis, and restrictive lung disease. These are defined by an FEV1 < 25% of its predictive value, a room air $PO_2 < 60$ mmHg with exercise desaturation $SaO_2 < 90\%$, >4 lower respiratory tract infections in the last 12 months, and/or moderate disease with progression [5].

Despite published data which indicates a 30% higher risk of allograft failure (mainly due to cardiovascular deaths), most transplant centers do not require that transplant recipients discontinue their smoking behavior prior to transplantation [48]. Patients do receive smoke cessation education and are encouraged to quit but only a minority discontinue and remain smoke free for any significant period of time.

Age

For most transplant centers in the United States there is no maximum age limit over which patients cannot be listed for renal transplantation. The overall ESKD population has increased dramatically in recent years but the largest proportional increase has been in the older (over 70 years) age group. More than half of the newly listed patients awaiting kidney transplantation in 2005 were older than 50 years, and 13% were older than 65 years. As waiting times for a deceased donor kidney increase, these older candidates are disadvantaged by rapidly deteriorating health, often resulting in death or removal from the waiting list before transplantation.

Consequently, some authorities suggest that older recipients may benefit from being listed for "expanded criteria donor" (ECD) kidneys [7]. An ECD kidney is defined as a kidney from a donor over 60 years; also, as a kidney from a donor aged between 50 and 59 with at least two of the following criteria: death as a result of a cerebrovascular accident, a history of hypertension or serum creatinine >1.5 mg/dL. These allografts are more likely to be affected by delayed graft function, with graft survival being shorter than kidneys from "standard criteria" donors. However, the waiting time is considerably shorter than for standard criteria kidneys.

When the complications associated with accumulated years on dialysis and the large differential in terms of quality of life are taken into consideration, transplantation with an ECD kidney may represent a very acceptable alternative for many older patients.

Despite advancing age and comorbidity, there is good evidence as to the survival benefit to transplantation in the older population. Registry data suggests that these recipients enjoy an overall 41% lower risk of death at 3 years compared with those of a similar age who are on a waiting list and on dialysis. In the same study, those receiving ECD kidneys had a 25% lower mortality risk at 3-year follow-up [49]. Similarly, while death with a functioning graft is a more common event in this recipient population, there appears to be little difference in graft survival between this and younger age groups. From the available data, patient selection on the basis of individual characteristics and comorbidities appears to be more important factors than age itself.

Diabetes Mellitus

Approximately, 40% of the ESKD population has diabetes and this proportion is progressively rising. The risks and benefits of dialysis vs. combined kidney and pancreas transplantation, vs. kidney transplantation alone, should be discussed with Type I diabetic patients at the time of progression to ESKD. For patients choosing transplantation, a kidney from a human leukocyte antigen (HLA) identical living donor is recommended as the treatment of choice.

Pancreas transplantation can offer freedom from the requirement for exogenous insulin and may additionally halt or reverse the consequences of long-term hyperglycemia. Those with brittle diabetes and hypoglycemic unawareness may gain the greatest benefit. Transplantation can take the form of pancreas transplant alone (PTA), pancreas transplant after kidney transplantation (PAK), or simultaneous pancreas–kidney transplantation (SPK). Islet cell transplantation is a potentially novel approach which is undergoing careful scrutiny in multicenter trials. SPK is the most commonly performed of these surgeries and, based on currently available data, appears to offer the best pancreas graft outcomes.

Certain complications of diabetes appear to improve more readily after pancreas transplantation. There is rapid improvement in sensory and motor nerve conduction velocities after pancreas transplantation. Recovery appears more complete in sensory nerves and can continue to improve for up to 5 years after transplantation. However, variable impact is observed on the progression of diabetic retinopathy. Progression of macrovascular disease on long-term follow-up appears to be significantly lower in SPK recipients compared with kidney transplant alone [50].

In a large observational cohort study from the United Network for Organ Sharing (UNOS) database, when compared to living donor kidney transplantation, SPK transplantation was associated with similar overall patient survival at 8 years. The SPK group had a greater early mortality risk (initial 18 months posttransplant) but the living donor kidney recipients showed a greater late mortality from that point onwards [51].

Malignancy

Cancer is responsible for 9–12% of deaths in renal transplant recipients. Patients with ESKD have, at baseline, a higher risk of malignancy than the general population of age-matched controls. Additional immunosuppressive treatment increases the risk of malignancy posttransplant approximately fourfold. However, those patients who are successfully treated for malignancy become suitable candidates after a defined waiting period to exclude recurrence. This is generally of the order of 2–5 years, dependent upon the particular tumor involved. Specific data on malignancies in transplant patients is available at the Israel Penn International Transplant Tumor Registry (http://www.ipittr.org/Home.htm). According to this registry, 54%

of cancer recurrences occurred in patients who had their pretransplant malignancies treated within 2 years of transplantation and 13% of recurrences occurred in patients treated more than 5 years before transplantation.

While these statistics may provide general guidelines, the risk of tumor recurrence has to be balanced against the benefits of renal transplantation.

A specialist oncology opinion may be helpful in individual cases. Suggested waiting times after common malignancies are given in Table 4.4.

All potential candidates should undergo age-appropriate cancer screening as part of their evaluation. Specific and frequent forms of cancer which deserve additional comment follow.

Cervical Cancer

The incidence in ESKD is 2–4 times higher than that of the general population. All female transplant candidates should undergo Papanicolaou smear as part of the initial evaluation and annually thereafter. For those with cervical carcinoma, a 6% recurrence rate is seen after transplantation and there is a high associated mortality. Transplantation can be performed right away in women with in situ cervical carcinoma while the optimal waiting time after invasive cervical carcinoma remains unclear.

Breast Cancer

The incidence of breast cancer does not appear to be significantly increased in ESKD patients. Its recurrence rate posttransplant is around 23% and has an associated mortality of up to 76%. As a result, it is recommended to wait at least 5 years posttreatment before undertaking renal transplantation. All female transplant candidates should undergo annual mammogram from age 40, or earlier if there is a positive family history of breast cancer.

Colorectal Cancer

There is no known increased incidence of colorectal carcinoma in ESKD patients but rates may increase markedly 10–20 years after successful transplantation. Most renal transplant candidates with a history of colorectal cancer should wait at least 5 years from successful treatment to transplantation, although a shorter waiting time of 2–5 years may be sufficient in patients with localized disease (Duke's stage A or B1). Recurrence is seen in up to 21% of patients transplanted before a 5-year disease-free interval, and the associated mortality rate is around 63%.

Colonoscopy screening of all transplant candidates from age 50 is recommended. This should be repeated every 10 years, with increased frequency in high-risk groups (positive family history, inflammatory bowel disease, previous endoscopic abnormalities, etc.).

Prostate Cancer

Screening should be carried out with digital rectal examination and checking prostate specific antigen annually on all men from age 50 and earlier in high-risk groups.

Those with known prostate cancer should wait for a 2–5-year disease-free interval after treatment prior to renal transplantation. Patients with disease localized to the prostate gland can undergo transplantation immediately following radical prostatectomy.

Bladder Cancer

Patients from high-risk groups, such as those with prior cyclophosphamide use, analgesic nephropathy, or aristolochic acid nephropathy should undergo screening cystoscopy prior to transplantation.

Renal Cell Carcinoma

Incidence of renal cell carcinoma is increased in patients with a history of smoking and in those suffering from acquired cystic renal disease and analgesic abuse nephropathy. This group of patients should undergo renal imaging procedures (ultrasound, CT scanning) during the evaluation process. Recurrent renal cancer after renal transplantation is rarely seen in those with a disease-free interval of 5 years prior to transplantation. However, when it occurs, it has an associated mortality rate of 80%. The 2001 American Society of Transplantation Clinical Practice Guidelines suggest that those with an initial tumor less than 5 cm in diameter can generally be safely transplanted 2 years after surgical removal provided follow-up imaging remains unremarkable.

Multiple Myeloma

Transplant candidates with clinical, biochemical, or radiological abnormalities suggestive of plasma cell dyscrasias should be screened with serum electrophoresis, immunoelectrophoresis, and serum free light chains testing.

In general, those with multiple myeloma are not suitable renal transplant candidates. It is recommended that they undergo treatment and be relapse free for 5 years prior to listing. However, myeloma recurrence is still seen in almost two thirds of transplanted patients with considerable associated mortality, almost 100% in one report. The risk of posttransplant infection appears markedly increased in these patients [52].

Preliminary single centers studies report good outcomes in a small number of patients with myeloma and ESKD who undergo combined nonmyeloablative allogeneic bone marrow and kidney transplant from an HLA identical sibling [53]. However, there is considerable morbidity and mortality associated with this approach and very few candidates are suitable.

Approximately, 1% of cases of monoclonal gammopathy of unknown significance (MGUS) develop myeloma or a related lymphoproliferative disorder with each year of follow-up. Transplantation should be deferred for at least 1 year after diagnosis. There are very limited data on expected outcomes in patients with stable MGUS. Rostaing et al. reported increases in monoclonal paraprotein in three of five patients with MGUS followed after transplantation. Two cases developed asymptomatic myeloma [54]. Those with stable MGUS have been considered suitable to proceed to transplant but it would appear that extreme caution is warranted on the basis of the limited available data.

Kaposi Sarcoma

Patients who had a Kaposi sarcoma with a prior allograft have a high likelihood of recurrence upon re-transplantation and further immunosuppression. It may be appropriate to check titers of HHV8 in patients who come from endemic areas, to estimate risk prior to transplantation.

Table 4.4 Malignant disease-free intervals recommended prior to renal transplantation

Malignancy	Recommended minimum disease-free period
Thyroid	2 years
Testicular	2 years
Cervical	Up to 5 years
Breast – ductal carcinoma in situ	2 years
Breast–invasive	5 years
Colorectal carcinoma – localized	2 years
Colorectal carcinoma	5 years
Liver cancer	Not recommended[a]
Lymphoma	2 years[b]
Leukemia	2 years
Lung cancer	2 years
Multiple myeloma	Not recommended
Prostate – focal disease	None
Prostate	2 years
Bladder – superficial	None
Bladder – invasive	2 years
Renal cell – incidental	None
Renal cell – invasive	2 years
Wilm's tumor	1 year
Malignant melanoma	5 years
Nonmelanoma skin cancers	None

[a]Renal transplantation only in the context of simultaneous liver transplantation
[b]Includes Hodgkin's lymphoma, non-Hodgkin's lymphoma, and posttransplant lymphoproliferative disorder (PTLD)

Urological Disease

The goal of the urologic work up is to ensure the absence of infection, calculi, or malignancy and to ensure a functional lower urinary tract. The involvement of a urologist experienced in dealing with transplant candidates and recipients is extremely helpful.

The urinary tract should have three essential features prior to transplantation:

- An adequate urinary reservoir to permit storage of an adequate volume of urine at low pressure.
- Continence.
- A consistent and reliable method of complete bladder evacuation: either voiding or clean intermittent self-catheterization.

Patients with remnant kidney function should have a urinalysis and urine culture.

Most patients with known bladder dysfunction can be managed without pretransplant urinary diversion or bladder augmentation. Studies comparing results of reimplantation into a defunctionalized bladder with maintenance of urinary diversions have demonstrated lower rates of complications in selected patients managed with reimplantation as compared with either maintenance or new creation of urinary diversion [55].

Clean intermittent self-catheterization is a suitable option for many, if not most, patients with defunctionalized bladders. Infection remains the major complication. However, long-term prophylactic antibiotics usually are not necessary and allograft function in general is not compromised. Unfortunately, there is little evidence in the literature to guide the management of patients requiring surgical intervention to ensure adequate urinary drainage and, therefore, treatment must be individualized on a case-by-case basis.

Consideration may need to be given to native nephrectomy in selected cases (see Table 4.5). Clearly, many of these indications are relative and potential benefits need to be balanced against the risks of removing residual renal function.

Table 4.5 Possible indications for pretransplant nephrectomy

• Large, painful polycystic kidneys
• Chronic parenchymal infection
• Infectious calculi
• Obstructive uropathy complicated by recurrent sepsis
• Congenital nephrotic syndromes
• Adults with nephrotic syndrome uncontrolled with medical management
• Congenital abnormalities associated with high risk of Wilm's tumors
• Poorly controlled hypertension
• Renal mass lesions

Infections

The purpose of pretransplant screening is to eliminate any infections that could potentially be reactivated and become life threatening in the posttransplant period. Therefore, it is critical to exclude latent or active infections. These include, among others, endovascular, periodontal, device-related, or deep seated intra-abdominal or genitourinary infections (see Tables 4.6 and 4.7). Transplantation should be deferred until these are appropriately managed.

Where possible, immunizations should be administered pre-engraftment and ideally prior to ESKD, for maximal efficacy.

The transplant candidate evaluation for infectious diseases involves a detailed medical and social history, with attention to high-risk behaviors, sexually transmitted infections, intravenous drug abuse, incarceration, travel history and especially consideration of exposure to endemic mycoses.

An assessment of the overall "net state of immunosuppression" of the candidate also needs to be made, not only to guide immunosuppressive therapy posttransplant but also to accurately estimate the risk of posttransplant infection. This includes review of prior immunosuppressive treatments which the patient received either with a prior allograft or for treatment of autoimmune conditions (systemic lupus, vasculitis, etc.) and/or one of the primary glomerulonephritides. Comorbid conditions such as diabetes, liver disease, immunoglobulin deficiencies, malnutrition, asplenia, prior history of substance abuse, or others which impair the host immune response, also need to be assessed and carefully reviewed as part of the transplant work up.

Finally, the frequency of hospitalizations, antibiotic exposure, the presence of prosthetic material (such as endovascular grafts), and details of methicillin-resistant staphylococcus aureous (MRSA) and vancomycin resistant enterococcus (VRE) colonization/infection are relevant data in terms of estimating the risk of antibiotic resistance or unusual infection in the posttransplant period.

Table 4.6 Pretransplant screening for infections

- Antibiotic allergies/adverse reactions
- Dental review
- Chest X-ray
- Urine culture
- PPD
- Viral and fungal serological studies

Table 4.7 Specific pretransplant infectious considerations

Infection	Screening	Significance/management
HIV	HIV I & II Ab	See text
HBV	HBsAg, HBcAb (IgM-IgG), HBsAb	Vaccinate if negative. See text
HCV	HCV IgG, HCV PCR	See text
CMV	CMV IgG	Posttransplant prophylaxis if positive recipient or donor
EBV	EBV IgG	Unclear. If negative, monitor for posttransplant seroconversion
VZV	VZV Ab	Vaccinate if negative
Tuberculosis	PPD & CXR	INH prophylaxis if latent infection
HSV	HSV 1 & 2	Consider posttransplant prophylaxis
HHV 8	HHV 8 Ab	Increased risk of development of Kaposi sarcoma
HTLV I & II	HTLV I & II Ab	Patients from endemic areas
Syphilis	RPR	Treatment as appropriate for stage
Strongyloides stercoralis	Stool for ova and parasites, ELISA serology	Patients from endemic areas
Coccidioides	IgM and IgG by EIA	Patients from endemic areas
Influenza	None	Annual vaccination
Pneumococcus	None	5 yearly vaccination
Tetanus	None	10 yearly booster

HIV

It is estimated that 0.5–2.5% of prevalent ESKD patients are HIV positive. HIV infection has traditionally been considered a relative contraindication to renal transplantation due to concerns for infectious complications and progression of AIDS (see Table 4.8). A recent review and meta-analysis looked at this issue and reported good outcomes overall. Higher rates of acute rejection were reported in the HIV positive recipients; however, this was generally responsive to therapy. Immunosuppressive drug dosing was more challenging due to interactions with antiretroviral medications. Of note, there were no excess infectious complications or AIDS-defining illnesses in the HIV positive transplant recipients [56].

Overall, there still remains a dearth of long-term data available as to whether transplantation is associated with improved outcomes in this particular cohort. An ongoing NIH sponsored multicenter study should provide, upon completion, the much needed guidelines.

BK Virus

Otherwise eligible patients who have lost a prior allograft to polyoma virus infection should be considered for re-transplantation. It has been suggested that re-transplantation should be delayed until urine and plasma viral loads have become negative, but there

Table 4.8 Requirements prior to listing of HIV positive patients for transplantation

• Undetectable viral load
• Demonstrated compliance with HAART regimen
• No opportunistic infections
• CD 4 count >300/mm^3

are few prospective data to support this recommendation. Short-term graft and patient survival with re-transplantation after a failed graft from BK virus (BKV) appear to be excellent. Long-term outcomes remain unknown [57]. The role of allograft nephrectomy prior to re-transplantation remains controversial. In certain reported series, a significant proportion of patients with graft loss after BKV nephropathy underwent allograft nephrectomy prior to re-transplant. However, recurrent disease has also been observed in this group, suggesting that nephrectomy is not necessarily protective.

Tuberculosis

All patients require a chest x-ray and purified protein derivative (PPD) skin testing as part of their pretransplant evaluation. Given the high prevalence of anergy in patients with end stage renal failure, careful review of clinical and radiographic history is essential. If there is a history of treated tuberculosis, duration and nature of therapy should be reviewed. Abnormalities on chest radiography may warrant more detailed investigation. Active tuberculous infection must be excluded prior to transplantation.

High-risk individuals include those from geographical areas of highly prevalent infection rates (e.g., the developing world), those with prior active disease or exposure, and those who have other immunosuppressing conditions. Peritransplant prophylaxis with Isoniazid may be indicated in these high-risk individuals or those with latent infection.

Liver Disease

Hepatitis B

All potential transplant candidates should be screened for Hepatitis B virus (HBV). Patients who are HBsAg negative should be vaccinated against HBV. HBV antibody status should be monitored and booster doses given when antibody concentrations fall below protective levels.

Patients who are HBsAg positive and are being assessed for renal transplantation require further investigation. Initially, they should undergo testing for active viral replication (i.e., HBV DNA, HBeAg). Serum transaminases should also be checked but as the sensitivity for active hepatitis is quite low, it is recommended that these patients undergo liver biopsy as part of their evaluation.

Based on the biopsy results, patients can be stratified. For those with established cirrhosis, renal transplantation is contraindicated. This group should be further assessed for a combined liver and kidney transplant as appropriate (see Table 4.9) [58]. Those with mild histological changes on liver biopsy can be further subdivided based on the presence or absence of viral replication; those with active replication should be treated with antivirals prior to renal transplantation, whereas those without evidence of viral replication can be put forward for kidney transplant. It is important to note that the absence of replication pretransplant does not preclude reactivation of HBV in the posttransplant period.

Data from a prior meta-analysis has shown that HBV infection is associated with worse outcomes posttransplant in terms of patient and kidney survival [59]. However, this is not a universal finding and there have also been small studies showing prolonged survival in HBV infected patients. Of note, many of the studies were carried out prior to the recognition of coinfection with HCV or hepatitis D, both of which are known to confer worse prognosis for liver disease postrenal transplant. In addition, the effect of antiviral therapy with Lamivudine, which is now being widely used, has not yet been studied in detail in this population.

However, liver disease remains an important cause of death in renal transplant recipients with HBV or HCV. Therefore, while HBV is not a contraindication to renal transplantation, the risks and benefits need to be discussed in detail with the individual patient and fully informed consent obtained.

Hepatitis C

Hepatitis C virus (HCV) remains prevalent in the ESKD population and patients should be screened as outlined earlier.

Renal transplantation in HCV infected patients represents a difficult management issue. There have been conflicting data in the literature as to their posttransplant outcomes. Overall, it appears that there is poorer patient and allograft survival than seen in non-HCV infected candidates. However, HCV infected dialysis patients appear to fare worse than their transplanted counterparts. Complications of HCV infection, which occur after renal transplantation, include increased viral proliferation, de novo or recurrent HCV-associated MPGN, cryoglobulinemia, and high rates of posttransplant diabetes mellitus. In terms of liver disease, there is a risk of progressive chronic hepatitis and of the development of fibrosing cholestatic hepatitis. Therefore, fully informed consent prior to undertaking renal transplantation is critical in this group.

As noted in HBV, transaminases may not be markedly elevated in dialysis patients and liver biopsy is recommended for full evaluation (the lack of correlation between liver function studies and histological findings is well known). Patients with mild chronic hepatitis can be safely transplanted whereas those with cirrhosis should not undergo transplant due to the risk of progressive liver failure. These patients may be more appropriately assessed for combined liver and kidney transplantation. Otherwise, they have better outcomes by remaining on hemodialysis.

Table 4.9 Indications for combined liver/kidney transplant

• ESKD with cirrhosis and portal hypertension
• ESLD and CKD (eGFR < 30 mL/min /1.73m^2) for 90 days
• ESLD with dialysis dependent AKI > 8 weeks
• ESLD and evidence of CKD with a kidney biopsy demonstrating >30% glomerulosclerosis or >30% fibrosis

Those patients with HCV infection who are suitable renal transplant candidates should be assessed for treatment of their HCV prior to engraftment. The Kidney Disease: Improving Global Outcomes (KDIGO) guideline for HCV in CKD recommends that these patients should be given a trial of interferon (IFN) therapy prior to wait-listing for renal transplant. However, the work group recommends that IFN should be stopped at 12 weeks if there is no early viral response, as the likelihood of successful treatment beyond that point is so low as to render it more beneficial to proceed with renal transplantation, rather than to undertake a protracted treatment course [60]. Posttransplantation treatment with IFN confers a high risk of severe and irreversible transplant rejection and is only recommended if the potential benefits to be derived outweigh the substantial risk to the allograft.

Gastrointestinal Disease

Diverticular Disease

Diverticular disease is relatively common in those on dialysis, particularly those with ADPKD, where it is seen in 40–80% of patients. Posttransplant colonic perforation is most frequently related to diverticulitis and has a high associated mortality, up to 43% in transplant recipients. Currently, pretransplant colonoscopy to screen for diverticulae is not recommended in most candidates (including ADPKD patients). However, patients with a history of acute diverticulitis should be assessed and it is recommended that consideration be given to elective partial colectomy in selected severe cases.

Peptic Ulcer Disease

Active peptic ulcer disease is a contraindication to renal transplantation. Early on, transplant recipients are at increased risk of peptic ulceration due to high dose steroids and infections such as CMV, HSV, Candida, and *H. pylori*. However, there is no benefit to screening with upper gastrointestinal (GI) endoscopy or *H. pylori* serology in asymptomatic individuals. Those transplant candidates with recurrent upper GI symptoms or a history of peptic ulcer disease may benefit from endoscopy and appropriate treatment prior to transplantation.

Cholelithiasis

There is controversy regarding the need for pretransplant elective cholecystectomy. There are conflicting data as to the effect of the treatment of asymptomatic gallstones upon outcomes posttransplant. However, in patients with suggestive symptoms or prior cholecystitis, screening ultrasound is recommended. If gallstones are present, these patients should be offered pretransplant cholecystectomy to minimize the risk of recurrence or sepsis posttransplant.

Pancreatitis

There are few data looking at the incidence of acute or chronic pancreatitis in transplant recipients. Pancreatitis is associated with significant morbidity and mortality in the posttransplant setting. As a result, certain authorities recommend deferring transplantation until 6 months after an episode of acute pancreatitis and 1 year after chronic pancreatitis has become quiescent.

Risk of Recurrence of Disease After Renal Transplantation

With few exceptions, most causes of ESKD can recur in the allograft (Table 4.10). However, graft loss from recurrent disease has traditionally been perceived as a relatively unusual event. It is difficult to accurately estimate the risk of recurrence for many of these diseases for several important reasons. Firstly, it is estimated that only 20% of patients with ESKD undergo native renal biopsy and, therefore, many of those who present with advanced CKD may be labeled with an inaccurate diagnosis. Secondly, there are differing triggers for transplant biopsies among different studies. Some report on protocol biopsies, others report on biopsies where there was clinical indication, which can give widely varying estimates of incidence. Thirdly, the incidence of recurrence observed is dependent upon length of follow-up, as many of these diseases only become apparent many years after engraftment.

With more detailed long-term follow-up data, it is now recognized that recurrent glomerular disease is the third most frequent cause of graft loss at 10 years [61]. However, there are no causes of ESKD that are absolute contraindications to a first renal transplant.

Risk factors that can be helpful to predict the likelihood of recurrence in the allograft include the rate of progression of primary disease to ESKD, age of onset, time period on dialysis prior to transplantation and, in certain situations, degree of HLA mismatching. These issues are of particular importance in discussions with potential living donors where, in certain situations, there exists a relatively high risk of graft loss due to recurrent disease. While this topic is covered more extensively in Chap. 3, there are several disease states which are not classically thought of as recurrent diseases posttransplantation but the presence of the disease does impact graft survival.

Table 4.10 Estimates of recurrent disease postrenal transplantation

Primary disease	Risk of recurrence	Risk of graft loss due to recurrence
IgA nephropathy	50%	15%
FSGS	20–50% (80% if prior graft loss)	50%
MPGN type I	20–50%	15%
MPGN type II	80–100%	15–30%
Membranous GN	10–30%	20–50%
Anti-GBM disease	Rare (if quiescent at time of transplant)	Rare
ANCA vasculitis	15–20%	6–8%
SLE	2–9%	2–4%
HUS/TTP	15–25%	50%
Diabetic nephropathy	100%	Rare
Immunoglobulin deposition diseases	50%	30%
Amyloidosis	40%	20%
Fabry disease	100%	Rare
Scleroderma	20%	50%
Oxalosis	100%	50%
Cystinosis	0%	0%

Diabetes Mellitus

Diabetic changes are frequently seen in the allograft. Up to 100% of cases will demonstrate some changes consistent with diabetic nephropathy by 3 years post-transplant. However, graft loss secondary to diabetic nephropathy is rare and patients should be managed in the usual manner with ACE inhibition, blood pressure control, and appropriate glycemic control.

Fabry's Disease

Transplant recipients with Fabry's disease consistently show histological reaccumulation of glycosphingolipid in the allograft but recurrent disease progresses slowly. Generally, these patients die with a functioning graft due to other complications of the disease. Recombinant α(alpha)-galactosidase is now commercially available but there are as yet no data as to its role in the posttransplant setting [61].

Oxalosis

Primary oxalosis is a rare cause of ESKD. It is an autosomal recessive condition characterized by deficiency of the hepatic enzyme alanine:glycoxylate aminotransferase. This leads to an increase in urinary excretion of calcium oxalate, recurrent urolithiasis, nephrocalcinosis and, ultimately, renal failure occurring in 50% by age 15. The resulting impaired urinary excretion of oxalate leads to total body overload, i.e., oxalosis. Liver transplantation is curative and these patients are frequently considered for combined liver and kidney transplantation. Aggressive hemodialysis should be used to reduce the oxalate load pretransplant. In addition, if renal transplantation is carried out in isolation, intensive medical management is crucial to prevent recurrent nephrolithiasis in the allograft.

Obesity

Similar to the trends observed in the general population, an increasing proportion of transplant candidates are obese, defined as BMI > 30 kg/m^2. Obese patients have a higher risk of delayed graft function, prolonged hospitalization, and postoperative complications, such as wound dehiscence and infection. In addition, the incidence of new onset diabetes mellitus and cardiovascular disease posttransplantation is higher in this group. Some studies have shown increased risk of renal allograft loss but this has not been a consistent finding. Obese recipients of combined pancreas and kidney transplants have been shown to have inferior graft survival for both organs.

For these reasons, it appears prudent to advise obese patients on weight management strategies to target a BMI < 30 kg/m^2. A multidisciplinary approach to helping such individuals with weight loss offers the greatest chance of success. The role of bariatric surgery in this patient population has not been established but limited registry data suggests higher postoperative mortality than in nonrenal operative candidates [62]. However, weight loss surgery may be considered in extreme cases.

There are no firm data to recommend a BMI at which candidates should be denied transplantation on the basis of weight alone and the associated risks must be balanced against those of remaining on long-term dialysis.

Thrombophilia

Approximately, 2% of renal allografts are lost to thrombosis. All patients should undergo standard coagulation testing but routine screening for prothrombotic states is expensive and of low yield. Those candidates with recurrent thrombotic events such as clotted vascular access sites, venous or arterial thromboses should be assessed in more detail. Suggested work up includes screening for Factor V Leiden, protein C and S levels, and prothrombin G20210A mutation. Transplant candidates with a history of systemic lupus erythematosus (SLE) should be screened for the presence of antiphospholipid antibodies.

Thrombophilia is not a contraindication to transplantation. If any of the above screens are positive, consideration should be given to perioperative anticoagulation to reduce thrombotic complications.

Psychosocial Issues

Given the critical nature of treatment compliance posttransplant, a detailed psychosocial assessment is an important aspect of the transplant evaluation. A skilled transplant social worker that is experienced in the evaluation of transplant candidates may screen the patients initially. Those individuals who may have potential problems can then be referred on to a psychologist or psychiatrist as needed.

Prior episodes of substance abuse and noncompliance are not always barriers to renal transplantation. In such cases, transplantation should be deferred for 6 months until patients have demonstrated freedom from substance abuse and appropriate compliance with dialysis and other treatments. All patients should be strongly encouraged to stop smoking.

Similarly, patients with developmental delay or cognitive impairment can be suitable candidates for renal transplantation and may benefit both in terms of longevity and also quality of life. Care needs to be taken to ensure consent is appropriately taken and there are adequate structures in place to support the patient after transplantation, in terms of administration of medications, attending for lab draws and clinic appointments, to ensure the optimal outcome. If the patient is deemed incompetent to give consent, a legally acceptable surrogate decision maker must be identified and provided with the appropriate information regarding the risks and benefits of kidney transplantation. Ideally, this surrogate should also be able to assume responsibility for the patient posttransplant to ensure compliance with medications and follow up.

Candidates with major psychiatric disease can be successfully transplanted if their symptoms are well controlled. However, perioperative events and immunosuppressive drugs, particularly high dose steroids, can destabilize such patients. The involvement of a dedicated psychiatric professional is invaluable in such situations. Where feasible, patients should be converted from nephrotoxic psychiatric medications, such as Lithium, prior to undergoing renal transplantation.

The financial implications of transplantation also need to be addressed at the time of evaluation. Despite Medicare and other insurance coverage, patients may still face considerable copayments and may need to devote a sizable portion of their income to payment for immunosuppressive medications. Taking time off work necessary to attend clinic appointments can also impact on the individual's earning potential. A social worker with expertise in dealing with transplant recipients plays a vital role in helping patients to understand and deal with these issues.

Management of Patients on the Deceased Donor Transplant Waiting List

Renal transplantation is a unique surgical procedure since it is an urgent procedure carried out in an elective population. As such, it is essential that candidates be medically stable for the duration of their time on the waiting list. Good communication between those providing ongoing care to these patients and the transplant center is vital. If a patient is called and proves medically unsuitable, this may result in either cancellation of a transplant or performance of a transplant under unnecessary or unrecognized risk.

In order to minimize such events and ensure ongoing suitability to undergo transplantation, most programs rescreen transplant candidates on a biannual basis. Repeat screening is primarily focused upon cardiovascular health as this often represents the greatest challenge to transplant candidacy.

References

1. Wolfe RA, Ashby VB, Milford EL, et al. Comparison of mortality in all patients on dialysis, patients on dialysis awaiting transplantation, and recipients of a first cadaveric transplant. N Engl J Med. 1999;341:1725–30.
2. Kasiske BL, Ramos EL, Gaston RS, et al. The evaluation of renal transplant candidates: clinical practice guidelines. Patient Care and Education Committee of the American Society of Transplant Physicians. J Am Soc Nephrol. 1995;6:1–34.
3. Steinman TI, Becker BN, Frost AE, et al. Guidelines for the referral and management of patients eligible for solid organ transplantation. Transplantation. 2001;71:1189–204.
4. Kasiske BL, Cangro CB, Hariharan S, et al. The evaluation of renal transplantation candidates: clinical practice guidelines. Am J Transplant. 2001;1 Suppl 2:3–95.
5. Knoll G, Cockfield S, Blydt-Hansen T, et al. Canadian Society of Transplantation: consensus guidelines on eligibility for kidney transplantation. CMAJ. 2005;173:S1–25.
6. Goldfarb-Rumyantzev A, Hurdle JF, Scandling J, et al. Duration of end-stage renal disease and kidney transplant outcome. Nephrol Dial Transplant. 2005;20:167–75.
7. Gaston RS, Danovitch GM, Adams PL, et al. The report of a national conference on the wait list for kidney transplantation. Am J Transplant. 2003;3:775–85.
8. Kiberd B, Boudreault J, Bhan V, Panek R. Access to the kidney transplant wait list. Am J Transplant. 2006;6:2714–20.
9. Lentine KL, Brennan DC, Schnitzler MA. Incidence and predictors of myocardial infarction after kidney transplantation. J Am Soc Nephrol. 2005;16:496–506.
10. Lentine KL, Schnitzler MA, Abbott KC, et al. De novo congestive heart failure after kidney transplantation: a common condition with poor prognostic implications. Am J Kidney Dis. 2005;46:720–33.
11. Lentine KL, Schnitzler MA, Abbott KC, et al. Incidence, predictors, and associated outcomes of atrial fibrillation after kidney transplantation. Clin J Am Soc Nephrol. 2006;1:288–96.
12. Kasiske BL, Maclean JR, Snyder JJ. Acute myocardial infarction and kidney transplantation. J Am Soc Nephrol. 2006;17:900–7.
13. Sharma R, Pellerin D, Gaze DC, et al. Dobutamine stress echocardiography and the resting but not exercise electrocardiograph predict severe coronary artery disease in renal transplant candidates. Nephrol Dial Transplant. 2005;20:2207–14.
14. De Lima JJ, Sabbaga E, Vieira ML, et al. Coronary angiography is the best predictor of events in renal transplant candidates compared with noninvasive testing. Hypertension. 2003;42:263–8.
15. Charytan D, Kuntz RE, Mauri L, DeFilippi C. Distribution of coronary artery disease and relation to mortality in asymptomatic hemodialysis patients. Am J Kidney Dis. 2007;49:409–16.
16. Gowdak LH, de Paula FJ, Cesar LA, et al. Diabetes and coronary artery disease impose similar cardiovascular morbidity and mortality on renal transplant candidates. Nephrol Dial Transplant. 2007;22:1456–61.
17. Gowdak LH, de Paula FJ, Cesar LA, et al. Screening for significant coronary artery disease in high-risk renal transplant candidates. Coron Artery Dis. 2007;18:553–8.

18. Patel RK, Mark PB, Johnston N, et al. Prognostic value of cardiovascular screening in potential renal transplant recipients: a single-center prospective observational study. Am J Transplant. 2008;8:1673–83.
19. EBPG Expert Group on Renal Transplantation. European best practice guidelines for renal transplantation. Section IV: long-term management of the transplant recipient. IV.5.1. Cardiovascular risks. Cardiovascular disease after renal transplantation. Nephrol Dial Transplant. 2002;17(Suppl 4):24–5.
20. K/DOQI Workgroup. K/DOQI clinical practice guidelines for cardiovascular disease in dialysis patients. Am J Kidney Dis. 2005;45:S1–153.
21. Klocke FJ, Baird MG, Lorell BH, et al. ACC/AHA/ASNC guidelines for the clinical use of cardiac radionuclide imaging – executive summary: a report of the American College of Cardiology/American Heart Association Task Force on Practice Guidelines (ACC/AHA/ASNC Committee to Revise the 1995 Guidelines for the Clinical Use of Cardiac Radionuclide Imaging). J Am Coll Cardiol. 2003;42:1318–33.
22. Cheitlin MD, Armstrong WF, Aurigemma GP, et al. ACC/AHA/ASE 2003 guideline update for the clinical application of echocardiography – summary article: a report of the American College of Cardiology/American Heart Association Task Force on Practice Guidelines (ACC/AHA/ASE Committee to Update the 1997 Guidelines for the Clinical Application of Echocardiography). J Am Coll Cardiol. 2003;42:954–70.
23. Koistinen MJ, Huikuri HV, Pirttiaho H, Linnaluoto MK, Takkunen JT. Evaluation of exercise electrocardiography and thallium tomographic imaging in detecting asymptomatic coronary artery disease in diabetic patients. Br Heart J. 1990;63:7–11.
24. Marwick TH, Steinmuller DR, Underwood DA, et al. Ineffectiveness of dipyridamole SPECT thallium imaging as a screening technique for coronary artery disease in patients with end-stage renal failure. Transplantation. 1990;49:100–3.
25. Dahan M, Viron BM, Faraggi M, et al. Diagnostic accuracy and prognostic value of combined dipyridamole-exercise thallium imaging in hemodialysis patients. Kidney Int. 1998;54:255–62.
26. Schmidt A, Stefenelli T, Schuster E, Mayer G. Informational contribution of noninvasive screening tests for coronary artery disease in patients on chronic renal replacement therapy. Am J Kidney Dis. 2001;37:56–63.
27. Reis G, Marcovitz PA, Leichtman AB, et al. Usefulness of dobutamine stress echocardiography in detecting coronary artery disease in end-stage renal disease. Am J Cardiol. 1995;75:707–10.
28. Bates JR, Sawada SG, Segar DS, et al. Evaluation using dobutamine stress echocardiography in patients with insulin-dependent diabetes mellitus before kidney and/or pancreas transplantation. Am J Cardiol. 1996;77:175–9.
29. Herzog CA, Marwick TH, Pheley AM, White CW, Rao VK, Dick CD. Dobutamine stress echocardiography for the detection of significant coronary artery disease in renal transplant candidates. Am J Kidney Dis. 1999;33:1080–90.
30. Budoff MJ, Shaw LJ, Liu ST, et al. Long-term prognosis associated with coronary calcification: observations from a registry of 25,253 patients. J Am Coll Cardiol. 2007;49:1860–70.
31. Goodman WG, Goldin J, Kuizon BD, et al. Coronary-artery calcification in young adults with end-stage renal disease who are undergoing dialysis. N Engl J Med. 2000;342:1478–83.
32. Herzog CA, Ma JZ, Collins AJ. Long-term outcome of renal transplant recipients in the United States after coronary revascularization procedures. Circulation. 2004;109:2866–71.
33. McFalls EO, Ward HB, Moritz TE, et al. Coronary-artery revascularization before elective major vascular surgery. N Engl J Med. 2004;351:2795–804.
34. Boden WE, O'Rourke RA, Teo KK, et al. Optimal medical therapy with or without PCI for stable coronary disease. N Engl J Med. 2007;356:1503–16.
35. Manske CL, Wang Y, Rector T, Wilson RF, White CW. Coronary revascularisation in insulin-dependent diabetic patients with chronic renal failure. Lancet. 1992;340:998–1002.
36. Patel AD, Abo-Auda WS, Davis JM, et al. Prognostic value of myocardial perfusion imaging in predicting outcome after renal transplantation. Am J Cardiol. 2003;92:146–51.

37. Kasiske BL, Malik MA, Herzog CA. Risk-stratified screening for ischemic heart disease in kidney transplant candidates. Transplantation. 2005;80:815–20.
38. Lewis MS, Wilson RA, Walker K, et al. Factors in cardiac risk stratification of candidates for renal transplant. J Cardiovasc Risk. 1999;6:251–5.
39. Eagle KA, Berger PB, Calkins H, et al. ACC/AHA Guideline Update for Perioperative Cardiovascular Evaluation for Noncardiac Surgery – Executive Summary. A report of the American College of Cardiology/American Heart Association Task Force on Practice Guidelines (Committee to Update the 1996 Guidelines on Perioperative Cardiovascular Evaluation for Noncardiac Surgery). Anesth Analg. 2002;94:1052–64.
40. Gill JS, Ma I, Landsberg D, Johnson N, Levin A. Cardiovascular events and investigation in patients who are awaiting cadaveric kidney transplantation. J Am Soc Nephrol. 2005;16:808–16.
41. Siedlecki A, Foushee M, Curtis JJ, et al. The impact of left ventricular systolic dysfunction on survival after renal transplantation. Transplantation. 2007;84:1610–7.
42. de Mattos AM, Siedlecki A, Gaston RS, et al. Systolic dysfunction portends increased mortality among those waiting for renal transplant. J Am Soc Nephrol. 2008;19:1191–6.
43. Burt RK, Gupta-Burt S, Suki WN, Barcenas CG, Ferguson JJ, Van Buren CT. Reversal of left ventricular dysfunction after renal transplantation. Ann Intern Med. 1989;111:635–40.
44. Sung RS, Althoen M, Howell TA, Merion RM. Peripheral vascular occlusive disease in renal transplant recipients: risk factors and impact on kidney allograft survival. Transplantation. 2000;70:1049–54.
45. Makisalo H, Lepantalo M, Halme L, et al. Peripheral arterial disease as a predictor of outcome after renal transplantation. Transpl Int. 1998;11 Suppl 1:S140–3.
46. Oliveras A, Roquer J, Puig JM, et al. Stroke in renal transplant recipients: epidemiology, predictive risk factors and outcome. Clin Transplant. 2003;17:1–8.
47. Ong AC. Screening for intracranial aneurysms in ADPKD. BMJ. 2009;339:b3763.
48. Kasiske BL, Klinger D. Cigarette smoking in renal transplant recipients. J Am Soc Nephrol. 2000;11:753–9.
49. Rao PS, Merion RM, Ashby VB, Port FK, Wolfe RA, Kayler LK. Renal transplantation in elderly patients older than 70 years of age: results from the Scientific Registry of Transplant Recipients. Transplantation. 2007;83:1069–74.
50. Biesenbach G, Konigsrainer A, Gross C, Margreiter R. Progression of macrovascular diseases is reduced in type 1 diabetic patients after more than 5 years successful combined pancreas-kidney transplantation in comparison to kidney transplantation alone. Transpl Int. 2005;18:1054–60.
51. Reddy KS, Stablein D, Taranto S, et al. Long-term survival following simultaneous kidney-pancreas transplantation versus kidney transplantation alone in patients with type 1 diabetes mellitus and renal failure. Am J Kidney Dis. 2003;41:464–70.
52. Heher EC, Spitzer TR, Goes NB. Light chains: heavy burden in kidney transplantation. Transplantation. 2009;87:947–52.
53. Spitzer TR, Sykes M, Tolkoff-Rubin N, et al. Long-term follow-up of recipients of combined human leukocyte antigen-matched bone marrow and kidney transplantation for multiple myeloma with end-stage renal disease. Transplantation 2011;91:672–6.
54. Rostaing L, Modesto A, Abbal M, Durand D. Long-term follow-up of monoclonal gammopathy of undetermined significance in transplant patients. Am J Nephrol. 1994;14:187–91.
55. Nguyen DH, Reinberg Y, Gonzalez R, Fryd D, Najarian JS. Outcome of renal transplantation after urinary diversion and enterocystoplasty: a retrospective, controlled study. J Urol. 1990;144:1349–51.
56. Landin L, Rodriguez-Perez JC, Garcia-Bello MA, et al. Kidney transplants in HIV-positive recipients under HAART. A comprehensive review and meta-analysis of 12 series. Nephrol Dial Transplant. 2010;25:3106–15.
57. Dharnidharka VR, Cherikh WS, Neff R, Cheng Y, Abbott KC. Retransplantation after BK virus nephropathy in prior kidney transplant: an OPTN database analysis. Am J Transplant. 2010;10:1312–5.

58. Eason JD, Gonwa TA, Davis CL, Sung RS, Gerber D, Bloom RD. Proceedings of consensus conference on simultaneous liver kidney transplantation (SLK). Am J Transplant. 2008;8:2243–51.
59. Fabrizi F, Martin P, Dixit V, Kanwal F, Dulai G. HBsAg seropositive status and survival after renal transplantation: meta-analysis of observational studies. Am J Transplant. 2005;5:2913–21.
60. Kidney Disease: Improving Global Outcomes (KDIGO). KDIGO clinical practice guidelines for the prevention, diagnosis, evaluation, and treatment of hepatitis C in chronic kidney disease. Kidney Int Suppl. 2008;(109):S1–99.
61. Mignani R, Feriozzi S, Schaefer RM, et al. Dialysis and transplantation in Fabry disease: indications for enzyme replacement therapy. Clin J Am Soc Nephrol. 2010;5:379–85.
62. Modanlou KA, Muthyala U, Xiao H, et al. Bariatric surgery among kidney transplant candidates and recipients: analysis of the United States renal data system and literature review. Transplantation. 2009;87:1167–73.

Chapter 5
Surgical Management of the Renal Transplant Recipient

Sayeed K. Malek and Stefan G. Tullius

Abstract The modern era of renal transplantation began in the 1950s with the first successful transplant of a kidney between identical twin brothers. Since then, kidney transplantation has become a common procedure performed worldwide with a low incidence of technical complications. The number of kidney transplants in the United States has increased steadily over the past decades, and in 2004 the number of deceased kidney donor transplants in the United States exceeded 10,000 for the first time. Despite these encouraging facts, both the number of patients on the wait list and the wait time for a deceased donor kidney have continued to increase. According to the United Network for Organ Sharing (UNOS) data, there are more than 72,000 patients on the decease donor kidney transplant waiting list in the United States. This chapter will discuss the surgical follow up and complications that may occur following renal transplantation.

Keywords Laproscopic donation • Surgical complications • Arterial thrombosis • Primary non-function • Lymphocele

Introduction

Kidney transplantation is well established as the treatment of choice for patients with end stage renal disease (ESRD). Compared with dialysis, it is associated with increased patient survival and improved quality of life, as well as being more cost effective [1]. In the first half of the twentieth century, with the advancement in vascular surgical techniques based on the work of Alexis Carrel, tremendous interest was generated in the field of organ transplantation. Initial attempts were, however,

S.K. Malek, MD (✉) • S.G. Tullius, MD, PhD
Division of Transplant Surgery, Brigham and Women's Hospital, Boston, MA, USA
e-mail: smalek@partners.org

A. Chandraker et al. (eds.), *Core Concepts in Renal Transplantation*,
DOI 10.1007/978-1-4614-0008-0_5, © Springer Science+Business Media, LLC 2012

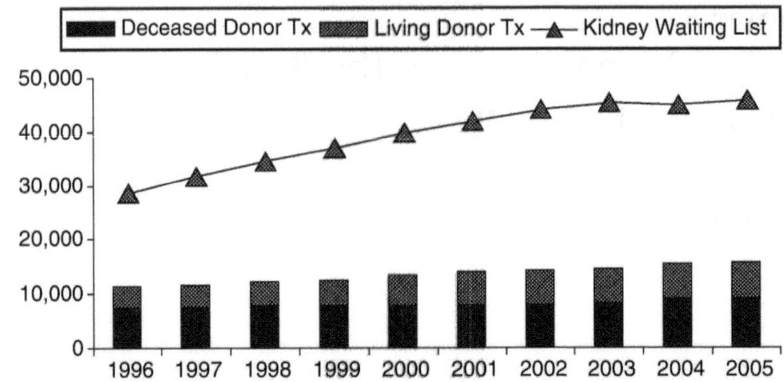

Fig. 5.1 Kidney transplants at a glance: number of transplants and size of waiting list. From Port et al. [10] used with permission

unsuccessful and it was only after World War II with progress in the field of immunology that interest in human transplantation was revived. The modern era of renal transplantation began in the 1950s with the first successful transplant of a kidney between identical twin brothers, on December 23, 1954, at the Peter Bent Hospital in Boston. Since then, kidney transplantation has become a common procedure performed worldwide with a low incidence of technical complications. The number of kidney transplants in the United States has increased steadily over the past decades, and in 2004 the number of deceased kidney donor transplants in the United States exceeded 10,000 for the first time. Despite these encouraging facts, the number of patients on the wait list and the wait time for a deceased donor kidney, have both continued to increase [2]. According to the United Network for Organ Sharing (UNOS) data, there are over 72,000 patients on the decease donor kidney transplant waiting list in the United States [3] (Fig. 5.1).

Pre-Transplant Evaluation

- In preparation for transplantation, patients undergo a detailed medical and surgical evaluation [4–7]. Selection criteria are much more liberal than in the past. The availability of more potent immunosuppression and improvements in human leukocyte antigen (HLA) typing and crossmatching have made it possible for immunologically high-risk patients to be considered candidates for transplantation. The two absolute contraindications for transplantation are untreated malignancy and active infection. Recommended initial studies are given in Table 5.1.

Screening for cardiovascular disease is a critical component in the evaluation of the renal transplant candidate. Cardiovascular disease is the leading cause of death after renal transplantation. Prior ischemic heart disease, cerebrovascular disease, and peripheral vascular disease predict postransplantation mortality. Cardiovascular

Table 5.1 Recommended initial studies before transplantantation

Medical, surgical, and family history	History of the original disease that led to renal failure, including biopsy history and reports
	Urologic disease
	Dialysis history, including adherence to dialysis
	History of cardiovascular and neoplastic disease
	Pregnancy history
	Current medications
	Previous transfusions
	Previous transplantation
	Detailed family history of ESRD, cardiovascular disease (including hypertension), cancer, diabetes mellitus, and liver disease
	Past surgical history of previous surgical procedures
Psychosocial and financial history	Education history
	Current and previous employment
	Disability status
	Recreational drug use
	Alcohiol consumption
	Smoking history
	Activity level (i.e., active or sedentary)
	History of adherence to the medical prescriptions
	Stress level
	Family dynamics
Physical examination of the patient	Standard format
	Assessment of the iliac arteries for decreased pulses or bruits
Diagnostic and screening tests	Complete blood count, serum electrolytes, blood urea nitrogen, serum creatinine, calcium, phosphorous, liver function tests, serum albumen, prothrombin time, INR, and PTT (partial thromboplastin time)
	Serologic tests for HIV, hepatitis, cytomegalovirus (CMV), varicella virus, herpes simplex virus, Epstein–Barr virus (EBV) and syphilis
	PPD
	Immunological profile, blood type (ABO), panel reactive antibody (PRA)
	HLA typing
	Urinalysis, urine culture
	Chest X-ray, EKG
	In selected patients
	Abdominal and renal ultrasound
	Echocardiogram and stress testing
	Cardiac catheterization
	Carotid duplex and peripheral arterial Doppler studies
	Urological assessment
	GI endoscopy
	Pulmonary function test
	Prostate specific antigen (male >50)
	Pap smear and breast examination (for females; mammogram if age >40 years or history of breast cancer)

(continued)

Table 5.1 (continued)

Histocompatibility testing	Blood group
	Tissue typing or HLA typing
	Mixed leukocyte culture (MLC) (or for cross-match procedure to determine the B cell reactivity between donor and recipient)
	T cell cross-match

risk factors need to be identified and appropriate treatment instituted in order to reduce the risk of postransplantation cardiovascular events. Initial assessment is with noninvasive tests, which may vary depending upon the expertise of the transplant center. In high-risk patients and in those with a positive noninvasive test, angiography may be required.

For patients with a suspected coagulation disorder, a hematologic workup is ordered to determine the need for anticoagulation at the time of transplant.

Increasingly, as older recipients are being considered for transplantation, a significant proportion of renal transplant recipients have peripheral vascular disease. The surgical evaluation should identify vascular problems that may complicate the transplant procedure. Preoperative imaging such as noninvasive Doppler studies or a computed tomography (CT) angiogram to evaluate aorto-iliac disease may be required. If aorto-iliac disease is severe, vascular reconstruction with an aorto-iliac or aorto-femoral bypass graft may be required prior to transplantation.

In addition to medical and surgical evaluation, a thorough psychosocial evaluation is necessary to ensure that the recipients understand the transplant procedure, demonstrate compliance, and have no social or financial barriers to transplantation.

A vital component of the preoperative transplant workup is the identification and evaluation of potential living donors. Living donors accounted for approximately 40% of kidneys transplanted in 2005. Living donor renal transplantation has several advantages over deceased donor kidney transplantation. It is associated with improved patient and graft survival [8] and a decreased incidence of delayed graft function. Surgery can be planned as an elective procedure and it avoids the prolonged waiting times for a deceased organ. The operation is safe, with reported mortality rates of 0.03–0.06% [9, 10]. More importantly, because of the limited number of deceased donor kidneys available, living kidney donation represents a valuable resource. The more frequent utilization of laparoscopic and hand-assisted donor nephrectomy, which have been shown to reduce hospital stay, decreases the use of analgesics, and a faster return to normal activity has resulted in increasing the number of living donor kidney transplants.

Donor Operation

The acute shortage of deceased donor organs and the exponential growth in the waiting list continue to pose challenges for the ESRD population. Identification and utilization of living donors is one method to increase the number of kidney

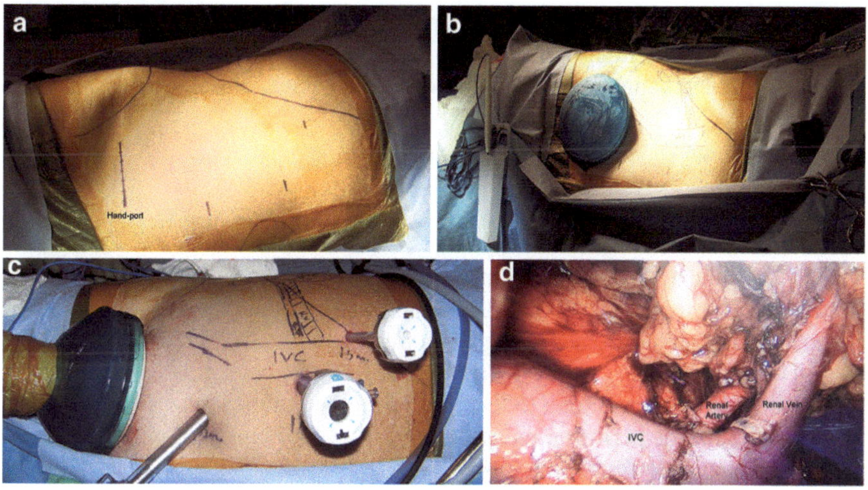

Fig. 5.2 (**a**) Skin markings for right-sided laparoscopic hand-assisted retroperitoneoscopic donor nephrectomy. (**b**) Right-sided laparoscopic hand-assisted retroperitoneoscopic donor nephrectomy with hand-port in place. (**c**) Right-sided laparoscopic hand-assisted retroperitoneoscopic donor nephrectomy with hand-port and laparoscopic ports in place. (**d**) Right-sided laparoscopic hand-assisted retroperitoneoscopic donor nephrectomy showing renal vessels and inferior vena cava (IVC)

transplants. Traditionally performed as an open operation using a flank incision it is now more commonly performed using a laparoscopic or a hand-assisted laparoscopic approach. Moreover, the open operation has been associated with significant morbidity in terms of postoperative pain, longer length of stay, and return to work. Advantages of the laparoscopic technique include a shorter length of stay, less postoperative pain, earlier return to normal activity, and improved cosmesis. A transperitoneal approach is commonly used with the patient in a modified lateral decubitus position. Alternatively, it can also be performed using a hand-assisted technique, either transperitoneally or via a retroperitoneal approach (Fig. 5.2). The hand-assisted approach has the advantage of maximizing tactile feedback and minimizing cold ischemia time as the kidney can be retrieved rapidly after division of the ureter and the vessels. It is particularly helpful for right-sided donor nephrectomies as it permits safe division of the right renal vein close to the inferior vena cava to maximize the length available to the recipient surgeon. Before proceeding with the surgery, precise knowledge of the renal vascular anatomy is essential and is most commonly performed using CT angiography. With rapid evolution in radiological techniques and instrumentation, spiral multidetector CT (MDCT) scans are being used which provide higher spatial and temporal resolutions; 20–25% of the donors may have more than one renal artery bilaterally which may require reconstruction at the time of surgery.

Live donor nephrectomy is a safe operation with a mortality of 0.03% and morbidity of 8–20%. Long-term risks to the donor are minimal but more registry data are needed to better define the long-term medical outcomes.

Renal Transplant Operation

Kidney transplants from living donors are elective surgical procedures but the majority of transplants from deceased donors require the patient to be admitted emergently and are performed at night or on weekends. It is important to limit the cold ischemia time to decrease the rate of delayed graft function. Ideally it is better to keep the cold ischemia time to less than 24 h, though the kidneys can be maintained on a pulsatile perfusion pump device for 48 h or longer. A complete blood count, serum electrolytes, prothrombin and partial prothrombin time, type and cross for ABO compatibility, are ordered. Chest X-ray and electrocardiogram are also obtained. Preoperative dialysis may be required when the last dialysis was greater than 24 h or when hyperkalemia ($K+ >5.5$) is present. Antibiotic prophylaxis is administered in the operating room prior to skin incision.

After induction of general anesthesia, a triple lumen Foley catheter and a central line are inserted. The kidney allograft is removed from its sterile container and examined on the back-table to define graft anatomy. Over the past decade many centers are using pulsatile perfusion pump devices to store and transport deceased donor kidneys. These devices are particularly being used for expanded criteria donor (ECD) kidneys and donation after cardiac death (DCD) kidneys. Perinephric fat is removed and the renal artery and vein are inspected. Polar arteries, if present, are identified. A small upper polar artery may be sacrificed but a polar artery to the lower pole should be preserved and reconstructed to prevent ureteral ischemia and the development of a ureteral stricture.

The technique of renal transplantation has changed little since the first transplant in 1954. The transplanted kidney is placed in a heterotopic location in the right or left lower quadrant, using a retroperitoneal approach. This approach allows easy access for an ultrasound-guided percutaneous biopsy. Commonly used incisions are either a lower abdominal hockey stick incision with minimal muscle-splitting or a Gibson incision, which extends from the midline one finger breadth above the symphysis pubis to a point two finger breadths medial to the anterior superior iliac. The right iliac fossa is usually chosen as the site of transplantation as the iliac vein follows a more superficial course on the right side. Some surgeons prefer to place the right donor kidney in the left iliac fossa of the recipient and vice versa. The left iliac fossa is also the preferred side when a simultaneous pancreas and kidney (SPK) transplant is being performed or when the patient is a candidate for a future pancreas after kidney (PAK) transplant. In the past, bilateral native nephrectomy was performed at many centers but it is rarely required now and the majority of transplant centers do not use it on a routine basis. The external oblique muscle is divided in the direction of its fibers, the internal oblique and transversalis muscles are split, and the properitoneal space is entered and developed by sweeping the peritoneum medially. The rectus sheath may also need to be incised medially to help expose the bladder. Division of the rectus muscle itself is rarely required. The inferior epigastric vessels at the lateral border of the rectus are identified and ligated. The spermatic cord in males is retracted medially and preserved and the round ligament in females is divided. The external iliac artery and vein are dissected and proximal and distal control obtained. A Bookwalter self-retaining retractor may be placed to facilitate retraction. The arterial and venous anastamoses are constructed using 5–0 or 6–0 monofilament suture. The end of the renal artery from the donor is anastamosed to the side of the external iliac artery of the recipient after making an arteriotomy of the appropriate length. Similarly, the end of the renal vein is sutured to the side of the external iliac vein. Upon completion of the anastamosis, the vascular clamps are removed and the kidney normally perfuses and pinks up almost immediately. It is vital for the patient to be adequately perfused and not have a low blood pressure. Hemostasis is secured and attention is then turned towards the ureter. Urinary continuity may be restored by a few different methods. The most common is the Lich-Gregoir or extra vesical technique. The donor ureter is spatulated and anastamosed to the recipient bladder mucosa using 5–0 polyglyconate sutures (ureteroneocystostomy) and to prevent reflux, the seromuscular layers is closed over it with interrupted sutures. An alternative method is the Leadbetter-Politano technique which requires an anterior cystostomy and creation of a submucosal tunnel. Placement of a double J stent to allow free drainage and to protect the anastamosis is not mandatory but is practiced by many centers. Post-operatively the stent is removed in 5–6 weeks and does not require general anesthesia. A Jackson-Pratt drain is usually placed in the retroperitoneal space prior to fascial closure.

Early Postoperative Management

Intensive care management is rarely required for kidney transplant patients and most are transferred to the floor after surgery once they recover from anesthesia in the post-anesthesia care unit (PACU). Initial assessment should focus on hemodynamic management and establishing cardio-respiratory stability. Volume status needs to be monitored closely. In patients who do not make any urine and are on dialysis, voluminous urine output after surgery is a sign of excellent graft function. However, in patients who have normal or near normal urine output, the presence of urine per se cannot be relied on as an indicator of graft function. Evaluation of blood flow to the kidney by ultrasound examination and determining the patency of the renal artery and vein is helpful in ruling out decreased perfusion or obstruction. The urinary catheter should be irrigated to rule out obstruction and to flush out blood clots. Central venous pressure is monitored to ensure adequate volume status. Half normal saline is the intravenous solution used to replace urine output because the sodium concentration of the urine from a transplant kidney is around 60–80 mEq/L. Delayed graft function occurs in 20–40% of deceased donor renal transplants.

It is more frequently encountered when the kidney is an ECD kidney or is procured as a DCD kidney. Once the patient is stable hemodynamically and has recovered from anesthesia, transfer to the floor is initiated.

Complications

Surgical complications after renal transplantation have an incidence of 5–10% and remain an important cause of graft loss. They may be vascular [11–14] or urologic [15, 16] in origin and usually present early after transplantation.

Graft Thrombosis

Graft thrombosis may be arterial or venous and usually occurs in the first 24–72 h. The incidence ranges from 0.5 to 5%. Renal artery thrombosis may present with sudden cessation of urine output and the diagnosis is made by Doppler ultrasound which shows the absence of arterial inflow and non-perfusion of the transplant kidney. Renal artery thrombosis is a catastrophic complication and almost invariably results in graft loss. Early graft loss is mainly a result of technical complications during surgery with unrecognized intimal injury. Although successful thrombectomy with recovery of graft function has been reported on rare occasions, most cases result in graft loss and the need for allograft thrombectomy.

With renal vein thrombosis the clinical presentation includes a sudden decrease in graft function, hematuria, pain, and swelling over the graft. Diagnosis is confirmed by Doppler ultrasound. Similar to thrombosis of the renal artery, renal vein thrombosis presents early and almost invariably results in the loss of the transplant kidney. With renal vein thrombosis the transplanted kidney becomes edematous because of outflow obstruction and the risk of rupture and hemorrhage from the transplant kidney is high. Urgent exploration and allograft thrombectomy is required.

Renal Artery Stenosis

Renal artery stenosis is the most common vascular complication seen after renal transplantation. The incidence of renal artery stenosis is reported to range from 2 to 10%. The presentation is late, from a few months to a year or two post-transplants. Patients may present with sudden onset of refractory hypertension associated with peripheral edema and graft dysfunction. The anastamotic site is the most common location. The cause is multifactoral and may be related to technique, kinking, or twisting of the anastomosis or from atheromatous changes in the recipient vessels. Initial screening is with Doppler studies followed by magnetic resonance angiogram or a CT angiogram. The gold standard for diagnosis remains the arteriogram. Treatment is with percutaneous transluminal angioplasty (PTA), with or without stent placement. Open surgical correction may sometimes be required in selected cases but carries with it the potential risk of graft loss with an increased risk of 5–10%.

Urologic Complications

Urological complications after kidney transplantation have an incidence of 2–10%. Close attention to detail and meticulous recovery of the donor kidney is critical in reducing the incidence of urological complications. It is important not to skeletonize the ureter during organ recovery as this may compromise its blood supply from the lower pole of the kidney and result in ischemic injury. To preserve the blood supply to the ureter during organ procurement, the tissue around the ureter and the pad of fat at the lower pole of the kidney should be removed enbloc. Hilar dissection should be minimal and the shortest possible length of ureter that permits a tension-free anastamosis to the bladder is utilized to create the neoureterocystostomy. Urologic complications may present either as urine leak or as urinary obstruction. Symptoms and signs may include pain and swelling over the graft, fever, decreased urine output, an elevated serum creatinine, and urine draining from the skin incision. Urine leaks usually occur early after transplantation. Analysis of fluid drainage from the wound showing elevated creatinine concentration of the fluid as compared to serum creatinine can help in establishing the diagnosis. An isotope scan or cystography with films taken in both anterior/posterior and oblique views may be required. Small leaks can be managed by placing a Foley catheter for bladder decompression. For larger leaks, open operative repair and drainage are usually required.

Obstruction of the urinary tract often presents with findings similar to acute allograft rejection with a fall in urine output, tenderness over the graft, and fever. Ultrasound examination is required to confirm the diagnosis which shows the typical finding of hydronephrosis. Early obstruction is commonly from technical errors and late obstruction is usually a result of ischemic strictures of the ureter. Treatment will depend on the etiology. A percutaneous nephrostomy is placed to relieve the obstruction and decompress the urinary system. Short–segment ureteral strictures can be treated with percutaneous endourological techniques such as balloon dilation of the stricture and double J stent placement. Stents are generally left in place for 6 weeks. If endoscopic techniques fail to resolve the obstruction then open surgical repair is indicated.

Lymphocele

The majority of lymphoceles are asymptomatic and are detected on routine ultrasound examination. The incidence of lymphoceles that are clinically significant ranges from 0.6 to 18.0% [17]. Lympoceles may form as a consequence of leakage

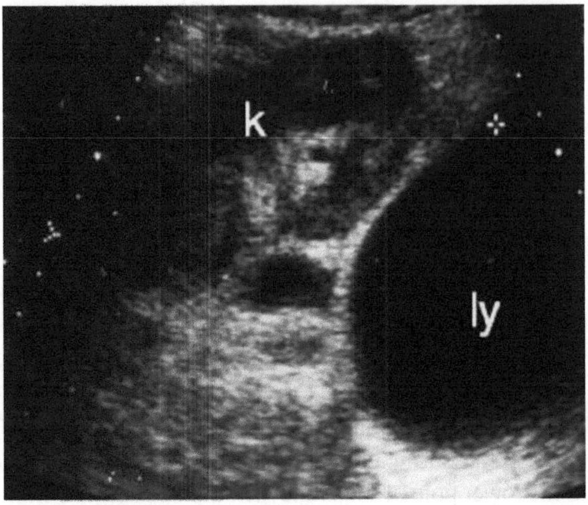

Fig. 5.3 Ultrasound of transplant kidney showing perinephric lymphocele

from transected lymph channels around the iliac vessels during dissection of the external iliac artery and vein or from lymphatics divided during kidney procurement in the perihilar tissue of the allograft. Clinically significant lymphoceles may present with fullness around the allograft (Fig. 5.3) or with signs of ureteral obstruction. Ipsilateral lower extremity swelling may also be a presenting feature. Percutaneous aspiration and placement of a catheter drain are initially employed with an overall success rate of 60–73%. Sclerosants such as tetracycline or povidone iodine have been used in an attempt to obliterate the cavity. They should be used cautiously as they may leak into the peritoneal cavity causing chemical peritonitis. Lymphoceles that do not respond to nonoperative measures are treated surgically using an open or a laparoscopic approach. This involves creation of a peritoneal window (intraperitoneal marsupalization) and has a primary success rate of 90%. A preoperative CT scan is performed to identify the precise location of the lymphocele.

Patient and Graft Survival

The improvement in post-transplant outcomes has been attributed to improvements in organ preservation, refinement of surgical technique, and the use of newer, more potent immunosuppressive agents.

Both patient and graft survival rates are now excellent with 1- and 5-year patient survival for living donors at 98 and 90%, and 96 and 83% for deceased donors, respectively. However, racial and ethnic disparities continue to persist, both in terms of access and listing for transplantation as well as for transplant outcomes. In the United States, frequencies of ESRD are 3.6, 1.8, and 1.4 times higher in African-Americans, Native Americans, and Asians, compared to Caucasians [2], and more than 50% of patient's waitlisted for kidney transplantation belong to ethnic minorities. African-American transplant recipients are disproportionately represented on the waiting list comprising 33% of those listed [18, 19]. Barriers exist at various stages of the transplant process and are responsible for inferior outcomes. Graft survival analyzed at different time points (3 months, 1, 5, and 10 years) shows that African-Americans had the lowest graft survival at each interval [20]. Both immunological and non-immunological factors have been identified. Research is needed to determine the reasons for this disparity. The etiology is multi-factorial and complex and will require a concerted effort on the part of the transplant community and policy makers to improve outcomes and eliminate disparity.

Conclusions

Renal transplantation is the preferred therapy for patients with ESRD. Patient and graft survival rates are excellent but long-term outcomes have not shown much change. The attrition rate of renal allografts remains a concern. This is true of both living and deceased donor transplants where the half-life has shown little change over the past decade. According to USRDS data, the graft survival half-life for deceased donor kidney transplants was 11.4 years in 1995 and 10.5 in 2002; for living donor transplants the rates were 18.4 and 19.1. At the same time the number of patients commencing or re-initiating dialysis as a consequence of a failed allograft has increased from 3,752 in 1995 to 5,156 in 2004. Shortage of organs remains the major challenge, with more than 70,000 (46,00 active, 24,000 inactive) patients waiting for a kidney transplant at the end of 2006. Continued efforts to increase the donor pool are needed to alleviate the donor shortage.

References

1. Wolfe RA et al. Comparison of mortality in all patients on dialysis, patients on dialysis awaiting transplantation, and recipients of a first cadaveric transplant. N Engl J Med. 1999;341:1725–30.
2. U.S. Renal Data System. 2006 Annual Data Report: Atlas of End-Stage Renal Disease in the United States. Bethesda: National Institute of Health, National Institute of Diabetes and Digestive and Kidney Diseases; 2006.
3. Port FK et al. The 2006 SRTR Report on the State of Transplantation: trends in organ donation and transplantation in the United States, 1996–2005. Am J Transplant. 2007;7(5):1319–26.
4. Kasiske BL, Ramon EL, Gaston RS, et al. The evaluation of renal transplant candidates: clinical practice guidelines. J Am Soc Nephrol. 1995;6:1.
5. Steinman TI, Becker BN, Frost AE, et al. Guidelines for the referral and management of patients eligible for solid organ transplantation. Transplantation. 2001;71:1189.
6. The evaluation of renal transplant candidates. Clincal practice guidelines. Am J Transplant. 2001;2(Suppl 1):5.
7. Ramos E, Brennan DC. The evaluation of the potential renal transplant recipient.UpToDate.com.

8. Cohen DJ, St Martin L, Christensen LL, et al. Kidney and pancreas transplantation in the United States, 1995–2004. Am J Transplant. 2006;(Part2):1153–69.
9. Davis CL. Evaluation of living kidney donor: current perspectives. Am J Kidney Dis. 2004;43:508–30.
10. Ellison MD, McBride MA, Edwards LB, et al. Living organ donation: mortality and early complications among 16,395 living donors in the US. Am J Transplant. 2003;3:517A, (abstr).
11. Osman Y, Shokeir A, Ali-el-Din B, et al. Vascular complications after live donor renal transplantation: study of risk factors and effects on graft and patient survival. J Urol. 2003;169:859–62.
12. Englesbe MJ, Punch JD, Armstrong DR, et al. Single-center study of technical graft loss in 714 consecutive renal transplants. Transplantation. 2004;78:623–6.
13. Fervenza FC, Lafayette RA, Alfrey EJ, et al. Renal artery stenosis in kidney transplants. Am J Kidney Dis. 1998;31:142–8.
14. Odland MD. Surgical technique/post-transplant surgical complications. Surg Clin North Am. 1998;78:55–60.
15. Streeter EH, Little DM, Cranston DW, et al. The urological complications of renal transplantation; a series of 1535 patients. BJU Int. 2002;90:627–34.
16. Kocak T, Nane I, Ander H, et al. Urological and surgical complications in 362 consecutive living related donor kidney transplantations. Urlo Int. 2004;72:252–6.
17. Burgos FJ, Teruel JL, Mayayo TL, et al. Diagnosis and management of lymphoceles after renal transplantation. Br J Urol. 1988;61:289–93.
18. Young CJ, Gaston RS. African Americans and renal transplantation; disproportionate need, limited access, and impaired outcomes. Am J Med Sci. 2002;323:94–9.
19. Calender CO, Miles PV. Institutionalized racism and end stage renal disease; is its impact real or illusionary? Semin Dial. 2004;17:77.
20. Fan PY, Ashby VB, Fuller DS, et al. Access and outcomes among minority transplant patients, 1999–2008, with a focus on determinants of kidney graft survival. Am J Transplant. 2010;10:1090.

Chapter 6
Overview of Immunosuppressive Therapies in Renal Transplantation

Steven Gabardi and Eric M. Tichy

Abstract The primary focus of the transplant practitioner is the optimal management of renal transplant recipients in order to achieve long-term patient and allograft. Short-term outcomes of transplantation have improved considerably in the recent years. This success is due in large part to a better understanding of the immune system and improvements in surgical techniques, organ procurement, immunosuppression and post-transplant care. Despite the success in improving short-term outcomes, late graft loss and the morbidity associated with long term immunosuppression remain major concerns. In order to improve outcomes in renal transplantation, it is critical that the knowledge base of transplant practitioners be expanded beyond understanding the basics of immunosuppressive therapies. It is imperative that clinicians are aware of the specific advantages and disadvantages of the available immunosuppressants, as well as the potential for adverse drug reactions and drug–drug interactions commonly seen with these agents. This chapter will review the currently available immunosuppressive agents used for induction and maintenance therapy and focus on their pharmacology, dosing, adverse event profile and clinical efficacy.

Keywords Induction • Maintenance immunosuppression • Pharmacokinetics • Acute rejection • Drug interactions

S. Gabardi, PharmD (✉)
Department of Medicine, Renal Division, Brigham and women's Hospital and Harvard Medical School, Boston, MA, USA
e-mail: sgabardi@partners.org

E.M. Tichy, PharmD
Department of Pharmacy, Yale New Haven Hospital, New Haven, CT, USA

A. Chandraker et al. (eds.), *Core Concepts in Renal Transplantation*,
DOI 10.1007/978-1-4614-0008-0_6, © Springer Science+Business Media, LLC 2012

Introduction

The primary focus of the transplant practitioner is the optimal management of renal transplant recipients (RTRs) in order to achieve long-term patient and allograft. Short-term outcomes of transplantation have improved considerably in the recent years. This success is due in large part to a better understanding of the immune system and improvements in surgical techniques, organ procurement, immunosuppression and post-transplant care. Despite the success in improving short-term outcomes, late graft loss and the morbidity associated with long-term immunosuppression remain major concerns.

In order to improve outcomes in renal transplantation, it is critical that the knowledge base of transplant practitioners be expanded beyond understanding the basics of immunosuppressive therapies. It is imperative that clinicians are aware of the specific advantages and disadvantages of the available immunosuppressants, as well as the potential for adverse drug reactions and drug–drug interactions (DDIs) commonly seen with these agents. This chapter will review the currently available immunosuppressive agents used for induction and maintenance therapy and focus on their pharmacology, dosing, adverse event profile and clinical efficacy.

Immunosuppressive Therapies

The common premise for immunosuppressive therapies in renal transplantation is to utilize multiple agents, which work on different immunologic targets. The use of a multi-drug regimen not only allows for pharmacologic activity at several key steps in the T-cell activation/replication process, but it also allows for lower doses of each individual agent, thereby, producing fewer drug-related toxicities.

In general, there are three stages of clinical immunosuppression: (1) induction therapy; (2) maintenance therapy; and (3) treatment of an established rejection episode. Immunosuppressive therapies used for each of these stages will be discussed in detail below.

Induction Therapy

The goal of induction therapy is to provide a high level of immunosuppression in the critical early post-transplant period, when the risk of acute rejection is highest. This stage of immunosuppression is often initiated intra-operatively or immediately post-operatively and is generally concluded within days following transplantation. Induction therapy is not an obligatory stage of recipient immunosuppression. However, since acute rejection is a major concern in RTRs and its impact on chronic rejection is undeniable, induction therapy is often considered essential to optimize outcomes. Induction therapy agents are pharmacologically classified as either monoclonal or polyclonal antibodies. However, mechanistically, they are more clearly delineated by categorizing them as either depleting (OKT3, antithymocyte globulins [ATGs], alemtuzumab) or non-depleting proteins (basiliximab, daclizumab).

There are several important reasons why induction therapy in utilized. First, the induction agents are highly immunosuppressive, allowing for a significant reduction in acute rejections rates and improved 1-year graft survival. Second, due to their unique pharmacologic effect, these agents are often considered essential for use in patients at high risk for poor short-term outcomes, such as those patients with preformed antibodies, history of previous organ transplants, multiple HLA mismatches or transplantation of organs with prolonged cold ischemic time or from expanded-criteria donors and donors after cardiac death. Induction therapy also plays an important role in preventing early onset calcineurin inhibitor (CNI) induced nephrotoxicity. With the use of induction agents, initiation of CNIs, the backbone of maintenance immunosuppression, can often be delayed until the graft regains some degree of function [1].

The improvements in short-term outcomes gained from the use of induction therapies cannot be denied. Despite these advances, studies detailing the impact of induction therapy on long-term allograft function or survival are lacking. On the other hand, when using these highly immunosuppressive agents, particularly the depleting proteins (also known as the antilymphocyte antibodies [ALAs]) the host defenses are often profoundly impaired, which increases the risk of opportunistic infections and malignancy.

It should be noted that declining worldwide use and the expense associated with manufacturing both OKT3 and daclizumab have led the makers of these agents to decide to discontinue their production. Given these decisions, this review will discuss only those induction therapy agents that will remain on the United States market in the foreseeable future (Table 6.1).

Non-depleting Protein (Basiliximab)

Pharmacology: Basiliximab is a monoclonal antibody that contains murine sequences in the variable region and has been termed a chimeric antibody, consisting of approximately 30% murine and 70% human sequences [2, 3]. This agent binds with high affinity to the alpha subunit of the IL-2 receptor, also known as CD25, where it acts as a receptor antagonist. Basiliximab functions by inhibiting IL-2 mediated activation of lymphocytes, which is important for clonal expansion of T-cells [2, 3].

Dosing: The dose of basiliximab is 20 mg given intravenous (IV) 2 h prior to transplant, followed by a second 20 mg dose on post-op day 4 [2, 3]. This dosing schedule can be used for both adults and children greater than or equal to 35 kg. In children less than 35 kg, two doses of 10 mg each should be used. Basiliximab remains bound to the CD25 subunit for approximately 5–8 weeks after transplantation. There are no dose adjustments needed in renal or hepatic impairment [2, 3].

Adverse Events: Safety is one of the most evident benefits of basiliximab, especially the absence of any increased risk of cytomegalovirus (CMV) infection or malignancy. The incidence of all adverse reactions with basiliximab was similar to placebo in clinical trials [2, 3].

Table 6.1 Biologic agents used in renal transplant [2, 18, 19]

Generic name (brand name)	Depleting/ non-depleting protein	FDA approval I	FDA approval AR	Dosing	Common adverse events
Basiliximab (Simulect®)	Non-depleting	Yes	No	20 mg IV × 2 doses	None reported compared to placebo
Antithymocyte globulin equine (ATGAM®)	Depleting	Yes	Yes	15 mg/kg/day IV × 3–14 days	Flu-like symptoms, GI distress, rash, back pain, myelosuppression
Antithymocyte globulin rabbit (Thymoglobulin®)	Depleting	No	Yes	1.5 mg/kg/day IV × 3–14 days	Flu-like symptoms, GI distress, rash, generalized pain, myelosuppression
Alemtuzumab (Campath®)	Depleting	No	No	30 mg IV × 1–2 doses	Flu-like symptoms, GI distress, dizziness, myelosuppression

If the common dose is weight based then a dose was calculated based on a 70-kg patient
AR acute rejection; *I* induction; *IV* intravenous

Although basiliximab is considered to be safe, severe acute hypersensitivity reactions have occurred after both initial exposure and re-exposure to this antibody [2, 3]. Hypotension, tachycardia, cardiac failure, dyspnea, wheezing, bronchospasm, pulmonary edema, respiratory failure, urticaria, rash and pruritus characterize this reaction. Hypersensitivity reactions are extremely rare, occurring in less than 1% of the patients, but are significant enough that the FDA required product labeling revisions to reflect this potential danger [2, 3].

Depleting Proteins (Antithymocyte Globulins)

Pharmacology: Polyclonal antibodies against human lymphoid tissue are prepared from the serum of animals immunized with human thymocytes [2, 4–6]. Currently, two ATG preparations are available. Antithymocyte globulin equine (eATG) is a purified, concentrated and sterilized antibody preparation derived from the hyperimmune serum of horses. This preparation reduces the number of circulating, thymus-dependent lymphocytes by several mechanisms. Equine ATG contains antibodies against several T-cell surface markers and after binding to these markers, eATG promotes T-cell depletion by either opsonization and complement-mediated lysis or clearance into the reticuloendothelial system. Cell recovery after depletion with eATG may take several months. Overall, this agent reduces the number of lymphocytes in the peripheral circulation, as well as in the thymus and spleen [1, 2, 4, 6].

Antithymocyte globulin rabbit (rATG) is also a cytolytic polyclonal antibody preparation [2, 5, 6]. It is a purified and pasteurized preparation of gamma immunoglobulin obtained by immunizing rabbits with human thymocytes. Possible mechanisms by which rATG induces immunosuppression in vivo include T-cell clearance from the circulation and modulation of T-cell activation, homing and cytotoxic activities. In vitro, rATG mediates T-cell suppressive effects via inhibition of proliferative responses to several mitogens. rATG is thought to induce T-cell depletion and modulation by a variety of methods, including Fc receptor-mediated complement-dependent lysis, opsonization and phagocytosis by macrophages, and immunomodulation leading to long-term depletion via apoptosis and antibody-dependent cell-mediated cytotoxicity. Immune reconstitution may take several months following a course of rATG [2, 5, 6]. One interesting analysis showed that T-cell recovery after rATG-induced depletion is associated with an expansion of cell subsets that are linked to suppressor function potentially resulting in long-term immunomodulation [7].

Dosing: The standard induction therapy dosing strategy for eATG is 10–30 mg/kg/day IV for 7–14 days [1, 2, 4, 6]. The first dose usually begins shortly before or after transplantation. However, the difficult outpatient administration and high cost of this agent make this prolonged course difficult in many instances. A shorter course of therapy is often used to counter these issues and consists of dosing eATG at 15 mg/kg/day for 7–10 days, stopping once the maintenance immunosuppressive regimen is optimized. Rabbit ATG is not FDA approved for induction therapy; however, many in the transplant community routinely use this antibody for induction therapy. When used in this capacity, rATG has been dosed at 1–4 mg/kg/day and is usually administered for 3–10 days after transplantation. The most common dosing schedule for this agent is four doses of 1.5 mg/kg/day, resulting in a total dosage of 6 mg/kg over the course of the therapy [2, 5, 6]. In many renal transplant centers, the initial dose is administered intra-operatively prior to the anastamosis of the renal artery to help reduce organ re perfusion injury [8].

Adverse Events: Regardless of the preparation used, cytokine release-related adverse events are common. The most frequently occurring of these include fever (63%), chills (43.2%), headache (34.6%), back pain (43.2%), nausea (28.4%), diarrhea (32.1%), dizziness (24.7%), malaise (3.7%), leukopenia (29.6%) and thrombocytopenia (44.4%) [2]. In order to lower the incidence of fever and chills during the infusion, pre-medication with an antihistamine and acetaminophen is recommended. The overall incidence of opportunistic infections is 27.2%, with CMV disease occurring in 11.1% of the patients. Anaphylactic reactions have occurred with the administration of eATG and the manufacturer strongly recommends the administration of a skin test prior to the first dose of eATG to assess the potential for an allergic reaction. The patient and injection site should be examined every 15–20 min for 1 h after the administration of the test dose. Unfortunately, a negative skin test does not completely rule out the potential for an allergic reaction. The strong recommendation of the skin test makes the use of eATG more difficult when compared to other antibody preparations [1, 2, 4].

The adverse events of rATG tend to be very similar to those seen with eATG and may include fever (63.4%), chills (57.3%), headache (40.2%), nausea (36.6%), diarrhea (36.6%), malaise (13.4%), dizziness (8.5%), leukopenia (57.3%), thrombocytopenia (36.6%) and generalized pain (46.3%) [2]. The incidence of infection is 36.6%, with CMV disease occurring in 13.4% of the patients. Pre-medication with an antihistamine and acetaminophen is recommended to lower the incidence of potential infusion-related reactions [2, 5].

Comparative Efficacy (eATG vs. rATG): The sentinel study comparing eATG to rATG was conducted by Brennan et al. [9]. In this analysis, 72 RTRs were randomly assigned rATG 1.5 mg/kg ($n=48$) or eATG 15 mg/kg ($n=24$) daily for up to 6 days. All patients were maintained on cyclosporine (CsA), azathioprine (AZA) and prednisone, or CsA, mycophenolate mofetil (MMF) and prednisone. There was no difference between rATG and eATG in patient survival and renal function at 12 months. At 1 year, graft survival was higher with rATG (98%) compared to eATG (83%; $p=0.020$) and acute rejection occurred more frequently with eATG (25%) compared to rATG (4.2%; $p=0.014$). An evaluation of the safety parameters revealed that leukopenia occurred more commonly with rATG (56.3%) than with eATG (4.2%; $p<0.0001$). Despite this, the incidence of CMV disease was lower in patients treated with rATG (10%) than eATG (33%; $p=0.025$) at 6 months. No patients in either arm developed post-transplant lymphoproliferative disease (PTLD) [9].

A 10-year follow-up of this study showed both event-free survival (48 vs. 29%; $p=0.011$) and the incidence of acute rejection (11 vs. 42%; $p=0.004$) favored rATG. Mean serum creatinine levels were higher (1.7+0.5 vs. 1.2+0.3 mg/dL; $p=0.003$) in the rATG group. There were 0.53 quality-adjusted life years gained from rATG induction [10].

Comparative Efficacy (Basiliximab vs. rATG): Given the differences in their mechanisms of immunosuppression, many have theorized that when using depleting protein one sacrifices a higher incidence of adverse events for improved efficacy vs. a non-depleting protein. Several studies have attempted to prove this by evaluating the differences between basiliximab and rATG for induction therapy in RTRs. The most applicable study was done by Brennan et al. [11]. Per protocol, event-free survival was defined as freedom from a composite endpoint (biopsy-proven acute rejection [BPAR], delayed graft function [DGF], graft loss and death). The patients were randomized to receive either rATG (1.5 mg/kg/day from Day 0 to Day 4; $n=141$) or basiliximab (20 mg/day on Days 0 and 4; $n=137$). Maintenance immunosuppression consisted of CsA-modified, MMF and corticosteroids. The composite endpoint was similar in both the groups at 12 months (rATG=50.4%, basiliximab=56.2%; $p=0.34$). However, the incidence of BPAR was lower with rATG (15.6%) vs. basiliximab (25.5%; $p=0.02$). Nearly 99% of the patients in both the groups experienced at least one adverse event. There were significantly more infectious complications associated with rATG than with basiliximab (85.8 vs. 75.2%; $p=0.03$); conversely, CMV infections were significantly more frequent in the basiliximab group (17.5 vs. 7.8%; $p=0.02$). Myelosuppression was seen in a significantly higher number of the rATG-treated patients. Five patients in the rATG group and one patient in the basiliximab group developed malignancy [11].

A recent meta-analysis of the IL-2 receptor antibodies has been completed [12]. When these agents were analyzed against the ATG preparations it was found that there was no difference in graft loss. Induction with ATG therapy lowered the rates of BPAR at 1 year (8 studies: RR 1.30 95% CI 1.01–1.67), but at the cost of a 75% increase in malignancy (7 studies: RR 0.25 95% CI 0.07–0.87) and a 32% increase in CMV disease (13 studies: RR 0.68 95% CI 0.50–0.93). Adverse events, including fever, cytokine release syndrome and myelosuppression were seen in a higher percentage of patients receiving ATG preparations [12].

Depleting Proteins (Alemtuzumab)

Pharmacology: Alemtuzumab is a recombinant DNA-derived monoclonal antibody that binds to the 21–28 kDa cell surface glycoprotein, CD52 [2, 13]. CD52 is present on the surface of almost all B- and T-lymphocytes, many macrophages, NK cells and a subpopulation of granulocytes. This agent's mechanism of action is believed to be antibody-dependent cell lysis following its binding to CD52 cell surface markers. Alemtuzumab produces a rapid and extensive lymphocyte depletion that may take several months to return to pre-transplant levels [13].

Dosing: Alemtuzumab has not been FDA approved for use in RTRs. There is no consensus on the appropriate dose of alemtuzumab for induction therapy. Some studies have demonstrated that a dose of 20–30 mg IV or SC on day 0 and again on either day 1 or 4 post-transplant to be effective in preventing acute rejection [14]. However, current studies are evaluating the use of a single 30 mg dose given on post-op day 0, figuring it will prove to be as effective, but better tolerated [13].

Adverse Events: Some of alemtuzumab's serious adverse reactions include anemia (47%), neutropenia (70%), thrombocytopenia (52%), headache (24%), dysthesias (15%), dizziness (12%), nausea (54%), vomiting (41%), diarrhea (22%), autoimmune hemolytic anemia (rare), infusion-related reactions (15–89%) and infection (37%; CMV viremia occurred in 15% of patients) [2]. The FDA recommends that pre-medication with acetaminophen and oral antihistamines is advisable to reduce the incidence of infusion-related reactions [2, 13].

Comparative Efficacy: Data exist on alemtuzumab's efficacy and safety in several observational studies while only a few randomized, controlled trials have been published to date in RTRs. These data show that alemtuzumab induction in combination with low-dose CNIs provides acceptable rates of rejection and infection while allowing important cost saving when compared with other induction agents.

Farney et al. conducted a prospective randomized single-center trial comparing alemtuzumab ($n = 113$) to rATG ($n = 109$) for induction therapy in adult renal and pancreas transplant recipients [15]. Allograft and patient survival were similar between the groups, but BPAR occurred less frequently with alemtuzumab (14 vs. 26%; $p = 0.02$). Infections and malignancy were similar between the two induction arms [15].

One potential concern of the profound immune depletion after alemtuzumab induction is the potential response associated with immune reconstitution. Although data are not available in renal transplantation, a study in multiple sclerosis demonstrated a profound IL-21-driven autoimmune response following lymphocyte depletion from alemtuzumab [16]. Further characterization of the immune system following alemtuzumab use in renal transplant recipients is needed to understand the full impact of using this agent as induction therapy.

Induction Therapy: Conclusion

Induction therapy with biological agents continued a 9-year trend of increasing utilization to 74% of kidney transplants in 2004–2005 [17]. However, there is no universal consensus on the optimal induction agent. The most recent analysis in 2005 demonstrated that rATG was the most frequently used induction agent in the United States. It was used in 39% of RTRs about whom information was available. In contrast, the IL-2 receptor antibodies were used in 28%, alemtuzumab in 9% and eATG or OKT3 in <2% of all RTRs [6, 17].

Maintenance Therapy

The goals of maintenance immunosuppression are to further aid in preventing acute rejection episodes and to optimize long-term patient and graft survival. Anti-rejection medications require careful selection and dosage titration to balance the risks of rejection with the risks of toxicities. The occurrence of some of the most notorious post-transplant adverse events (i.e., infection, malignancy) is associated with the net state of immunosuppression; therefore, it is essential that the degree of immunosuppression is gradually reduced over time.

During the early years of renal transplantation, there were few choices for maintenance immunosuppression, with AZA and corticosteroids being the cornerstones of therapy. In the early 1980s, the development of CsA revolutionized renal transplant by dramatically reducing rejection rates and improving 1-year graft survival. The evolution of maintenance immunosuppressants in the 1990s saw several new options become available to further prevent rejection and improve outcomes. These agents in combination with antibody therapy have made it possible to attain acute rejection rates at or below 10% and increase 1-year graft survival to greater than 90%.

The common maintenance immunosuppressive agents can be divided into four classes (Table 6.2):

- CNIs (CsA and tacrolimus [TAC]).
- Target of Rapamycin (ToR) Inhibitors (sirolimus and everolimus).
- Antiproliferatives (AZA and the mycophenolic acid [MPA] derivatives).
- Co-stimulation Blockade (belatacept).
- Corticosteroids.

Maintenance immunosuppression is generally achieved by combining two or more medications from the different classes to maximize efficacy by specifically targeting unique components of the immune response. This method of medication

Table 6.2 Maintenance immunosuppressive medications [2, 18, 19]

Generic name (brand name)	Generics available	Common oral dosage	Common adverse effects
CsA (Sandimmune®, Neoral®, Gengraf®)	Yes	4–5 mg/kg by mouth twice a day	Neurotoxicity, gingival hyperplasia, hirsutism, hypertension, hyperlipidemia, glucose intolerance, nephrotoxicity, electrolyte abnormalities
TAC (Prograf®)	Yes	0.05–0.075 mg/kg by mouth twice a day	Neurotoxicity, alopecia, hypertension, hyperlipidemia, glucose intolerance, nephrotoxicity, electrolyte abnormalities
AZA (Imuran®)	Yes	1–2.5 mg/kg by mouth once a day	Myelosuppression, gastrointestinal disturbances, pancreatitis
MMF (CellCept®)	Yes	0.5–1.5 g by mouth twice a day	Myelosuppression, gastrointestinal disturbances
EC-MPA (Myfortic®)	No	720 mg by mouth twice a day	Myelosuppression, gastrointestinal disturbances
Sirolimus (Rapamune®)	No	1–10 mg by mouth once a day	Hypertriglyceridemia, myelosuppression, mouth sores, hypercholesterolemia, gastrointestinal disturbances, impaired wound healing, lymphocele, pneumonitis
Everolimus (Zortress®)	No	0.75 mg by mouth twice a day	Hypertriglyceridemia, myelosuppression, mouth sores, hypercholesterolemia, gastrointestinal disturbances, impaired wound healing, lymphocele, pneumonitis
Belatacept (Nulojix®)	No	10 mg/kg/dose IV on post-op days 1 and 5 and at the end of post-op weeks 2, 4, 8 and 12.5 mg/kg/dose given every 4 weeks starting at the end of post-op week 16.	Anemia, leukopenia, peripheral edema, gastrointestinal disturbances, headache
Prednisone (Deltasone®)	Yes	Maintenance: 2.5–20 mg by mouth once a day	Mood disturbances, psychosis, cataracts, hypertension, fluid retention, peptic ulcers, osteoporosis, muscle weakness, impaired wound healing, glucose intolerance, weight gain, hyperlipidemia

selection also helps to minimize individual drug-related adverse events. Immunosuppressive regimens vary between transplant centers, but most often they include a CNI with an adjuvant agent, with/without corticosteroids. Selection of appropriate immunosuppressive agents should be patient specific and, in doing so, transplant practitioners must assess the immunosuppressive medication's pharmacologic properties, adverse event profile and potential for DDIs, as well as the patients' co-morbidities and medication requirements.

CNIS (Cyclosporine and Tacrolimus)

Pharmacology: The CNIs illicit their immune response by complexing with cytoplasmic proteins, cyclophilin (CsA) and FK binding protein-12 (FKBP-12; TAC) [2, 18, 19]. This drug–protein complex then binds to and inhibits calcineurin phosphatase, which prevents the dephosphorylation and translocation of nuclear factor of activated T-cells (NFAT). Inhibition of NFAT's passage through the nuclear membrane hampers the expression of several key cytokine genes that promote T-cell activation and expansion, including IL-2, IL-4, interferon-gamma (INF-γ) and tumor necrosis factor-alpha (TNF-α). The end result of calcineurin inhibition is a reduction in cytokine synthesis with a subsequent decline in lymphocyte proliferation [2, 18, 19].

Pharmaceutics and Dosing: The FDA first approved CsA in 1983, but the original, oil-based formulation had bile-dependent absorption and was associated with variable inter- and intra-patient oral bioavailability. A newer formulation, CsA-modified was introduced in 1994 and has more reliable bioavailability [20]. Cyclosporine modified is the formulation of choice for transplant centers that utilize CsA-based maintenance therapy. It is important to note that the two formulations are not interchangeable.

The labeled initial oral adult dose of CsA after renal transplant is 15 mg/kg/day (range of 8–18 mg/kg/day) given in two divided doses [2, 18, 19]. The appropriate selection of a starting dose is impacted by the patients' immunologic risk, co-morbidities and other immunosuppressive agents utilized. The use of CsA therapeutic drug monitoring (TDM) for dose adjustments is necessary to ensure efficacy and prevent toxicities.

Cyclosporine and CsA-modified are both available as 25 and 100 mg individually blister-packed capsules and oral solutions (100 mg/mL) [2]. An IV formulation is also available, but it is used infrequently due to its high risk of nephrotoxicity and potential incompatibilities with other IV infusions. The high incidence of nephrotoxicity with the IV formulation may be attributable to the inherent poor bioavailability of oral CsA. If used, the IV formulation must be infused over at least 2 h, although a continuous infusion is recommended. Cyclosporine IV solutions should be diluted in D5W and contained in non-PVC container to maximize stability. When converting a patient from oral to IV, the dose should be reduced to approximately one-third of the total daily oral dose [2, 19]. Generic formulations are available for both CsA and CsA-modified, and are considered, by FDA standards, to be bioequivalent to their innovator products.

The recommended adult oral dose of TAC after renal transplant is 0.2 mg/kg/day (range of 0.1–0.3 mg/kg/day) given in two divided doses [2, 18, 19]. The first dose should be administered within 24 h of transplantation in patients not receiving induction therapy. However, when induction therapy is used, TAC dosing may be delayed until kidney function has recovered. The appropriate selection of a starting dose is impacted by the patients' immunologic risk, race, co-morbidities and concomitant immunosuppressants [2, 18, 19].

Tacrolimus for transplantation is commercially available in 0.5, 1, and 5 mg capsules and as an injectable [2]. A once daily, extended-release TAC formulation is available in the international market and may be made available in the US. In rare instances, oral TAC may also be given sublingually to avoid first pass metabolism [21, 22]. The IV formulation is usually avoided due to the risk of anaphylaxis, secondary to its hydrogenated castor oil component [2]. If used, the IV formulation must be diluted prior to administration and should be infused over at least 2 h, although a continuous infusion is preferred. Tacrolimus solutions can be diluted with either D5W or NS, but should be contained in a non-PVC container to maximize stability. When converting a patient from oral to IV, the dose should be reduced to approximately one-third to one-fifth of the total daily oral dose [2, 19]. Generic formulations of TAC are available.

Therapeutic Drug Monitoring: The measurement of CsA and TAC blood levels is essential to the management of RTRs. TDM is imperative given the great variation in inter- and intra-patient metabolism of these agents [23–25]. There is a relationship, although inconsistent, between CNI blood levels and outcomes. Cyclosporine therapeutic trough concentrations (C_0; blood levels drawn immediately preceding a dose) may range 50–400 ng/mL, depending on the patient's degree of immunologic risk and the time elapsed since the transplant. Steady-state concentrations are generally achieved after 3–4 days. Dose adjustments are made to achieve these target concentrations, but doses may also be adjusted to alleviate adverse events. Target level recommendations are institution- and patient specific [23–25].

Although C_0 has been the standard monitoring parameter for the management of patients taking CsA, it has been shown that trough concentrations do not have the best correlation with either efficacy or toxicity [24–26]. Newer studies suggest that monitoring blood concentrations of CsA-modified at 2 h (+15 min) post-dose (C_2) correlates better with toxicity and efficacy when compared to C_0. A typical range for C_2 levels is 800–1,500 ng/mL [24, 25]. The long-term benefits garnered by C_2 monitoring are unclear, but using this measurement may provide an initial improvement in renal function and reduce the frequency and severity of CsA-induced hypertension compared with traditional C_0 monitoring.

Trough concentrations are the mainstay of TAC TDM, based on the evidence that these levels are a good reflection of the overall drug exposure [23, 24]. Trough monitoring should begin after the initial doses of TAC due to the wide inter-patient metabolic variability, however, steady-state concentrations are generally achieved after 3–4 days. The manufacturer of TAC recommends that C_0 should be monitored and maintained between 4 and 20 ng/mL, depending on the degree of the patients' immunologic risk and the time elapsed since the transplant [2]. Many practitioners have argued that the manufacturer's recommendations for the upper limit of the trough concentration are very high and contemporary studies have shown excellent efficacy and tolerability with TAC trough concentrations of no greater than 12 ng/mL [24]. Dosing modifications are made to achieve these target concentrations, but may also be made when TAC-induced toxicities are evident.

Adverse Events: One of the major drawbacks of the CNIs is their extensive adverse event profile, with most of the toxicities being dose dependent. One of the most dubious effects of the CNIs is their ability to cause acute and chronic nephrotoxicity [27]. Acute nephrotoxicity, a result of vasoconstriction at the afferent arteriole, has been correlated with high doses and is usually reversible. Chronic toxicity, however, is typically irreversible and is linked to chronic drug exposure [27]. Table 6.3 expands upon the more common CNI-induced adverse events and provides recommendations for managing these issues [18, 19].

Comparative Efficacy: It is not clear which CNI should be used preferentially in renal transplantation. Several studies have assessed the clinical efficacy and safety of CsA vs. TAC.

Table 6.3 Management of common adverse events associated with the CNIs [2, 18, 19]

Adverse event	Most likely offending CNI	Monitoring parameters	Therapeutic management options
Alopecia	TAC	Patient complaints of excessive hair loss	Reduce TAC dose (if possible) Hair growth treatments (i.e., minoxidil, finasteride for males only) Change from TAC to CsA or sirolimus
CNS toxicities[a]	TAC	Fine hand tremor Headache Mental status changes	Reduce TAC dose (if possible) Change from TAC to CsA or sirolimus
Electrolyte imbalance	Either	K (usually ↑) Mg (usually ↓) PO4 (usually ↓)	Treat electrolyte imbalance (i.e., Mg replacement) Reduce CI dose (if possible) Modify regimen (add or change to non-CI containing regimen)
GI distress[a]	TAC	Patient complaints of nausea, vomiting or diarrhea	GI distress is often blamed on mycophenolate and this agent may be dose reduced prior to changing the TAC dose Reduce TAC dose (if possible) Change from TAC to CsA or sirolimus
Gingival hyperplasia	CsA	Patient complaints of excessive gum growth Recommendations for therapy from the patient's dentist	Reduce CsA dose (if possible) Oral surgery (gum resection) Change from CsA to TAC or sirolimus
Hematologic	Either	White blood cell count Platelets Hemoglobin Hematocrit Symptoms of anemia	Reduce CI dose (if possible) Modify regimen (add or change to non-CI containing regimen; although hematologic risk are high for all meds except steroids)

(continued)

Table 6.3 (continued)

Adverse event	Most likely offending CNI	Monitoring parameters	Therapeutic management options
Hepatotoxicity	Either	Liver function tests	Reduce CI dose (if possible) Modify regimen (add or change to non-CI containing regimen)
Hirsutism	CsA	Patient complaints of excessive hair growth or male-pattern hair growth	Reduce CsA dose (if possible) Cosmetic hair removal Change from CsA to TAC or sirolimus
Hyperglycemia[a]	TAC	Blood glucose (fasting and non-fasting) HgA1c	Diet modifications Reduce steroids (if patient is taking them and if possible) Reduce TAC dose (if possible) Initiate patient-specific glucose-lowering therapy (insulin or oral therapy) Change from TAC to CsA or sirolimus
Hyperlipidemia[b]	CsA	Fasting lipid panel	Initiate patient-specific cholesterol-lowering therapy Reduce CsA dose (if possible) Change from CsA to TAC
Hypertension[b]	CsA	Blood pressure Heart rate	Initiate patient-specific antihypertensive therapy Reduce CsA dose (if possible) Change from CsA to TAC or sirolimus
Hyperuricemia	CsA	Uric acid levels Patient complaints of a gout flare	Initiate hyperuricemia treatment (allopurinol, probenecid, colchicines for a gout flare) Avoid NSAID use, if possible, for symptomatic relief of a gout flare Reduce CsA dose (if possible) Change from CsA to TAC or sirolimus
Nephrotoxicity	Either	Serum creatinine BUN Urine output Biopsy-proven CI-induced nephrotoxicity	Reduce CI dose (if possible) Use of CCB for HTN control Modify regimen (add or change to non-CI containing regimen)

CCB calcium channel blocker; *CI* CNI; *HTN* hypertension; *K* potassium; *Mg* magnesium; *NSAID* non-steroidal anti-inflammatory drugs; PO_4 phosphate

[a]CsA is also associated with CNS toxicities, GI distress and hyperglycemia, but to a lower extent compared to TAC

[b]TAC is also associated with hyperlipidemia and hypertension, but to a lower extent compared to CsA

In 2005, a meta-analysis was published in an attempt to differentiate the relative efficacy and safety of CsA and TAC in RTRs [28]. This report evaluated 30 randomized controlled trials with more than 4,100 patients. It showed that at 6 months post-transplant TAC was associated with a significantly reduced rate of allograft loss (RR 0.56; 95% CI=0.36–0.86). This benefit prolonged for 3 years post-transplant, but was diminished in patients where higher TAC concentrations were targeted. This advantage over CsA was independent of the type of CsA formulation used. Tacrolimus was also shown to have a 12-month benefit on the incidence of rejection (RR 0.69; 95% CI=0.60–0.79) and steroid-resistant rejection (RR 0.49; 95% CI=0.37–0.64). The safety profiles of the two CNIs were also compared and this analysis demonstrated that TAC was associated with a higher risk of PTDM, neurologic effects and gastrointestinal (GI) disorders. Cyclosporine treated patients complained of more cosmetic-related adverse events and more hyperlipidemia [28].

Most of the available data are difficult to interpret and apply given the variability concerning the formulations of CsA used and differences in drug dosing, trough concentrations, concurrent immunosuppressive agents used (induction and maintenance), indications for transplantation and co-morbid disease states. Overall, no study has determined what the ideal CNI is for the long-term management of RTRs. Selection of the most appropriate CNI should be based on patient-specific factors and the expected adverse event profile for each of the agents.

Target of Rapamycin Inhibitors: Sirolimus and Everolimus

Pharmacology: Sirolimus and everolimus are macrolide antibiotics that inhibit lymphocyte activation and proliferation [29–31]. Intracellularly, both agents complex with FKBP-12, which subsequently binds to and modulates the activity of the mammalian ToR. ToR is a key regulatory kinase in cytokine-dependent cellular proliferation. Inhibition of ToR results in the arrest of the cell-division cycle in the G_1-to-S phase. Both ToR inhibitors also affect hematopoietic and nonhematopoietic cells [29–31].

Pharmaceutics and Dosing: Sirolimus is available in oral formulation only [30]. For initiation of sirolimus in de novo renal transplant recipients who are at low to moderate immunologic risk, it is recommended that a sirolimus loading dose of 6 mg be given, followed by a 2-mg/day maintenance dose [30]. Although maintenance doses of 5 mg/day, after a 15-mg loading dose, have been studied for this indication, no efficacy advantage over the 2 mg/day dose has been established. For sirolimus dosing in RTRs at high immunologic risk, a recommended loading dose of 15 mg is recommended followed by a maintenance dose of 5 mg/day [30]. Everolimus is only indicated for prevention of rejection in low to moderate risk RTRs when given in conjunction with basiliximab induction, reduced-dose CsA and corticosteroids [29, 31]. The recommended starting dose of everolimus is 0.75 mg twice daily without the need for a loading dose.

Therapeutic Drug Monitoring: An excellent correlation exists between whole-blood C_0 and the area under the time-concentration curve (AUC) for sirolimus [32]. Sirolimus C_0 ranges from 5 to 24 mg/mL, depending on institution-specific protocols [30, 32]. The manufacturer has recommended goal concentrations in specific populations. In low to moderate immunologic risk patients where cyclosporine therapy is to be withdrawn, whole blood C_0 range is 16–24 ng/mL within the first year post-transplantation [30]. Thereafter, the target sirolimus concentrations should be 12–20 ng/mL. In high immunologic risk patients, it is recommended that sirolimus doses be adjusted to obtain C_0 within the range of 10–15 ng/mL. Additional therapeutic ranges for various immunosuppression strategies can be found in the package insert. However, due to dose-dependent side effects often associated with sirolimus, higher therapeutic ranges of sirolimus are not encouraged. Of note, sirolimus has a half-life of approximately 62 h. Utilization of the loading dose generally helps achieve steady-state C_0 within 24 h for de novo renal transplant recipients. However, in maintenance patients requiring dose adjustments a new steady state will not be achieved for several days, therefore, C_0 should be monitored 5–7 days after the dosage adjustment. For everolimus, the recommended C_0 goal is 3–8 ng/mL [29, 31]. With a significantly shorter half-life, everolimus steady state can be reached in 90–150 h.

Adverse Events: Some of the most frequently reported adverse events with sirolimus include hematologic toxicities, musculoskeletal and metabolic disturbances, particularly, hypertriglyceridemia, and gastrointestinal disorders [29, 30]. Early post-transplant complications of sirolimus, particularly the potential to prolong or increase the incidence of DGF, as well as poor wound healing, lymphocele formation, pneumonitis, and mucositis, have limited the de novo use of this agent [29, 30]. Everolimus is indicated for de novo use despite the potential to have a similar toxicity profile. Proteinuria and glomerulonephropathy have been reported with the ToR inhibitors, especially after conversion from a CNI [33–38]. Other important, yet rare, adverse events with these agents include hemolytic uremic syndrome/thrombotic microangiopathy and liver dysfunction [31].

Comparative Efficacy: Sirolimus has been studied extensively as an immunosuppressant. Early studies focused on its use as an adjunct agent in combination with CsA. Newer studies have focused on its use as a primary immunosuppressant to be used in place of CNIs.

An evaluation of the ToR inhibitors was done in a meta-analysis of 33 sirolimus and/or everolimus trials for initial maintenance immunotherapy in RTRs [39]. Four different ToR inhibitor based immunosuppressive algorithms were assessed:

- When ToR inhibitors were substituted for CNIs, there was no difference in patient survival, allograft survival and BPAR rates at up to 2 years post-transplant [39]. The ToR inhibitors were associated with significantly lower serum creatinine concentrations and improved glomerular filtration rates (GFRs). The safety analysis revealed no difference in the incidence of malignancies, but patients receiving a ToR inhibitor had significantly more myelosuppression [39].

- When ToR inhibitors were substituted for the antimetabolites, the ToR inhibitors were associated with a reduced acute rejection rate and a lower incidence of CMV infections [39]. There were no differences in patient and allograft survival. However, patients receiving sirolimus or everolimus had significantly higher serum creatinine concentrations. ToR inhibitor therapy was linked with a higher overall incidence of hypercholesterolemia and thrombocytopenia, although the prevalence of malignancies was comparable [39].
- Comparison of low-dose ToR inhibitors vs. high-dose ToR inhibitors given along with standard-dose CNI and corticosteroid therapy demonstrated a significantly higher acute rejection rate in patients treated with low-dose sirolimus or everolimus [39]. Renal function, measured by calculated GFR, was considerably worse in the high-dose ToR inhibitor groups. High-dose ToR inhibitor therapy was also associated with a higher incidence of hypercholesterolemia and myelosuppression [39].
- When comparing low-dose ToR inhibitors with standard-dose CNI therapy vs. high-dose ToR inhibitors with low-dose CNI therapy, it was shown that low-dose sirolimus or everolimus was associated with not only a significantly lower acute rejection rate, but also a lower GFR. There were no differences in the observed safety parameters between the two groups [39].

Overall, an accurate analysis of the risks and benefits of ToR inhibitor therapy is a difficult undertaking given the multitude of possible immunosuppressive combinations that these agents have been studied with. Sirolimus appears to have a potential role in patients with severe adverse events from the CNIs or malignancy, especially skin cancers, lymphoma and renal cell carcinoma. Further analysis is needed with the ToR inhibitors to delineate their exact role in renal transplantation.

Antiproliferatives

The antiproliferative agents are generally considered to be adjuvant to the CNIs. The primary agents included in this class are AZA and the MPA derivatives, although other antiproliferatives, such as cyclophosphamide and leflunomide, have been used in transplantation.

Antiproliferatives (Azathioprine)

Pharmacology: Azathioprine is a pro-drug for 6-mercaptopurine (6-MP), which is a purine analog [2, 18, 19]. 6-MP acts as an antimetabolite after its incorporation into the cellular DNA where it alters the synthesis and function of RNA with a resultant reduction in T-cell proliferation. Azathioprine also inhibits the proliferation of promyelocytes, which can, in turn, reduce the number of circulating monocytes [2, 18, 19].

Pharmaceutics and Dosing: Azathioprine was originally FDA approved in 1968 as an immunosuppressant for use in RTRs. Prior to the advent of CsA, the combination of AZA and corticosteroids was the mainstay of immunosuppressive therapy. Over the past 10–15 years, the use of AZA has declined markedly, due in large part to the success of the MPA derivatives, which are more specific inhibitors of T-cell proliferation.

Azathioprine is available in oral and intravenous (IV) dosage forms [2]. The typical oral dose of AZA for transplantation is 1–5 mg/kg once a day, depending on whether it is used as the primary immunosuppressant or in conjunction with a CNI. The bioavailability of the oral preparation is approximately 50%; therefore, the appropriate conversion of IV to oral dosing would be doubling the dose; however, some practitioners feel a 1:1 conversion is appropriate. Dose reductions due to severely impaired renal function may be necessary since 6-MP and its metabolites are renally eliminated [2].

Therapeutic Drug Monitoring: TDM is not necessary with AZA therapy.

Adverse Events: Myelosuppression is a frequent, dose-dependent and dose-limiting complication (>50% of patients) that often necessitates dose reductions [2]. Other common adverse events include hepatotoxicity (2–10%) and GI distress (10–15%). Importantly, pancreatitis and veno-occlusive disease of the liver occur in less than 1% of the patients [2].

Antiproliferatives (Mycophenolic Acid)

Pharmacology: Mycophenolate mofetil is a pro-drug that is rapidly hydrolyzed to MPA, mostly by the liver, after oral absorption [2, 18, 19, 40]. Enteric-coated MPA (EC-MPA) is absorbed in the intestine as the active moiety. MPA acts by inhibiting inosine monophosphate phosphate deydrogenase, a vital enzyme in the de novo pathway of guanosine nucleotide synthesis. Inhibition of this enzyme prevents the proliferation of most cells that are dependent upon the de novo pathway for purine synthesis, including lymphocytes. Other rapidly dividing cell lines are capable of purine synthesis via the salvage pathway, which is not affected by MPA [2, 18, 19, 40].

Pharmaceutics and Dosing: Mycophenolate mofetil was FDA approved in 1995 and EC-MPA in 2004. Mycophenolate mofetil is available in 250 and 500 mg capsules, an oral suspension (200 mg/mL; in cherry syrup) and as an injectable [2]. The recommended dose of MMF in RTRs is 2,000 mg/day in two divided doses. The bioavailability of the oral dosage forms of MMF exceeds 90%; therefore, conversion between oral and IV MMF is 1:1. The administration of food with the oral formulations of MMF has been discouraged because of a 40% reduction in the maximum concentration of MPA. However, the extent of MPA absorption is not affected by food indicating that MMF may be administered with or without food [2, 18, 19]. Generic formulations are available for MMF.

Enteric-coated MPA is available in 180 and 360 mg tablets [2]. The recommended starting dose of EC-MPA is 720 mg given twice daily, as this dose provides the equivalent equimolar MPA concentrations seen with MMF 1,000 mg twice daily [2, 40]. Converting between the two different MPA preparations has been proven to be safe and will be discussed later [40]. Administration of EC-MPA can be done without regard to food [2]. There are no generic forms of EC-MPA.

Therapeutic Drug Monitoring: MPA has a very complex pharmacokinetic profile; therefore, interpretation of therapeutic concentrations is difficult [41]. The exact role of TDM for patients receiving MPA is uncertain as there are conflicting results regarding actual improvement in efficacy and safety outcomes when using MPA TDM. MPA AUC has shown good correlation with efficacy in patients who are also receiving non-depleting protein induction therapy and CsA [41]. In one analysis, a MPA AUC of 30–60 mg·h/L was correlated with lower acute rejection rates when compared to an AUC level of <30 mg·h/L [42].

In a prospective analysis by Le Meur et al., RTRs were randomized to receive either fixed-dose MMF ($n=65$) or TDM-dosed (AUC=40 mg·h/L) MMF ($n=65$) [43]. All the patients also received basiliximab induction therapy, along with CsA-modified and corticosteroids. The prevalence of treatment failures was significantly lower in the TDM-dosed arm compared to the fixed-dose arm (29.2 vs. 47.7%; $p=0.03$). The safety analysis revealed comparable rates of adverse events between the two groups [43].

Some practitioners may consider MPA TDM to be useful in high immunologic risk patients, but there is no evidence to support this practice. Overall, the use of MPA TDM in RTRs is not routinely recommended [41].

Adverse Events: The most common side effects associated with MPA are GI adverse events (18–54%) and myelosuppression (20–40%) [2, 40, 44].

Enteric-coated MPA was developed in an attempt to improve the upper GI adverse event profile associated with MMF [40]. Both medications have been studied head-to-head in de novo and stable RTRs. Most notably, there were no significant differences in GI side effects between the two formulations [40].

Comparative Efficacy: MPA derivatives have largely replaced AZA and are widely used because they are effective in combination with other immunosuppressive agents, relatively easy to use without monitoring, and do not cause nephrotoxicity. The large multi-center studies comparing MMF to AZA show superior acute rejection rates with mycophenolate [45]. While some of those studies are not entirely consistent with current practice since they did not use contemporary immunosuppression (i.e., comparisons were made using CsA and not CsA modified or TAC), more recent data showing that MPA and AZA provide comparable rates of acute rejection have not been able to reverse the dominant role MPA derivatives has established as the antiproliterative of choice in modern transplant practice.

Costimulation Blockade: Belatacept

Pharmacology: Belatacept (LEA29Y) is a newly approved, intravenous biologic indicated for long-term maintenance immunosuppressive therapy in RTRs [46, 47]. This agent works by binding to CD80 and CD86 on APCs and blocking the CD28-mediated costimulation of T-cells, which is a critical component of the three-signal transplant model of T-cell activation [46, 47].

Pharmaceutics and Dosing: Belatacept represents a major paradigm shift in transplant immunosuppression, as this is the first FDA-approved intravenous maintenance immunosuppressant. This medication is administered in two distinct phases, the initial phase and the maintenance phase [47, 48]. In the initial phase, belatacept is administered at a dose of 10 mg/kg given on post-operative days 1 and 5, then again at the end of post-operative weeks 2, 4, 8, and 12. The maintenance phase begins at the end of week 16 following transplantation at a dose of 5 mg/kg. This dose is administered every 4 weeks (±3 days) thereafter. The manufacturer recommends that doses should be based on the patient's actual body weight at the time of transplantation and should not be modified during the course of therapy, unless there is a change in body weight of greater than 10%. The manufacturer also recommends that the final dose be evenly divisible by 12.5 in order for the dose to be prepared accurately. Every dose should be infused over 30 min [48].

Therapeutic Drug Monitoring: One of the benefits of belatacept is the absence of required TDM. In clinical trials, over the course of post-operative months 3–36 belatacept trough concentrations remained constant [47, 48]. Moreover, belatacept clearance is not affected by patient age, gender, race, renal or hepatic function or presence or absence of diabetes. These factors suggest that TDM is unnecessary [47, 48].

Adverse Events: The adverse event profile of belatacept has been shown to be similar or improved compared to CNI therapy [48–50]. However, belatacept carries a black-box warning regarding the risk of developing post-transplant lymphoproliferative disorder (PTLD), predominantly involving the central nervous system [46, 47]. In potential transplant recipients who have not been exposed to Epstein–Barr virus (EBV), the risk for PTLD is particularly high. The manufacturer recommends using belatacept only in patients who are EBV seropositive. The most common adverse events seen in clinical trials (≥20% frequency) included anemia, leukopenia diarrhea, constipation, nausea, vomiting, urinary tract infections, peripheral edema, cough, headache, and hyperkalemia [46, 47]. Infusion-related reactions have been noted to occur infrequently and, in general, infusions have been well tolerated, with only 18 infusion reactions (2%) reported in clinical trials [51–53]. Rare cases of progressive multifocal leukoencephalopathy (PML) have been reported. However, both cases of PML were in patient receiving doses that are much higher than the currently approved doses [51–53].

Comparative Efficacy: Belatacept has been studied in two phase III trials against CsA-modified, with one study in standard or living donor allografts and the second study in expanded criteria donors [48, 49]. In both the studies, the patients received basiliximab, MMF, and coriticosteroids. Acute rejection rates in the first study were higher in all belatacept groups, but in the extended criteria donor study acute rejection rates were similar across all the groups. In both the studies, belatacept-treated patients had significantly higher measured GFRs and lower rates of chronic allograft nephropathy compared to those receiving CsA. The higher GFRs were even seen in the belatacept patients who experienced acute rejection episodes. Belatacept is also associated with fewer metabolic and cardiovascular adverse events [48, 49].

The superior renal function and reduction in allograft damage in the belatacept vs. CNI-treated patients in these studies imply the potential of non-nephrotoxic immunosuppression to improve long-term outcomes. In addition, the improved cardiovascular profile may bode well for survival advantages associated with reduced complications of cardiovascular disease. However, these studies employed cyclosporine as opposed to tacrolimus which is the preferred CNI at most transplant centers, and these studies did not explore the use of rATG induction or steroid withdrawal. Moreover, in addition to the higher rates of rejection, more cases of PTLD were also seen in the belatacept arms. Long-term results and additional studies will be important to help establish the role of belatacept in kidney transplantation.

Corticosteroids

Pharmacology: Corticosteroids have various therapeutic effects. Their exact mechanism of immunosuppression is not fully understood, but it is believed that they provide an effective blockade against cytokine gene expression, as well as having several non-specific immunosuppressant effects [2, 18, 19]. Their most critical effect is blocking T-cell and APC-derived cytokine expression and inhibiting dendritic cell function. They do all this by binding to heat shock proteins, which then translocate into the nucleus and bind to glucocorticoid response elements resulting in inhibition of cytokine gene transcription. The end result is inhibition of the expression of IL-1, IL-2, IL-3, IL-6, INF-γ(gamma) and TNF-α(alpha). In a more non-specific manner, corticosteroids cause general anti-inflammatory effects that affect monocyte migration [2, 18, 19].

Pharmaceutics and Dosing: The most commonly used corticosteroids in transplantation are methylprednisolone (IV and oral) and prednisone (oral), although prednisolone and dexamethasone have also been shown to be effective immunosuppressants. There is no consensus on the optimal dose or maintenance schedule of steroids following renal transplantation. Corticosteroid doses vary according to center-specific protocols and patient characteristics. A typical taper would include a bolus of IV methylprednisolone 100–500 mg at the time of transplant, then tapered over 5–7 days to a maintenance dose of prednisone 10–20 mg/day. Further dose reductions occur over subsequent weeks and months post-transplant. Doses of 2.5–5 mg/day are commonly used for long-term maintenance therapy. Steroid avoidance and

Table 6.4 Common adverse events associated with corticosteroids [2, 18, 19]

Body system	Adverse event
Cardiovascular	Hyperlipidemia, hypertension
Central nervous system	Anxiety, insomnia, mood changes, psychosis
Dermatologic	Acne, diaphoresis, ecchymosis, hirsutism, impaired wound healing, petechiae, thin skin
Endocrine/metabolic	Cushing's syndrome, hyperglycemia, sodium and water retention
Gastrointestinal	Gastritis, increased appetite, nausea, vomiting, diarrhea, peptic ulcers
Hematologic	Leukocytosis
Neuromuscular/skeletal	Arthralgia, impaired growth, osteoporosis, skeletal muscle weakness
Ocular	Cataracts, glaucoma
Respiratory	Epistaxis

sparing protocols have been reported in the literature and will be briefly discussed later in the chapter.

Therapeutic Drug Monitoring: TDM for the corticosteroids is not employed.

Adverse Events: Corticosteroids are associated with a variety of acute and chronic toxicities. The most common adverse events have been summarized in Table 6.4. Not only do these adverse events impact patient morbidity and quality of life, but they also have financial ramifications. One analysis estimated the cost of corticosteroid-related adverse events to be $5300 (1996 US dollars) per patient per year [54]. Due to these issues, many newer transplant protocols have focused on corticosteroid sparing or avoidance.

Steroid Withdrawal Regimens: There have been two schools of thought associated with corticosteroid withdrawal (CSWD) supported in the literature: late withdrawal (steroid discontinuation greater than 3 months post-transplant) and early withdrawal (steroid discontinuation within 30 days of transplant). Selected studies from each of the withdrawal regimens will be briefly discussed below.

Late Withdrawal Data: Ahsan et al. describe a late prednisone withdrawal trial [55]. Patients were randomized to receive prednisone withdrawal (tapered over 8 weeks beginning at 3 months post-transplant) or maintenance prednisone (10 mg/day). The study was halted early due to excess rejection in the steroid withdrawal group (30.8 vs. 9.8% in the steroid arm). It was noted by the authors that the risk of rejection was higher in blacks (39.6%) than in non-blacks (16%). Despite the higher rates of rejection, the two groups had comparable rates of patient and graft survival at 12 months. Prednisone withdrawal was associated with a higher serum creatinine, lower cholesterol level and less need for antihypertensive medication use [55].

Early Withdrawal Data: Woodle et al. reported the outcomes of a randomized, double-blind, placebo-controlled trial of early CSWD (7 days post-transplant; $n=191$) vs. chronic low-dose corticosteroid therapy (CCS; $n=195$) in RTRs [56]. At 5 years, the incidence of the primary endpoint (death, graft loss or BPAR) was similar between the groups. However, individual analysis of BPAR revealed that the rates were higher in the CSWD group ($p=0.04$). Despite this, renal function in the two groups was similar at 5 years. An evaluation of the adverse event profiles revealed that early CSWD did provide an improvement in cardiovascular risk factors (i.e., triglycerides, hyperglycemia, weight gain) [56].

Steroid Avoidance Regimens: The FREEDOM trial was an open-label, multicenter study that randomized RTRs to receive no corticosteroids ($n=112$), early CSWD at post-op day 7 ($n=115$) or CCS therapy ($n=109$) with basiliximab induction therapy, CsA modified and EC-MPA [57]. At 12 months, renal function was similar among all groups. However, at this time point, the incidence of BPAR, graft loss or death was 36.0% in the corticosteroid-free group ($p=0.007$ vs. CCS), 29.6% with CSWD ($p=$ns vs. CCS) and 19.3% with CCS. Notably, steroid avoidance or withdrawal was associated with a reduction in the use of antidiabetic and lipid-lowering medication, triglycerides and weight gain vs. CCS [57].

Evaluation of the literature on steroid withdrawal and avoidance regimens shows that nearly all of the contemporary randomized trials show trends towards higher rates of rejection in patients withdrawn from corticosteroids when compared to those maintained on corticosteroid therapy. Although theoretic benefits exist with steroid withdrawal in terms of the incidence of adverse events, some practitioners believe that steroid minimization (2.5–5 mg/day) produces similar overall adverse events without the increased immunologic risks. Additional research is needed to assess steroid withdrawal and avoidance in more contemporary transplant regimens containing depleting protein induction therapy with TAC and mycophenolate maintenance therapy.

Treatment of Acute Rejection

The key to the effective management of acute rejection is an accurate and timely diagnosis and prompt administration of potent immunosuppression. Ideally, a balance must be struck between reversing the rejection episode and limiting excessive impairment of the host defenses. Currently, corticosteroids and rATG are the main components of antirejection therapy.

Corticosteroids

High-dose corticosteroids have been the mainstay of acute cellular rejection therapy since the inception of their use in transplantation. Oral corticosteroids (rejection reversal rates of 56–72%) have been successfully employed for the treatment of acute rejection, but IV methylprednisolone (rejection reversal rates of 60–76%) remains the treatment of choice [58, 59]. Pulse dose methylprednisolone therapy consists of administration of 250–1,000 mg/day for 3–4 days. One study demonstrated that the high doses were associated with a greater improvement in renal function, while the lower doses were linked to a lower prevalence of infectious complications [60].

Antithymocyte Globulins

The ATG agents have been shown to successfully reverse more than 90% of acute rejection episodes [61]. In comparison with the corticosteroids, use of the ATG preparations for treatment of acute rejection has resulted in a more rapid reversal of rejection, fewer repeat rejection episodes and better long-term graft survival [61, 62]. Gaber et al. studied rATG and eATG for the treatment of acute rejection in RTRs [63]. Patients received a 7–14-day course of either rATG (1.5 mg/kg/day; $n = 82$) or eATG (15 mg/kg/day; $n = 81$), which was initiated within a day of BPAR. The successful response rate for rATG was significantly greater than that for eATG (rATG = 87.8%; eATG = 76.3%). rATG was found to increase the duration of subsequent rejection-free graft survival for those who successfully achieved initial response ($p = 0.011$). Adverse event rates were similar in both the groups [63].

Future Immunosuppressive Agents

The immunosuppressant armamentarium is expanding with novel small molecules (i.e., AEB and the Janus-Kinase 3 inhibitors) and biological agents (i.e., IL-15 inhibitors) currently in clinical development [64]. These newer agents appear promising and may represent the emergence of novel immunosuppressive agents that can deliver immunosuppression without the long-term toxicities. Everolimus and belatacept are the closest of these agents to reaching clinical approval and the clinical data will be briefly reviewed below.

Drug–Drug Interactions

As the number of medications that a patient takes increases, so does the potential for DDIs. Disease severity, patient age and organ dysfunction are all risk factors for increased DDIs. In general, DDIs can be broken down into two categories: (1) pharmacokinetic and (2) pharmacodynamic interactions.

- Pharmacokinetic interactions result when one drug alters the absorption, distribution, metabolism or elimination of another drug.
- Pharmacodynamic interactions include additive, synergistic or antagonistic interactions that affect efficacy or toxicity.

Pharmacokinetic Interactions

Given the large number of medications consumed by RTRs, it is no surprise that this patient population is at high risk for DDIs. Pharmacokinetic DDIs pose a major dilemma with the maintenance immunosuppressants. Pharmacokinetic interactions can either result in increased concentrations of one or more agents with an increased risk for drug-induced toxicities or lowered drug concentrations, possibly leading to allograft rejection. As mentioned above, pharmacokinetic DDIs can be further categorized into interactions of absorption, distribution, metabolism and elimination.

Interactions of Absorption

Most DDIs due to altered absorption occur within the intestines. There are a variety of potential mechanisms through which the absorption of the maintenance immunosuppressants is altered, including:

- Gut metabolism ("Interactions of Metabolism" will be discussed below).
- Alteration in active transport.
- Changes in intestinal motility
- Chelation.

Active transporters play an important role in drug interactions. P-Glycoprotein (P-gp), a plasma membrane transport protein, is present in the gut, brain, liver and kidneys [67, 68]. This protein provides a biological barrier, eliminating toxic substances and xenobiotics that may accumulate in these organ systems. P-gp plays an important role in the absorption and distribution of many medications. In the GI tract, P-gp is located in the brush borders of mature enterocytes. The colon has the largest percentage of P-gp. P-gp affects the absorption of CsA, TAC and sirolimus. Some medications can alter the activity of P-gp (inhibit or induce its activity) Medications that are cytochrome P450 (CYP) 3A4 substrates, inhibitors or inducers also tend to affect P-gp; therefore, the potential exists for several DDIs with the immunosuppressants by this mechanism (see Table 6.5) [67, 68]. For example, medications that inhibit P-gp activity will increase the concentrations of CsA, TAC and sirolimus due to a reduction in P-gp-dependent drug elimination from the hepatic circulation.

When looking at the ability of drugs that change intestinal motility and their effects on the maintenance immunosuppressants, you can see notable interactions between the prokinetic agents and the CNIs. Cisapride and metoclopramide have been shown to increase the absorption of CsA and TAC by enhancing gastric mobility and emptying [69].

Most of the interactions with MMF and EC-MPA are due to reductions in intestinal absorption. Aluminum, magnesium and calcium containing products decrease the peak level of MPA [2]. If these agents are required, they must be administered at least 2 h before or 1 h after MPA. Of note, iron does not interact with the MPA preparations [70].

Table 6.5 Examples of medications with documented or potential for DDIS with CsA, TAC or sirolimus mediated through the CYP3A4 isozyme and/or P-GP [2, 68, 71]

Substrates[a]
Alfentanil, Alprazolam, Amiodarone, Amlodipine, Atorvastatin, Cilostazol, Cisapride, Chlorpromazine, Clonazepam, Cocaine, Cortisol, Cyclophosphamide, Dantrolene, Dapsone, Diazepam, Disopyramide, Dronedarone, Enalapril, Estradiol, Estrogen, Etoposide, Felodipine, Flutamide, Lidocaine, Loratadine, Lovastatin, Nevirapine, Nicardipine, Nifedipine, Omeprazole, Paclitaxel, Propafenone, Progesterone, Quetiapine, Quinidine, Sertraline, Simvastatin, Tamoxifen, Testosterone, Triazolam, Venlafaxine, Vinblastine, Warfarin, Zolpidem
Inducers[b]
Carbamazepine, Dexamethasone, Ethosuximide, Isoniazid, Nevirapine, Phenobarbital, Phenytoin, Prednisone, Rifabutin, Rifampin
Inhibitors[c]
Azithromycine, Cimetidine, Clarithromycin, Clotrimazole, Delavirdine, Diltiazem, Erythromycin, Fluconazole, Fluoxetine, Fluvoxamine, Grapefruit Juice, Indinavir, Itraconazole, Ketoconazole, Methylprednisolone, Miconazole, Nefazodone, Nelfinavir, Posaconazole, Ritonavir, Saquinavir, Troleandomycin, Verapamil, Voriconazole, Zafirlukast

[a]Substrates of the CYP3A4 isozyme and/or P-gp will compete with CsA, TAC and sirolimus for metabolism and/or drug transport; therefore, concentrations of all medications will be increased (usually by <20%)

[b]Inducers of the CYP3A4 isozyme and/or P-gp will enhance the metabolism and/or drug transport of CsA, TAC and sirolimus; therefore, concentrations of CsA, TAC and sirolimus will be decreased

[c]Inhibitors of the CYP3A4 isozyme and/or P-gp will decrease the metabolism and/or drug transport of CsA, TAC and sirolimus; therefore, concentrations of CsA, TAC and sirolimus will be increased

Interactions of Distribution

Interactions of distribution tend to occur with drugs that are highly protein bound. A drug that is extensively bound to plasma proteins can be displaced from its binding site by another agent that has greater affinity for the same binding site, thereby raising free concentrations of the displaced drug. MPA is the only highly protein bound (97% bound to albumin) maintenance immunosuppressant with a reported DDI by this mechanism. However, the adverse sequelae of this drug interaction have not been assessed and the clinical relevance may be relatively minor.

Interactions of Metabolism

Oxidative metabolism by CYP isozymes is the primary method of drug metabolism [71]. The purpose of drug metabolism is to make drugs more water soluble so they can be more easily eliminated. Cyclosporine, TAC and sirolimus are all substrates of the CYP3A isozyme system. The majority of CYP-mediated metabolism takes place in the liver; however, CYP is also expressed in the intestine, lungs, kidneys and brain. Two types of interactions usually occur with medications metabolized via the CYP enzyme system, inhibitory interactions and inducing interactions. Enzyme inhibition occurs when there is enzyme inactivation or mutual competition of substrates at a catalytic site. This usually results in a reduction of drug metabolism leading to increased concentrations of all medications involved. Enzyme induction interactions are just the opposite and occur when there is increased synthesis or decreased degradation of CYP enzymes. This type of interaction can produce decreased concentrations of medications [71]. Being CYP3A substrates, it would be anticipated that CsA, TAC and sirolimus would all experience similar pharmacokinetic DDIs. Table 6.5 details the clinically relevant DDIs that occur with the CNIs and sirolimus due to inhibition or induction of the CYP isozyme system.

Not all metabolic DDIs occur through the CYP system. Azathioprine has a considerable interaction with allopurinol that is not mediated through CYP [72, 73]. Allopurinol inhibits xanthene oxidase, which is the enzyme responsible for metabolizing 6-MP to inactive 6-thiouricate. Combining these agents can result in 6-MP accumulation and severe toxicities, particularly myelosuppression. It is recommended that concomitant therapy with AZA and allopurinol be avoided, but if necessary, AZA doses must be reduced to one-third or one-fourth of the current dose [73].

Interactions of Elimination

There are very few interactions of elimination with the maintenance immunosuppressants. However, the major interaction through this process involves MPA. MPA is metabolized to MPA-glucuronide (MPAG) via hepatic glucuronosyltransferase [2, 40]. MPAG is excreted in the bile for elimination in the gut. Deconjugation of MPAG back to MPA by intestinal flora results in a secondary absorption of MPA several hours after its administration [2, 40]. Several medications have been shown to interfere with the biliary excretion of MPAG, thereby eliminating its reabsorption in the intestines and lowering the overall exposure to MPA. Cyclosporine has been shown to reduce the overall exposure to the MPA derivatives through competitive inhibition of MPAG enterohepatic recirculation [74]. MPA levels are lower when it is administered in CsA-based immunosuppression regimens compared to TAC-based regimens. The bile acid sequestrants (i.e., cholestyramine, colestipol, colesevelam) has also been shown to decrease the overall MPA exposure through a similar mechanism [75, 76].

Pharmacodynamic Interactions

In addition to the pharmacokinetic interactions seen with the maintenance immunosuppressants, the possibility for pharmacodynamic interactions also exists. An in-depth review of pharmacodynamic interactions with maintenance immunosuppressive agents goes beyond the scope of this chapter. Pharmacodynamic interactions are common when immunosuppressive therapies that employ multiple medications with different mechanisms of action result in additive immunosuppression. Unfortunately, pharmacodynamic interactions can also be problematic, such as when medications with similar adverse events are used concomitantly. For example, nephrotoxic agents, such as amphotericin B, aminoglysides antibiotics and non-steroidal anti-inflammatory drugs may potentiate the nephrotoxic effects of the CNIs [2].

The potential exists for multiple pharmacodynamic interactions in transplant recipients due to the complexity of their medication regimens. Practitioners must be diligent in reviewing all medications for potential DDIs. In addition to reviewing prescription medications, it is essential to question the patients about the use of both nonprescription, complementary and alternative medicine, as these products also have the potential for significant interactions.

Outcome Evaluation

Successful outcomes in renal transplantation are generally measured by several endpoints. The short-term goals after renal transplantation revolve around reducing the incidence of acute rejection episodes and attaining a high graft survival rate. By accomplishing these goals, transplant clinicians hope to attain good allograft function that allows for an improved quality of life. These goals can be achieved through the appropriate use of clinical immunosuppression and scrutinizing over the therapeutic and toxic-monitoring parameters associated with each medication employed.

The long-term goals after organ transplant are to maximize the functionality of the allograft and prevent the complications of immunosuppression, which lead to improved patient survival. Clinicians must play multiple roles in the long-term care of transplant recipients; as, not only must the patient be followed from an immunologic perspective, but practitioners must also be focused on identifying and treating the adverse sequelae associated with life-long immunosuppression, including cardiovascular disease, malignancy, infection and osteoporosis, among others. The importance of limiting drug misadventures and assuring adherence with the therapeutic regimen is of the utmost importance.

References

1. Nashan B. Antibody induction therapy in renal transplant patients receiving calcineurin-inhibitor immunosuppressive regimens: a comparative review. BioDrugs. 2005;19:39–46.
2. Micromedex® Healthcare Series, (electronic version). Greenwood Village: Thomson Healthcare; 2010.
3. Ramirez CB, Marino IR. The role of basiliximab induction therapy in organ transplantation. Expert Opin Biol Ther. 2007;7:137–48.
4. Kirk AD. Induction immunosuppression. Transplantation. 2006;82:593–602.

5. Hardinger KL. Rabbit antithymocyte globulin induction therapy in adult renal transplantation. Pharmacotherapy. 2006;26:1771–83.
6. Beiras-Fernandez A, Thein E, Hammer C. Induction of immunosuppression with polyclonal antithymocyte globulins: an overview. Exp Clin Transplant. 2003;1:79–84.
7. Lopez M, Clarkson MR, Albin M, Sayegh MH, Najafian N. A novel mechanism of action for anti-thymocyte globulin: induction of CD4+ CD25+ Foxp3+ regulatory T cells. J Am Soc Nephrol. 2006;17:2844–53.
8. Goggins WC, Pascual MA, Powelson JA, et al. A prospective, randomized, clinical trial of intraoperative versus postoperative Thymoglobulin in adult cadaveric renal transplant recipients. Transplantation. 2003;76:798–802.
9. Brennan DC, Flavin K, Lowell JA, et al. A randomized, double-blinded comparison of Thymoglobulin versus Atgam for induction immunosuppressive therapy in adult renal transplant recipients. Transplantation. 1999;67:1011–8.
10. Hardinger KL, Rhee S, Buchanan P, et al. A prospective, randomized, double-blinded comparison of thymoglobulin versus Atgam for induction immunosuppressive therapy: 10-year results. Transplantation. 2008;86:947–52.
11. Brennan DC, Daller JA, Lake KD, Cibrik D, Del Castillo D. Rabbit antithymocyte globulin versus basiliximab in renal transplantation. N Engl J Med. 2006;355:1967–77.
12. Webster AC, Ruster LP, McGee R, et al. Interleukin 2 receptor antagonists for kidney transplant recipients. Cochrane Database Syst Rev. 2010;1(1):CD003897.
13. Morris PJ, Russell NK. Alemtuzumab (Campath-1H): a systematic review in organ transplantation. Transplantation. 2006;81:1361–7.
14. Ciancio G, Burke 3rd GW. Alemtuzumab (Campath-1H) in kidney transplantation. Am J Transplant. 2008;8:15–20.
15. Farney AC, Doares W, Rogers J, et al. A randomized trial of alemtuzumab versus antithymocyte globulin induction in renal and pancreas transplantation. Transplantation. 2009;88:810–9.
16. Jones JL, Phuah CL, Cox AL, et al. IL-21 drives secondary autoimmunity in patients with multiple sclerosis, following therapeutic lymphocyte depletion with alemtuzumab (Campath-1H). J Clin Invest. 2009;119:2052–61.
17. Andreoni KA, Brayman KL, Guidinger MK, Sommers CM, Sung RS. Kidney and pancreas transplantation in the United States, 1996–2005. Am J Transplant. 2007;7:1359–75.
18. Halloran PF. Immunosuppressive drugs for kidney transplantation. N Engl J Med. 2004;351:2715–29.
19. Hardinger KL, Koch MJ, Brennan DC. Current and future immunosuppressive strategies in renal transplantation. Pharmacotherapy. 2004;24:1159–76.
20. International Neoral Renal Transplantation Study Group. Cyclosporine microemulsion (Neoral) absorption profiling and sparse-sample predictors during the first 3 months after renal transplantation. Am J Transplant. 2002;2:148–56.
21. Reams BD, Palmer SM. Sublingual tacrolimus for immunosuppression in lung transplantation: a potentially important therapeutic option in cystic fibrosis. Am J Respir Med. 2002;1:91–8.
22. Reams D, Rea J, Davis D, Palmer S. Utility of sublingual tacrolimus in cystic fibrosis patients after lung transplantation. J Heart Lung Transplant. 2001;20:207–8.
23. Sukhpreet P. Therapeutic drug monitoring of immunosuppressants: An overview. Indian J Pharmacol. 2007;39:66–70.
24. Schiff J, Cole E, Cantarovich M. Therapeutic monitoring of calcineurin inhibitors for the nephrologist. Clin J Am Soc Nephrol. 2007;2:374–84.
25. Knight SR, Morris PJ. The clinical benefits of cyclosporine C2-level monitoring: a systematic review. Transplantation. 2007;83:1525–35.
26. Levy GA. C2 monitoring strategy for optimising cyclosporin immunosuppression from the Neoral formulation. BioDrugs. 2001;15:279–90.
27. Chapman JR, O'Connell PJ, Nankivell BJ. Chronic renal allograft dysfunction. J Am Soc Nephrol. 2005;16:3015–26.

28. Webster AC, Woodroffe RC, Taylor RS, Chapman JR, Craig JC. Tacrolimus versus ciclosporin as primary immunosuppression for kidney transplant recipients: meta-analysis and meta-regression of randomised trial data. BMJ. 2005;331:810.
29. Micromedex® Healthcare Series, (electronic version). In. Greenwood Village: Thomson Healthcare; 2010.
30. Morath C, Arns W, Schwenger V, et al. Sirolimus in renal transplantation. Nephrol Dial Transplant. 2007;22 Suppl 8:viii61–viii5.
31. Gabardi S, Baroletti SA. Everolimus: a proliferation signal inhibitor with clinical applications in organ transplantation, oncology, and cardiology. Pharmacotherapy. 2010;30:1044–56.
32. Franco AF, Martini D, Abensur H, Noronha IL. Proteinuria in transplant patients associated with sirolimus. Transplant Proc. 2007;39:449–52.
33. Pinheiro HS, Amaro TA, Braga AM, Bastos MG. Post-rapamycin proteinuria: incidence, evolution, and therapeutic handling at a single center. Transplant Proc. 2006;38:3476–8.
34. Rangan GK. Sirolimus-associated proteinuria and renal dysfunction. Drug Saf. 2006;29:1153–61.
35. Ruiz JC, Campistol JM, Sanchez-Fructuoso A, et al. Increase of proteinuria after conversion from calcineurin inhibitor to sirolimus-based treatment in kidney transplant patients with chronic allograft dysfunction. Nephrol Dial Transplant. 2006;21:3252–7.
36. van den Akker JM, Wetzels JF, Hoitsma AJ. Proteinuria following conversion from azathioprine to sirolimus in renal transplant recipients. Kidney Int. 2006;70:1355–7.
37. Letavernier E, Pe'raldi MN, Pariente A, Morelon E, Legendre C. Proteinuria following a switch from calcineurin inhibitors to sirolimus. Transplantation. 2005;80:1198–203.
38. Flechner SM, Goldfarb D, Modlin C, et al. Kidney transplantation without calcineurin inhibitor drugs: a prospective, randomized trial of sirolimus versus cyclosporine. Transplantation. 2002;74:1070–6.
39. Webster AC, Lee VW, Chapman JR, Craig JC. Target of rapamycin inhibitors (sirolimus and everolimus) for primary immunosuppression of kidney transplant recipients: a systematic review and meta-analysis of randomized trials. Transplantation. 2006;81:1234–48.
40. Gabardi S, Tran JL, Clarkson MR. Enteric-coated mycophenolate sodium. Ann Pharmacother. 2003;37:1685–93.
41. Shaw LM, Figurski M, Milone MC, Trofe J, Bloom RD. Therapeutic drug monitoring of mycophenolic acid. Clin J Am Soc Nephrol. 2007;2:1062–72.
42. van Gelder T, Hilbrands LB, Vanrenterghem Y, et al. A randomized double-blind, multicenter plasma concentration controlled study of the safety and efficacy of oral mycophenolate mofetil for the prevention of acute rejection after kidney transplantation. Transplantation. 1999;68:261–6.
43. Le Meur Y, Buchler M, Thierry A, et al. Individualized mycophenolate mofetil dosing based on drug exposure significantly improves patient outcomes after renal transplantation. Am J Transplant. 2007;7:2496–503.
44. Hardinger KL, Brennan DC, Lowell J, Schnitzler MA. Long-term outcome of gastrointestinal complications in renal transplant patients treated with mycophenolate mofetil. Transpl Int. 2004;17:609–16.
45. Knight SR, Russell NK, Barcena L, Morris PJ. Mycophenolate mofetil decreases acute rejection and may improve graft survival in renal transplant recipients when compared with azathioprine: a systematic review. Transplantation. 2009;87:785–94.
46. Martin ST, Tichy EM, Gabardi S. Belatacept: a novel biologic for maintenance immunosuppression after renal transplantation. Pharmacotherapy. 2011;31:394–407.
47. Nulojix [package insert]. Princeton: Bristol-Myers Squibb; 2011.
48. Vincenti F, Charpentier B, Vanrenterghem Y, et al. A phase III study of belatacept-based immunosuppression regimens versus cyclosporine in renal transplant recipients (BENEFIT study). Am J Transplant. 2010;10:535–46.
49. Durrbach A, Pestana JM, Pearson T, et al. A phase III study of belatacept versus cyclosporine in kidney transplants from extended criteria donors (BENEFIT-EXT study). Am J Transplant. 2010;10:547–57.

50. Ferguson R, Grinyo J, Vincenti F, et al. Immunosuppression with belatacept-based, corticosteroid-avoiding regimens in de novo kidney transplant recipients. Am J Transplant. 2011;11:66–76.
51. Vincenti F, Charpentier B, Vanrenterghem Y, et al. A phase III study of belatacept-based immunosuppression regimens versus cyclosporine in renal transplant recipients (BENEFIT study). Am J Transplant. 2010;10:535–46.
52. Durrbach A, Pestana JM, Pearson T, et al. A phase III study of belatacept versus cyclosporine in kidney transplants from extended criteria donors (BENEFIT-EXT study). Am J Transplant. 2010;10:547–57.
53. Vincenti F, Larsen C, Durrbach A, et al. Costimulation blockade with belatacept in renal transplantation. N Engl J Med. 2005;353:770–81.
54. Veenstra DL, Best JH, Hornberger J, Sullivan SD, Hricik DE. Incidence and long-term cost of steroid-related side effects after renal transplantation. Am J Kidney Dis. 1999;33:829–39.
55. Ahsan N, Hricik D, Matas A, et al. Prednisone withdrawal in kidney transplant recipients on cyclosporine and mycophenolate mofetil – a prospective randomized study. Steroid Withdrawal Study Group. Transplantation. 1999;68:1865–74.
56. Woodle ES, First MR, Pirsch J, Shihab F, Gaber AO, Van Veldhuisen P. A prospective, randomized, double-blind, placebo-controlled multicenter trial comparing early (7 day) corticosteroid cessation versus long-term, low-dose corticosteroid therapy. Ann Surg. 2008;248:564–77.
57. Vincenti F, Schena FP, Paraskevas S, Hauser IA, Walker RG, Grinyo J. A randomized, multicenter study of steroid avoidance, early steroid withdrawal or standard steroid therapy in kidney transplant recipients. Am J Transplant. 2008;8:307–16.
58. Mussche MM, Ringoir SM, Lameire NN. High intravenous doses of methylprednisolone for acute cadaveric renal allograft rejection. Nephron. 1976;16:287–91.
59. Gray D, Shepherd H, Daar A, Oliver DO, Morris PJ. Oral versus intravenous high-dose steroid treatment of renal allograft rejection. The big shot or not? Lancet. 1978;1:117–8.
60. Kauffman Jr HM, Stromstad SA, Sampson D, Stawicki AT. Randomized steroid therapy of human kidney transplant rejection. Transplant Proc. 1979;11:36–8.
61. Filo RS, Smith EJ, Leapman SB. Therapy of acute cadaveric renal allograft rejection with adjunctive antithymocyte globulin. Transplantation. 1980;30:445–9.
62. Shield 3rd CF, Cosimi AB, Tolkoff-Rubin N, Rubin RH, Herrin J, Russell PS. Use of antithymocyte globulin for reversal of acute allograft rejection. Transplantation. 1979;28:461–4.
63. Gaber AO, First MR, Tesi RJ, et al. Results of the double-blind, randomized, multicenter, phase III clinical trial of Thymoglobulin versus Atgam in the treatment of acute graft rejection episodes after renal transplantation. Transplantation. 1998;66:29–37.
64. Yabu JM, Vincenti F. Novel immunosuppression: small molecules and biologics. Semin Nephrol. 2007;27:479–86.
65. Vincenti F, Charpentier B, Vanrenterghem Y, et al. A phase III study of belatacept-based immunosuppression regimens versus cyclosporine in renal transplant recipients (BENEFIT study). Am J Transplant. 2010;10:535–46.
66. Durrbach A, Pestana JM, Pearson T, et al. A phase III study of belatacept versus cyclosporine in kidney transplants from extended criteria donors (BENEFIT-EXT study). Am J Transplant. 2010;10:547–57.
67. Aszalos A. P-glycoprotein-based drug-drug interactions: preclinical methods and relevance to clinical observations. Arch Pharm Res. 2004;27:127–35.
68. DuBuske LM. The role of P-glycoprotein and organic anion-transporting polypeptides in drug interactions. Drug Saf. 2005;28:789–801.
69. Prescott Jr WA, Callahan BL, Park JM. Tacrolimus toxicity associated with concomitant metoclopramide therapy. Pharmacotherapy. 2004;24:532–7.
70. Gelone DK, Park JM, Lake KD. Lack of an effect of oral iron administration on mycophenolic acid pharmacokinetics in stable renal transplant recipients. Pharmacotherapy. 2007;27:1272–8.
71. Lynch T, Price A. The effect of cytochrome P450 metabolism on drug response, interactions, and adverse effects. Am Fam Physician. 2007;76:391–6.

72. Aronson J. Serious drug interactions. Practitioner. 1993;237:789–91.
73. Baroletti S, Bencivenga GA, Gabardi S. Treating gout in kidney transplant recipients. Prog Transplant. 2004;14:143–7.
74. Gregoor PJ, de Sevaux RG, Hene RJ, et al. Effect of cyclosporine on mycophenolic acid trough levels in kidney transplant recipients. Transplantation. 1999;68:1603–6.
75. Bullingham RE, Nicholls AJ, Kamm BR. Clinical pharmacokinetics of mycophenolate mofetil. Clin Pharmacokinet. 1998;34:429–55.
76. Mignat C. Clinically significant drug interactions with new immunosuppressive agents. Drug Saf. 1997;16:267–78.

Chapter 7
Allograft Dysfunction: Diagnosis and Management

Colm C. Magee

Abstract Despite improvements in surgical techniques, histocompatability testing and immunosuppressive regimens, allograft dysfunction remains the most common complication of renal transplantation. The causes of allograft dysfunction depend on the time period after transplantation, allowing a rational diagnostic and therapeutic approach in many cases. The time periods for discussing graft dysfunction are classified into immediately, early (1–12 weeks), and late (>3 months) posttransplant. At these different time points the cause of graft dysfunction varies widely. By approaching the patient in a systematic way, the cause of graft dysfunction can be quickly diagnosed and addressed. In particular some causes of immediate graft dysfunction, such as renal vein thrombosis or hyperacute rejection, need to be diagnosed and treated within a very short time period to have any possibility of saving the allograft.

Keywords Acute rejection • Chronic allograft dysfunction • Nephrotoxicity • Delayed graft function • Donor disease

Introduction

Despite improvements in surgical techniques, histocompatability testing and immunosuppressive regimens, allograft dysfunction remains the most common complication of renal transplantation. The causes of allograft dysfunction depend on the time period after transplantation, allowing a rational diagnostic and therapeutic approach in many cases. Time periods are classified into immediately, early (1–12

C.C. Magee, MD, MPH FRCPI (✉)
Beaumont Hospital, Dublin, Ireland
e-mail: cmagee99@gmail.com

A. Chandraker et al. (eds.), *Core Concepts in Renal Transplantation*,
DOI 10.1007/978-1-4614-0008-0_7,

weeks), and late (>3–6 months) posttransplant, but there is obviously some overlap in causes between these periods.

Allograft Dysfunction in the Immediate Posttransplant Period: Delayed Graft Function and Slow Graft Function

Delayed graft function (DGF) is usually defined as failure of the renal allograft to function immediately posttransplant, with the need for at least one dialysis session within the first week. It is important to note that this is a clinical diagnosis. Using the requirement for dialysis as the sole criterion for diagnosis excludes some patients with residual native kidney function, however. Reported rates of DGF vary widely by region; in the United States overall, they are about 20% for standard-criteria deceased donor allografts [1]. Although ischemic acute tubular necrosis (ATN) is by far the most common cause of DGF, the two terms are not synonymous. There are several other causes of DGF (Table 7.1); in addition, ischemic and immunological injury may coexist. Slow graft function (SGF) is defined as a slow fall in creatinine in the first week, without the need for dialysis [2]; in general, its causes and management are similar.

Risk factors for DGF include recipient factors such as male sex, black race, longer duration on dialysis, higher panel-reactive antigen (PRA) status, and greater degree of human leukocyte antigen (HLA) mismatching; donor factors such as use of deceased donor kidneys (especially if extended criteria (ECD) or with cardiac death), greater donor age, and longer cold or warm ischemia times. Most of these factors mediate their effects via ischemia–reperfusion injury and immunologic mechanisms [3]. As Fig. 7.1 shows, the type of allograft used has a huge influence on the risk of DGF. Older studies suggested that calcineurin inhibitors (CNIs) prolonged and/or worsened DGF; this is probably less of an issue with currently employed doses. About 2% of deceased donor allografts and 1% of living donor allografts never function: these are said to have primary nonfunction [1].

Clinical, radiological, and often histological findings are used to diagnose the underlying causes of DGF. An algorithm for the management of transplant kidney

Table 7.1 Causes of DGF in renal transplantation

Prerenal
• Severe hypovolemia/hypotension
• Renal artery or vein thrombosis (rare)
• Acute cyclosporine/tacrolimus nephrotoxicity (±ATN)
Intrarenal
• Ischemic ATN
• Hyperacute rejection
• Accelerated or acute rejection superimposed on ATN
Postrenal
• Urinary tract obstruction/leakage

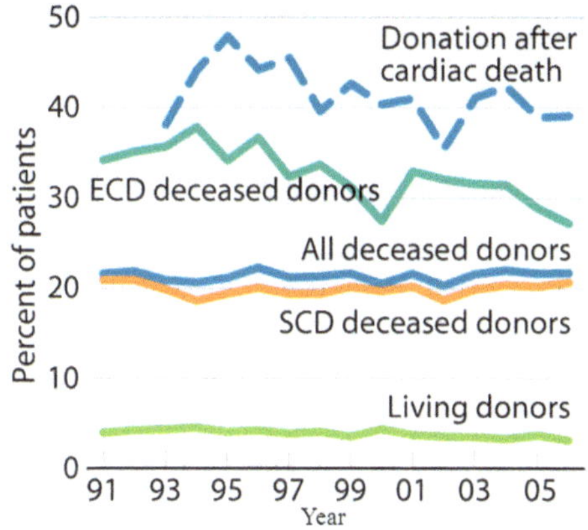

Fig. 7.1 Rates of DGF in recipients >18 years of age. *ECD* extended criteria donor; *SCD* standard criteria donor. From USRDS [1]

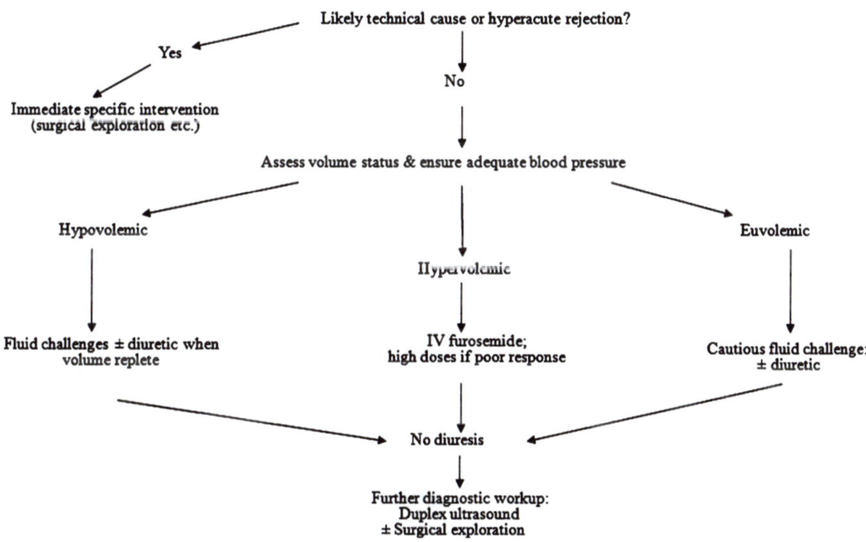

Fig. 7.2 Management of allograft nonfunction/oliguria in the immediate posttransplant period

nonfunction/oliguria immediately after surgery is shown in Fig. 7.2. The donor history and the retrieval and transplantation process must be carefully reviewed as they often provide clues to the etiology of DGF. Note that interpretation of the urine output requires knowledge of the pretransplant native kidney output. Prerenal and postrenal causes (including simple problems such as urinary catheter malposition or obstruction) must always be considered. Response to a fluid challenge implicates prerenal factors. If optimization of volume status and administration of diuretics fails to improve renal function, further investigations are required; the urgency of

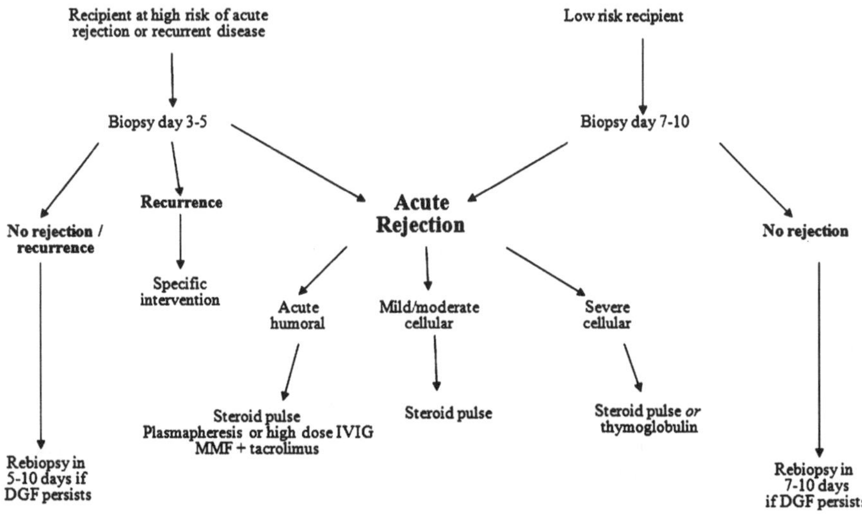

Fig. 7.3 Management of persistent DGF

which will depend on the individual case. For example, persistent oliguria of a living donor kidney despite administration of intravenous (IV) fluids and high-dose diuretics requires immediate radiological evaluation of renal blood flow (typically by ultrasound) or even immediate surgical re-exploration since the cause of impaired function is more likely to be a major surgical complication than ATN. On the other hand, an ECD allograft with prolonged ischemia times might be expected to suffer some delayed function from ischemic ATN (see below).

Ultrasound evaluation is very useful as it is inexpensive, noninvasive, and effective in excluding postrenal causes. Doppler flow studies are useful for assessing renal arterial and venous blood flow (and thus excluding thrombosis) but cannot reliably distinguish intrarenal causes based on changes in intrarenal vascular resistance. Isotope renography may provide additional information. It is sometimes used to confirm the absence of renal blood flow noted on duplex ultrasound. Occasionally, leakage or obstruction of the urinary tract are detectable by renography but not by initial ultrasonography. Although changes are seen on the radionuclide scan with intrarenal insults such as ATN or rejection, reliably distinguishing these is again not possible.

In many cases, prerenal and postrenal causes are excluded and the radiological abnormalities are consistent with an intrarenal insult. Definitive diagnosis requires allograft biopsy but biopsy is often deferred until at least 3–5 days posttransplant. The decision to biopsy will depend mainly on the duration of DGF, the likelihood of the underlying cause being ATN and the risk of rejection. An algorithm for diagnostic biopsy and treatment of persistent DGF is shown in Fig. 7.3. Specific treatment of DGF will obviously depend on the underlying cause (see below).

Table 7.2 Causes of ischemic damage to the deceased donor kidney

1. Preretrieval donor state • Shock syndromes • Endogenous and exogenous catecholamines • Brain injury • Nephrotoxic drugs
2. Organ retrieval surgery • Hypotension • Trauma to renal vessels
3. Organ transport and storage • Prolonged storage (cold ischemia time) • Pulsatile perfusion injury
4. Transplantation of recipient • Prolonged second warm ischemia time • Trauma to renal vessels • Hypovolemia/hypotension
5. Postoperative period • Acute heart failure (MI etc.) • Hemodialysis

Ischemic Acute Tubular Necrosis

Ischemic ATN is the most common cause of DGF in deceased donor kidney transplant recipients. As noted above, ATN is unusual in living donor allografts. The etiology of ATN in transplanted kidneys is presumed to be similar to that in native kidneys. At multiple steps during the surgical transplantation procedure, the deceased donor kidney is at risk of ischemic damage (Table 7.2). Reperfusion injury via direct endothelial trauma, oxygen-free radical damage, and leukocyte activation may also be important [3]. Spontaneous resolution of ATN usually occurs from 5 to 10 days posttransplant but ATN may persist for weeks. As is the case with acute renal failure in native kidneys, transplant ATN should be a diagnosis of exclusion. Several of the risk factors identified in Table 7.2 may be present. Radiologic studies confirm intact allograft perfusion and are consistent with an intrarenal insult (a high resistive index by ultrasound or slow clearance of radiotracer by renography). Histology, if available, shows tubular cell damage and necrosis.

Treatment is essentially supportive: avoidance of fluid overload, control of electrolyte abnormalities, and dialysis as needed. Minimum anticoagulation protocols should be used during hemodialysis. Care should be taken to avoid intradialytic hypotension which could worsen allograft damage. Peritoneal dialysis is probably best avoided in the first week posttransplant because of the risk of peritonitis or leakage of dialysis fluid into the wound area.

A major concern is that new surgical or medical complications involving the allograft are not easily detectable in the setting of ATN. Radiological evaluation of the allograft should be repeated regularly to detect new urinary or vascular complications.

In most centers, core kidney biopsies are repeated in patients with prolonged ATN (Fig. 7.3). The frequency with which they are repeated will depend on the clinical suspicion for superimposed insults such as rejection.

In the case of DGF secondary to ischemic ATN, an initial induction immunosuppression regimen incorporating antilymphocyte antibodies and low-dose CNI is often used. This has the presumed benefit of minimizing early CNI nephrotoxicity while reducing the risk of occult rejection.

Hyperacute Rejection

Besides ABO blood group incompatibility, hyperacute rejection is caused by preformed recipient anti-HLA class I antibodies cross-reacting with antigens on the endothelial surface of the allograft and hence activating the complement and coagulation cascades. These alloantibodies are formed in response to previous transplantation, blood transfusion, or pregnancy. Within minutes to hours after creating the vascular anastomosis there is cyanosis and mottling of the kidney, anuria, and sometimes disseminated intravascular coagulopathy. Radiological studies confirm absent or minimal renal perfusion, in contrast to ATN where blood supply is relatively well maintained. Histology shows widespread small vessel endothelial damage and thrombosis, usually with neutrophil polymorphs incorporated into the thrombus. There is no effective treatment and transplant nephrectomy is indicated. Fortunately, hyperacute rejection is now very rare because of very careful screening of the donor for antibodies against donor ABO and donor class I HLA antigens (the presence of the latter is often referred to as positive T-cell cross-match). Rare cases still occur because of clerical errors or due to the presence of other preformed antibodies which are not detected by routine screening methods.

Accelerated Rejection Superimposed on Acute Tubular Necrosis

Accelerated acute rejection refers to rejection episodes occurring between days 2 and 5 posttransplant. Pretransplant sensitization of the recipient to donor alloantigens is thought to be an important cause. Accelerated acute rejection may be superimposed on ischemic ATN in which case there may be no signs of rejection or it may occur in an initially functioning allograft. Patients with presumed ischemic ATN who are at high risk (e.g., very highly sensitized to HLA) of developing this form of rejection should undergo biopsy 3–5 days after transplantation. Diagnosis is made by renal biopsy and analysis of the serum for donor-specific antibody (DSA). Histology usually shows evidence of predominantly antibody rather than T-cell-mediated immune damage. The diagnosis and management of these two forms of rejection are discussed in detail below.

Acute Calcineurin Inhibitor Nephrotoxicity Superimposed on ATN

Both CNIs (tacrolimus and cyclosporine) cause a dose-dependent and reversible acute decrease in glomerular filtration rate (GFR) by renal vasoconstriction, particularly of the afferent glomerular arteriole. This might exacerbate ATN, particularly if doses and blood concentrations are high. This is discussed in more detail below.

Vascular and Urological Complications of Surgery

Renal vessel thrombosis, urinary leaks, and obstruction are rarer but important causes of DGF. These complications may also cause allograft dysfunction in the early postoperative period and are discussed briefly below.

Significance of Delayed and Slow Graft Function

Patients with DGF and SGF have longer hospitalization, more interventional studies and are at higher risk of occult rejection or other undiagnosed insults to the graft. Although the majority of patients become independent of dialysis, most studies have demonstrated that recipients with DGF have poorer long-term outcomes compared to those without immediate function [2, 3]. Those with SGF tend to have intermediate outcomes [2]. Measures to limit the incidence and duration of DGF and SGF are therefore very worthwhile. Strategies include optimization of donor status and maintenance of adequate volume status and blood pressure in the recipient. Meticulous surgical technique, rapid transport of retrieved allografts, and use of optimum preservation solutions are obviously very important [3]. There is accumulating evidence that machine perfusion of retrieved kidneys is more effective than simple cold storage in preventing DGF; in the best performed, prospective study to date, machine perfusion benefited recipients of all forms of deceased donor allografts [4]. As discussed above, induction antibodies are often prescribed, to allow "safe" use of low-dose CNIs initially, thus reducing the potential for CNI nephrotoxicity. Overall, there is no convincing evidence that administration of calcium channel blockers or dopamine to the recipient is of benefit. The role of anti-inflammatory and antioxidant drugs remains experimental [3].

Allograft Dysfunction in the Early Posttransplant Period

Table 7.3 shows the causes of allograft dysfunction during the early (1–12 weeks) posttransplant period. There is obviously some overlap between the causes of delayed and early allograft dysfunction. Despite its known limitations, the primary

Table 7.3 Causes of allograft dysfunction in the early postoperative period

Prerenal
• Hypovolemia/hypotension
• Renal vessel thrombosis
• CNIs
• Transplant renal artery stenosis (rare)
Intrarenal
• Acute rejection
• Acute CNI nephrotoxicity
• Toxic/ischemic ATN
• Recurrence of primary disease
• Acute pyelonephritis
• Acute allergic interstitial nephritis
• Acute thrombotic microangiopathy
Postrenal
• Urinary tract obstruction/leakage

Note: BK-nephritis is an important cause of allograft dysfunction but tends to occur later

measure of early and late transplant function remains the plasma creatinine; thus allograft dysfunction is typically defined as a persistent increase in plasma creatinine. Again, prerenal and postrenal failure should always be excluded. An algorithm for the management of dysfunction during this period is shown in Fig. 7.4.

Prerenal Dysfunction

Hypovolemia may occur due to bleeding (usually from the transplant site) or excess diuresis or diarrhea. Angiotensin-converting enzyme (ACE) inhibitors and nonsteroidal anti-inflammatory drugs (NSAIDs) should generally be avoided in the early posttransplant period because of the risk of functional prerenal failure; this risk may be enhanced by the renal vasoconstrictive effects of CNIs.

Renal Vessel Thrombosis

Renal artery or renal vein thrombosis usually occurs in the first 72 h but may be delayed for up to 10 weeks posttransplant. Risk factors for this condition are shown in Table 7.4. Acute vascular thrombosis is the most common cause of allograft loss in the first posttransplant week. Renal artery thrombosis presents with abrupt onset of anuria (unless there is a native urine output), rapidly rising plasma creatinine but often little localized allograft pain or discomfort. Doppler ultrasound shows absent arterial and venous blood flow. Isotope renography shows absent perfusion and absent visualization of the transplanted kidney. Removal of the infarcted kidney is indicated.

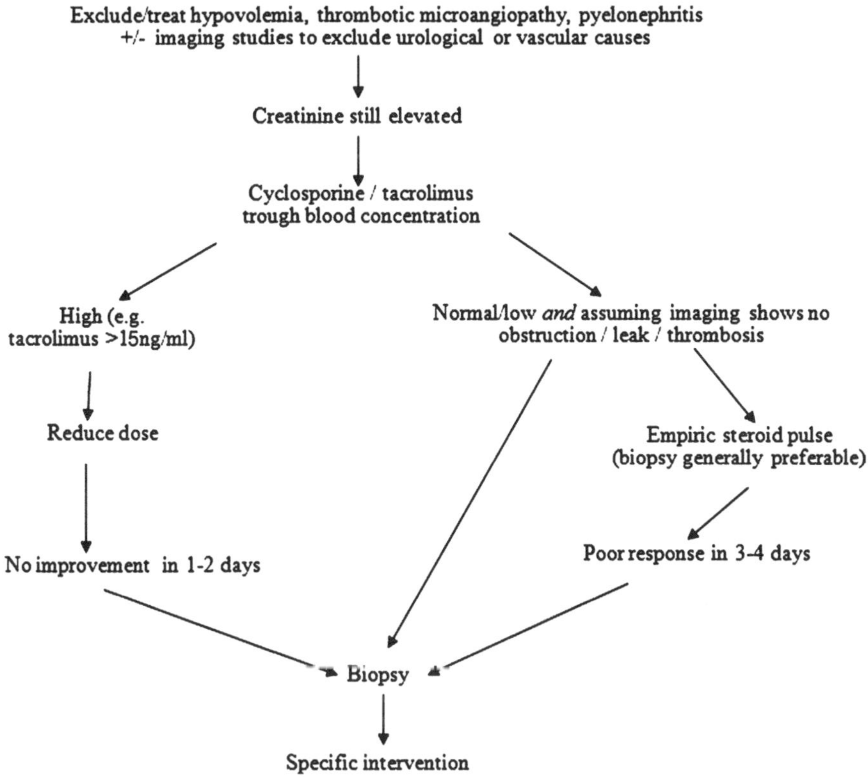

Fig. 7.4 Management of allograft dysfunction in the early posttransplant period. Again, the threshold for biopsy will be lower in the high risk patient

Table 7.4 Risk factors for renal vessel thrombosis

Risk factor	Comment
Pediatric donor	Especially if <6 years; reflects technical difficulties
Pediatric recipient	Especially if <6 years; reflects technical difficulties
History of thromboembolism or multiple unexplained access thromboses	Should always be sought in the pretransplant evaluation
Antiphospholipid antibody syndrome and other thrombophilic states	The presence of antiphospholipid antibodies or laboratory abnormalities alone does not necessarily increase risk

Renal vein thrombosis also presents with anuria and rapidly increasing creatinine. Pain, tenderness, and swelling in the allograft and hematuria are usually more pronounced than in renal artery thrombosis. Severe complications such as embolization or allograft rupture/hemorrhage may occasionally occur. Doppler studies show absent renal venous blood flow and characteristic highly abnormal renal arterial signals.

Table 7.5 Differences between pure forms (there can be overlap) of acute T-cell-mediated rejection and acute antibody-mediated rejection (AMR)

	T-cell-mediated rejection	Acute AMR
Typical clinical onset (days)	≥5	≥3
Donor-specific antibody in serum	Usually absent	Usually detectable
Tubulitis	Present	Absent
Neutrophil polymorphs in glomerular and peritubular capillaries	Absent	Present
C4d staining of peritubular capillaries	Absent	Present
Primary therapy	Pulse steroids	Pulse steroids; plasmapheresis or IVIg

Again, transplant nephrectomy is indicated. If the venous thrombosis extends beyond the renal vein, anticoagulation is necessary to reduce the risk of embolization. There are case reports of salvaging renal function after early diagnosis of renal vessel thrombosis and intervention with thrombolysis or thrombectomy. In almost all cases however, infarction occurs too quickly to make this treatment worthwhile. Thrombolysis is a high-risk strategy soon after transplantation because of the high risk of allograft-related bleeding.

Meticulous surgical technique and avoidance of recipient hypovolemia will minimize the incidence of this devastating complication.

Intrarenal Dysfunction

Acute Rejection

Acute rejection is defined as an acute deterioration in renal allograft function associated with specific pathological changes in the graft. The reported incidence of acute rejection has fallen over the last 30 years; with the newer immunosuppressive regimens incorporating mycophenolate mofetil (MMF), tacrolimus, steroids (and induction antibody), rates of rejection have fallen below 20% in the first year [5, 6]. Acute rejection is presumed to be due to both cellular and antibody-mediated immune responses but traditionally, evidence of T-cell-mediated responses have predominated on biopsies. However, in centers performing transplants in immunologically high-risk recipients, acute antibody-mediated rejection (AMR) is common. Differences between acute T-cell-mediated rejection (TCMR) and acute AMR are summarized in Table 7.5.

In addition to an increasing plasma creatinine, clinical signs may include allograft pain/tenderness and oliguria. Fever and severe allograft pain are very rare however, unless the rejection is very severe (these symptoms are more suggestive of a urine leak or pyelonephritis). Renal imaging is usually abnormal in acute rejection but the changes are not specific enough to exclude other causes. Definitive diagnosis requires biopsy but where there is a high likelihood of uncomplicated acute rejection, empirical treatment is often instituted before the biopsy.

Table 7.6 Updated BANFF 2007 classification of renal allograft pathology [7]

1. Normal
2. Antibody-mediated damage (acute or chronic active)
3. Borderline changes ("suspicious" for acute rejection). Foci of mild tubulitis only
4. T-cell-mediated rejection (acute or chronic active)
5. Interstitial fibrosis and tubular atrophy
6. Other (changes not considered to be due to rejection)

Note: a given biopsy may show features of >1 category

The BANFF classification (Table 7.6) is a widely used schema for grading histological signs of renal allograft rejection [7]. The classical histological findings in acute TCMR are: (i) edema and mononuclear cell infiltration of the interstitium, mainly with CD4+ and CD8+ T lymphocytes but also with some macrophages and plasma cells, and (ii) tubulitis (infiltration of tubular epithelium by lymphocytes). More severe acute TCMR is characterized by endothelialitis. Here, mononuclear cells undermine endothelium and the endothelial cells are swollen and detached. Endothelialitis is frequently a focal process and may therefore be easily missed on biopsy. It is important to note that focal infiltrates of mononuclear cells without endothelialitis or tubulitis may occur in the presence of stable allograft function.

Uncomplicated acute TCMR is usually treated with a short course of high-dose steroids – so-called "pulse" treatment. Typically 500–1,000 mg/day of methylprednisolone are given IV for 3–5 days. There is an approximate 70% response rate to this regimen. The main complication of such high-dose steroid therapy is an increased risk of infection. Doses of MMF and the CNI should be increased if they were low. Thymoglobulin or OKT3 are highly effective in treating first rejection episodes, reversing them in approximately 90% of cases. Because of cost and toxicity, these agents are usually reserved for steroid-resistant cases or where there is severe cellular rejection on the initial biopsy.

Steroid-resistant TCMR, defined somewhat arbitrarily as failure of improvement in urine output or plasma creatinine within 5 days of starting pulse treatment, is usually treated with thymoglobulin. If steroid treatment was based on an empirical rather than histological diagnosis of acute TCMR, a biopsy is strongly recommended before anti-T-cell antibody treatment to confirm this diagnosis. The response rate in these situations is fairly high. The most important adverse effects of thymoglobulin/OKT3 therapy are the increased risk of life-threatening infections and lymphoproliferative disease; therefore, the risks and benefits of such therapies should be carefully considered for each patient.

Acute Antibody-Mediated Rejection

Acute AMR is increasingly recognized as a cause of allograft dysfunction. This probably reflects: better diagnostic tools (in particular the C4d stain and for detecting DSAs), more awareness of acute AMR, better prevention of TCMR, and more transplantation across HLA or ABO incompatibilities. Diagnosis of acute AMR requires allograft dysfunction and at least two of the following: (i) neutrophil polymorphs or mononuclear cells or thrombi in peritubular or glomerular capillaries, (ii) diffuse positive staining of peritubular capillaries for C4d, (iii) serological evidence of antibody against donor HLA or ABO antigens [7]. Acute AMR typically occurs early after transplantation but can also occur late, especially in the setting of reduced immunosuppression or noncompliance. Acute AMR may occur alone or with acute TCMR.

Until recently, the prognosis of acute AMR was considered poor. Now, good short–medium term outcomes have been reported with protocols that typically include the following: pulse steroids, tacrolimus, MMF, plasmapheresis, or high-dose IV Ig. Rituximab is sometimes used as an adjunct in severe cases although randomized controlled trials are lacking.

Significance of Acute Rejection

Although acute rejection is frequently reversed (at least as assessed by plasma creatinine), retrospective studies show that it remains a major predictor of the development of chronic allograft dysfunction and poorer allograft survival. Poorer outcome has also correlated with the severity of rejection, the number of rejection episodes, and with resistance to steroid therapy. Whatever the outcome, treatment involves exposing the patient to additional and potentially life-threatening immunosuppression. Reducing the risk of acute rejection has been a major goal in transplantation. Unfortunately, although rates of acute rejection have fallen substantially, a concomitant increase in long-term allograft survival has been difficult to demonstrate [6].

Acute Calcineurin Inhibitor Nephrotoxicity

The CNIs, especially in high doses, causes an acute reversible decrease in GFR by renal vasoconstriction, particularly of the afferent glomerular arteriole. This is manifested clinically as dose-dependent and blood level-dependent acute reversible increases in plasma creatinine. As acute CNI nephrotoxicity is mainly vasomotor/prerenal, the histological changes in this setting may be unimpressive. With high blood levels, direct tubular damage and dysfunction may occur; biopsy may show vacuolization of tubular cells.

Distinguishing Acute Calcineurin Inhibitor Nephrotoxicity and Acute Rejection

Unfortunately, even with the aid of blood drug levels, distinguishing acute CNI nephrotoxicity and acute rejection clinically can be difficult. Low and high CNI blood levels in the presence of deteriorating renal function suggest but do not imply rejection and drug nephrotoxicity, respectively. Both syndromes may coexist. Pointers toward a diagnosis of acute CNI nephrotoxicity are signs of extrarenal toxicity such as severe tremor, a "moderate" increase in plasma creatinine (<50% over baseline) and high CNI whole blood levels (e.g., >15 ng/mL for tacrolmus). Pointers toward a diagnosis of acute rejection are fever, allograft pain, and swelling; rapid, nonplateauing increases in plasma creatinine and low CNI levels. Oliguria occurs in severe acute rejection but is rarely a predominant feature of CNI toxicity. Fever and symptoms localized to the allograft do not occur in CNI toxicity but by no means imply rejection: infections such as acute pyelonephritis must be considered. Acute CNI-induced allograft dysfunction is reversible even if it persists for several days but delaying appropriate treatment of acute rejection may compromise both short- and long-term allograft outcomes.

The threshold for biopsy to more firmly establish the diagnosis varies between centers. An algorithm for approaching this common clinical problem is shown in Fig. 7.4. One common strategy is to institute a "trial of therapy" and, if the clinical response to this is unsatisfactory, to proceed to biopsy within 48–96 h. For example, if acute CNI nephrotoxicity was suspected, the CNI dose would be reduced which should lead to rapid improvement in renal function, if this diagnosis was correct. A presumptive diagnosis of acute rejection would mean empirical treatment with a steroid pulse. Lack of response after several days of antirejection treatment because of resistant rejection, CNI nephrotoxicity, or another cause would be diagnosed by biopsy. The threshold for biopsy is lower in "high-risk" patients: those who are highly sensitized, have previously rejected an allograft or are at high risk of severe early recurrent primary renal disease (see below). Biopsy results alone should not dictate management; rather the constellation of clinical and histological findings should be used to shape a treatment plan.

It has been suggested that measuring the serum or urine levels of cytokines, adhesion molecules, or other inflammatory markers might be useful in diagnosing acute allograft rejection. A sufficiently sensitive and specific serum or urinary marker might obviate the need for biopsy or aid the follow-up of treated rejection. These markers have yet to be validated in large-scale multicenter human studies, however. Core kidney biopsy with appropriate histology remains the gold standard for diagnosing intrarenal causes of allograft dysfunction.

Acute Pyelonephritis

Urinary tract infections (UTIs) may occur at any time period but are most frequent shortly after transplantation because of catheterization, stenting, and aggressive immunosuppression. Other risk factors are anatomical urological abnormalities and neurogenic bladder. Fortunately, severe acute pyelonephritis is now much less common since the widespread use of prophylactic trimethoprim-sulfamethoxazole (TMP-SMX). Fever, allograft pain and tenderness, and raised peripheral blood white cell count are usually more pronounced in acute pyelonephritis than in acute rejection. Diagnosis requires urine culture and/or biopsy but empiric antimicrobial therapy is started immediately. Recurrent cases of pyelonephritis require investigation to rule out underlying urologic abnormalities.

Acute Allergic Interstitial Nephritis

Distinguishing acute allergic interstitial nephritis (AIN) and acute rejection is difficult. Histological findings are similar and eosinophilic infiltration of the transplanted kidney may occur with either condition. Extrarenal manifestations such as rash and eosinophilia suggest AIN but, in practice, these are rare. Both conditions usually respond to steroids. Drugs suspected to cause the AIN should be permanently stopped.

Acute Thrombotic Microangiopathy

Acute thrombotic microangiopathy (TMA) after renal transplantation is a rare but serious complication [8]. Causes include CNIs, OKT3, acute AMR (additional pathological findings are present, however), viral infections such as cytomegalovirus (CMV) and recurrence of primary disease (see below). The presence of hepatitis C and anticardiolipin antibodies may increase the risk [9]. Onset is usually in the early posttransplant period. The classic laboratory findings are increasing plasma creatinine and lactate dehydrogenase, thrombocytopenia, falling hemoglobin, schistocytosis and low haptoglobin. The hematologic features of TMA may be easily missed, however. For example, drugs such as thymoglobulin or MMF can depress platelet and red blood cell counts, although by different mechanisms. Allograft biopsy shows damaged endothelium and, in severe cases, thrombosis of glomerular capillaries and arterioles.

In severe cases, the long-term prognosis for the allograft is usually poor. There are no controlled trials of therapy for TMA posttransplant. Suggested measures are cessation of CNIs and other implicated drugs and control of any hypertension present. The benefit of plasma exchange is unclear.

Early Recurrence of Primary Disease

Several renal diseases may recur early and cause acute allograft dysfunction (diseases that recur later are discussed below). These are summarized in Table 7.7. Primary focal segmental glomerulosclerosis (FSGS) is reviewed in more detail here because of its propensity to cause severe allograft injury.

Primary Focal Segmental Glomerulosclerosis

Primary FSGS has a reported recurrence rate of about 30% and causes allograft loss in a high percentage of such cases (familial FSGS rarely recurs) [10]. Risk factors for recurrence include white recipient, younger recipient, rapidly progressive FSGS in the recipient's native kidneys, and recurrence of disease in a previous allograft.

Table 7.7 Diseases that may recur in the renal allograft

Condition	Risk of recurrence	Comments
Early recurring		
Primary FSGS	High especially if recurred in previous allograft	Recurrence can rapidly lead to nephrotic syndrome and allograft loss
Anti-GBM disease	Low if persistently anti-GBM negative for at least 6 months before transplant	Follow urine dipstick after transplant
Alport syndrome	This does not recur but see comments	Recipients may form anti-GBM antibodies and develop an associated glomerulonephritis
HUS/TTP – diarrhea-associated	Low	Defer transplantation until the disease is quiescent for at least 6 months
HUS/TTP – nondiarrhea-associated	High	Defining abnormalities of the complement system is useful as the risk of severe recurrence can be quantified
Primary hyperoxaluria	High	Combined liver-kidney transplantation prevents recurrence
Late recurring		
IgA glomerulonephritis	High over the long term	Clinical severity of recurrence varies but is often mild. Role of extra immunosuppression unclear; control of BP and proteinuria is probably best therapy
Type I MPGN (idiopathic)	Fairly high	Exclude secondary causes such as HCV infection and transplant glomerulopathy. Role of extra immunosuppression unclear; control of BP and proteinuria is probably best therapy
Type II MPGN (idiopathic)	Fairly high	Role of extra immunosuppression unclear; control of BP and proteinuria is probably best therapy
Lupus nephritis	Low if SLE is clinically quiescent for at least 12 months before transplant	If the patient is anticoagulated for antiphospholipid antibody syndrome, resume anticoagulation after transplant
ANCA-associated vasculitis	Fairly low if the vasculitis is clinically quiescent for at least 6–12 months before transplant	Renal and extrarenal recurrence is possible. ANCA titer at time of transplant does not predict relapse
Membranous nephropathy (idiopathic)	Fairly high	De novo membranous nephropathy can also occur but tends to have a more slowly progressive course. Role of extra immunosuppression unclear; control of BP and proteinuria is probably best therapy
Diabetic nephropathy	Not well studied but probably high over the medium–long term	New onset diabetes mellitus may also affect the allograft

Top panel shows diseases that tend to recur early; *bottom panel* those that tend to recur later

Most cases become manifest (as proteinuria) hours to weeks after transplant. This rapidity of recurrence suggests the presence of a pathogenic circulating plasma factor. Patients with FSGS should be monitored after transplantation for new-onset proteinuria. Early biopsy is indicated in those who develop proteinuria; this may not show FSGS lesions per se, but electron microscopy will demonstrate diffuse effacement of foot processes. Treatment options include plasmapheresis or immunoadsorption, high-dose CNIs, ACE-inhibitors, high-dose glucocorticoids and rituximab, but controlled studies are lacking. Those at high risk of recurrence should probably be offered deceased rather than living donor kidneys.

Hemolytic-Uremic Syndrome/Thrombotic Thrombocytopenia Purpura

The causes of TMA after renal transplant have been discussed above. Recurrence of atypical (nondiarrhea-associated) hemolytic-uremic syndrome/thrombotic thrombocytopenia purpura (HUS/TTP), particularly if inherited, is common [8]. Certain genetic disorders of complement regulation (such as Factor H or Factor I disorders) are associated with high risks of severe recurrence so it is very useful to define these – if possible – before proceeding with transplant (if at all). Some have advocated the fairly radical procedure of combined liver-kidney transplantation in this setting [11]. In general, the prognosis for the allograft is poor if there is recurrence.

Postrenal Dysfunction

The incidence of serious urological complications and associated morbidity in transplant recipients has decreased significantly over the last 20 years. Allograft loss from urological complications is now rare. Most urological complications are secondary to technical factors at the time of transplant and manifest themselves in the early postoperative period but immunological factors may play a role in some cases.

Urine Leaks

Urine leaks usually occur in the first few weeks after transplantation. It is important to note that the clinical features may mimic those of acute rejection – treatment is radically different, however. Treatment usually involves surgical exploration and repair. Selected patients may do well with endourologic treatment. Whenever urine leakage is suspected, a bladder catheter should be immediately inserted to decompress the urinary tract. The type of repair will depend on the level of the leak and the tissue viability.

Urinary Tract Obstruction

Urinary tract obstruction can cause allograft dysfunction at any time period after transplantation but is most common in the early postoperative period. The main intrinsic causes are poor implantation of the ureter into the bladder, intraluminal blood clots or slough material, and fibrosis of the ureter due to ischemia or rejection. The main extrinsic cause is an enlarged prostate in elderly men (causing bladder outlet obstruction); less common is compression by a lymphocele or other fluid collection. Rarely, calculi cause transplant urinary tract obstruction.

Typical clinical features are rising plasma creatinine without localizing symptoms (unless there is prostate-related obstruction). In severe cases, high pressure within the urinary tract may result in rupture and leakage (see above). Ultrasound usually demonstrates hydronephrosis. Because some dilation of the transplant urinary collecting system is often seen in the early postoperative period, serial scans showing worsening hydronephrosis may be needed to confirm the diagnosis. Isotope renograpy with diuretic washout is useful in equivocal cases. Percutaneous antegrade pyelography is the best radiologic technique for determining the site of obstruction and can be combined with interventional endourologic techniques. In expert hands, endourologic techniques (e.g., balloon dilation, stenting) may be effective in treating ureteric stenosis and stricture. More complicated cases require open surgical repair. Extrinsic compression requires specific intervention such as draining of the lymphocele. Obstruction in the early postoperative period due to an enlarged prostate should be managed with bladder catheter drainage and drugs such as tamsulosin. Prostate surgery may be required later.

Acute Allograft Dysfunction in the Late Posttransplant Period

The causes and evaluation of late (>3–6 months posttransplant) acute allograft dysfunction are broadly similar to those of early acute dysfunction. Acute prerenal failure may occur at any time, and the causes are similar to those seen with native kidneys, such as shock syndromes and ACE-I or NSAID hemodynamic effects. Urinary tract obstruction must also be considered in the differential diagnosis. At this point, the causes of obstruction are similar to those associated with native kidney disease, including stones, bladder outlet obstruction, and neoplasia. Ureteric obstruction due to BK virus infection has also been described. Several causes of late acute allograft dysfunction are reviewed in more detail below.

Late Acute Rejection

With standard immunosuppressive protocols, acute rejection is uncommon after the first 6 months. Late acute rejection should alert the physician to prescription of inadequate immunosuppression or patient noncompliance [12]. Transplant physicians

Table 7.8 Commonly used drugs which may induce acute renal failure in renal transplant recipients

Drug	Pathophysiology	Comment
NSAIDs	Functional prerenal failure; rarely interstitial nephritis	Avoid where possible
Acyclovir (high dose), foscarnet (high dose)	Crystal deposition in tubules causing obstruction and damage; also ATN	Hydration prevents crystal deposition
ACE-I, ARB	Functional prerenal failure – particularly if hypovolemia or renal artery stenosis present	Monitor renal function carefully after starting these drugs; avoid in early posttransplant period
SMX-TMP	High dose TMP impairs tubular secretion of creatinine (no effect on GFR); rarely interstitial nephritis	In general, drug is well tolerated in transplant recipients
Amphotericin	Proximal and distal tubular damage; cumulative dose effect	Lysosomal preparation is less nephrotoxic but expensive
Interferon-alpha	Immune stimulating effects promote acute rejection; other nephrotoxic effects reported	Risk/benefit of using interferon-alpha must be determined for individual patient
Erythromycin, verapamil, diltiazem, ketoconazole, voriconazole	Inhibit metabolism of CNIs	Monitor CNI concentrations carefully
Statins	Concentrations increased with concomitant cyclosporine therapy, increasing risk of rhabdomyolysis	Use lowest dose initially; monitor plasma creatine kinase

should be alert to the possibilities of poor compliance in all their patients. Cessation of steroids or CNIs by the physician – while sometimes appropriate – can lead to late acute rejection, therefore plasma creatinine must be carefully monitored when these drugs are stopped. Late acute rejection usually has a large cellular component but there may be superimposed acute AMR (C4d staining and testing for donor reactive antibodies should be routinely performed).

In general, treatment is the same as for early acute rejection (whether TCMR or acute AMR or both), as discussed above. Unfortunately, complete reversibility is difficult and registry data show that late acute rejection has a more negative impact on allograft survival than early acute rejection or DGF.

Late Acute CNI Nephrotoxicity

Although lower doses of CNIs are generally prescribed after the first 6–12 months, acute CNI toxicity may occur at any time after transplant. Intake of medications that impair metabolism of the CNIs (see Table 7.8) may induce acute deterioration in renal function, but this should be reversible with appropriate drug adjustment.

Transplant Renal Artery Stenosis

Transplant renal artery stenosis can arise at any time after transplantation. The reported incidence varies widely [13]. Luminal narrowing >70% is probably required to render a stenosis functionally significant. The stenosis may occur in the donor or recipient artery or at the anastomotic site. Stenosis of the recipient iliac artery may also compromise renal arterial flow. Causes include operative trauma to these vessels, atherosclerosis of the recipient vessels, and possibly immunologic factors. Features suggestive of functionally significant stenoses include resistant hypertension, fluctuating plasma creatinine especially with hypovolemia or ACE inhibition, peripheral vascular disease, and new bruits over the allograft [13].

The gold standard for diagnosis is renal angiography but this is invasive. Both MR angiography and duplex sonography are used as screening tests but the latter is very operator-dependent [13]. MR angiography has the advantage of better imaging the iliac arteries and identifying anatomy before angioplasty; its major disadvantage is that use of gadolinium is contraindicated in patients with GFR <30 mL/min (and caution is advised in those with GFR <60 mL/min).

"Mild" cases are often treated conservatively with antihypertensives, aspirin, etc. Percutaneous transluminal angioplasty (PTA) has been the treatment of choice for more severe cases. In most series, PTA was technically successful with few major complications. Early reports suggest stenting reduces recurrence. Surgical repair is reserved for severe cases, not amenable to PTA/stenting. Measures to minimize contrast nephropathy are discussed below.

BK Virus Infection

Over the last 10 years, BK virus has been increasingly recognized as an important cause of renal allograft dysfunction and loss [14]. This probably reflects more recognition and reporting of the disease, but more importantly the effects of more powerful maintenance immunosuppression, especially MMF and tacrolimus. Acute and chronic allograft dysfunction due to BK virus infection can occur from the first 2–6 months onwards. The allograft dysfunction is usually due to interstitial nephritis, although ureteric stenosis has been described. Diagnosis of BK virus nephritis requires allograft biopsy. As the histopathological changes may be patchy, two cores are recommended for analysis [15]. The presence of intranuclear tubule cell inclusions by light microscopy should raise suspicion; usually there is associated necrosis of tubular cells and interstitial inflammation. Diagnosis is confirmed by immunohistochemistry. Blood PCR quantification of viral load further confirms the diagnosis.

The most important therapy for established BK virus nephritis is major reduction in immunosuppression – to augment host mechanisms of viral clearance. Other therapies which have been reported in small series to be effective include leflunomide, low-dose cidofovir (high doses are nephrotoxic), and IVIg. It can be difficult to distinguish viral infection alone from infection plus superimposed rejection; such cases are sometimes managed with pulse steroids and reduction in other immunosuppression.

Many transplant centers now screen all new transplant recipients for subclinical infection – the idea being to reduce immunosuppression before severe nephritis occurs. Blood PCR quantification of viral load is commonly used. Positive screening tests trigger reduction in immunosuppression and – if the creatinine is increased – an allograft biopsy [14].

Drug and Radiocontrast Nephrotoxicity

A variety of drugs can cause acute dysfunction of the renal allograft. In many cases, the offending agent is a well-recognized cause of injury in native kidneys. However, a number of drug-related nephrotoxic effects are more common in the setting of transplantation (see Table 7.8). Many of these are due to interaction with the CNIs. Diltiazem, verapamil, macrolide antibiotics –particularly erythromycin – and the azole antifungals impair CNI metabolism and may lead to acute CNI nephrotoxicity unless there is concomitant reduction of the CNI. High-dose SMX-TMP may cause an acute increase in plasma creatinine by inhibiting tubular secretion of creatinine (in this case GFR is not affected and plasma creatinine decreases days after stopping SMX-TMP). Not surprisingly, ACE inhibitors or angiotensin II receptor antagonists have been implicated in precipitating ARF in the presence of transplant renal artery stenosis. Overall, if carefully prescribed, these agents are well tolerated.

Drugs with known nephrotoxic effects such as aminoglycosides, amphotericin, or NSAIDs probably have enhanced toxicity when used concomitantly with a CNI. Nevertheless, they are sometimes required in transplant recipients. Use of the lysosomal preparation of amphotericin is preferable because it is less nephrotoxic than the standard preparation.

Statins are commonly prescribed to renal transplant recipients. These drugs are generally well tolerated; however, there is an increased risk of rhabdomyolysis when they are used with cyclosporine (especially if an inhibitor of the cytochrome P450 system such as diltiazem is also administered).

The risk of acute renal failure after administration of radiocontrast to renal transplant recipients has not been well defined. Presumably, risk factors for contrast nephrotoxicity are similar to those in nontransplanted patients. Thus, the same preventive measures should be used.

Late Chronic Allograft Dysfunction (>6 Months)

Although short-term outcomes have improved, chronic allograft dysfunction and loss remain significant problems in renal transplantation [1, 6]. The principle causes of late chronic allograft dysfunction (after the first 6–12 months) are shown in Table 7.9. Traditionally, the main cause(s) of chronic injury was labeled "chronic allograft nephropathy" but this is a very general term. Recent consensus meetings have developed guidelines for establishing more accurate and discriminating diagnoses [16]. In practice, the clinical and histological picture often suggests a

Table 7.9 Causes of late chronic allograft dysfunction

Prerenal
• Transplant renal artery stenosis
• Heart failure
Intrarenal
• Chronic active antibody-mediated rejection
• Chronic active T-cell-mediated rejection (chronic allograft arteriopathy)
• Interstitial fibrosis and tubular atrophy, no specific etiology
• CNI toxicity
• Donor-related disease and/or perioperative injury
• Hypertension
• Chronic BK virus nephritis
• Recurrence of primary disease
• New disease
Postrenal
• Urinary tract obstruction

Note: More than one cause is frequently seen on biopsy

combination of causes – both immunological and nonimmunological. Determining the "most important" cause can be difficult. For example, the biopsy may show features of chronic rejection and chronic CNI toxicity: does this mean that CNI doses should be increased or decreased?

Chronic Rejection

This may be antibody-mediated or T-cell-mediated or both. There is growing evidence that antibody-mediated injury is an important cause of chronic dysfunction [17]. Clinical features are often not specific. However, there may be a history of acute rejection and/or noncompliance. Proteinuria may be prominent if there is transplant glomerulopathy (a feature of chronic AMR). The diagnostic criteria for late/chronic AMR include: (i) light microscopic changes such as transplant glomerulopathy or multilayering of peritubular capillaries or fibrointimal thickening of arteries with duplication of the internal elastica, (ii) diffuse C4d deposition in peritubular capillaries, and (iii) DSA in the serum [16]. Chronic active TCMR is characterized by arterial intimal fibrosis with mononuclear cell infiltration in the fibrosis and formation of neo-intima [16].

Chronic Calcineurin Inhibitor Toxicity

Just as in nonrenal solid organ transplantation, CNIs cause significant renal injury over the long term. Typical clinical features include months to years of exposure to CNIs, hypertension, slowly rising plasma creatinine, and bland urinalysis (obviously these are very nonspecific). Histology shows hyalinization of arterioles and interstitial fibrosis/tubular atrophy, either in striped or diffuse form [16].

Hypertension

Histologically, this is characterized by (i) fibrointimal thickening of arterial walls with reduplication of the elastica and (ii) interstitial fibrosis/tubular atrophy. Usually these changes are superimposed on other disease processes such as chronic rejection.

Interstitial Fibrosis/Tubular Atrophy: No Clear Etiology

In some cases of chronic dysfunction, allograft biopsy shows interstitial fibrosis/tubular atrophy but with no clear evidence of other associated injury (such as chronic rejection) [16]. A careful history may suggest contributors to this such as donor-related disease or severe perioperative ischemic damage (see below).

Donor-Related Disease/Perioperative Injury/Hyperfiltration

"Donor disease" such as hypertensive arteriosclerosis, glomerulosclerosis, or interstitial fibrosis/tubular atrophy can be an important contributor to chronic dysfunction. Not surprisingly, these changes become more severe with increasing donor age and use of ECD allografts [18]. Perioperative ischemic injury (clinically manifested as DGF) causes further damage and is associated with more chronic dysfunction [3, 18]. Determining the severity of "donor disease" is easy if a "time zero" biopsy has been performed – by definition the changes seen reflect only the effects of the donor's health and the organ retrieval/surgery. Where a "time zero" biopsy has not been performed, determining the degree of histological change due to donor conditions is more difficult, especially beyond the first 6 months. However, several aspects of the history can provide important clues: the donor's condition (age, predonation renal function) and the function of the donor's other transplanted kidney.

There is speculation that whatever the initial cause of chronic allograft dysfunction, inadequate "dosing" of nephrons (due to the single kidney state, donor disease, and/or posttransplant injury) leads to nephron overwork (hyperfiltration) and exhaustion. The degree to which hyperfiltration exacerbates allograft dysfunction is difficult to estimate in an individual patient, however.

Late Recurrence of Primary Disease

Late recurrence of primary disease is summarized in Table 7.7 and Fig. 7.5. The incidence of late recurrence is difficult to estimate: the original cause of ESRD is sometimes unknown, transplant kidney biopsies are not always performed and most

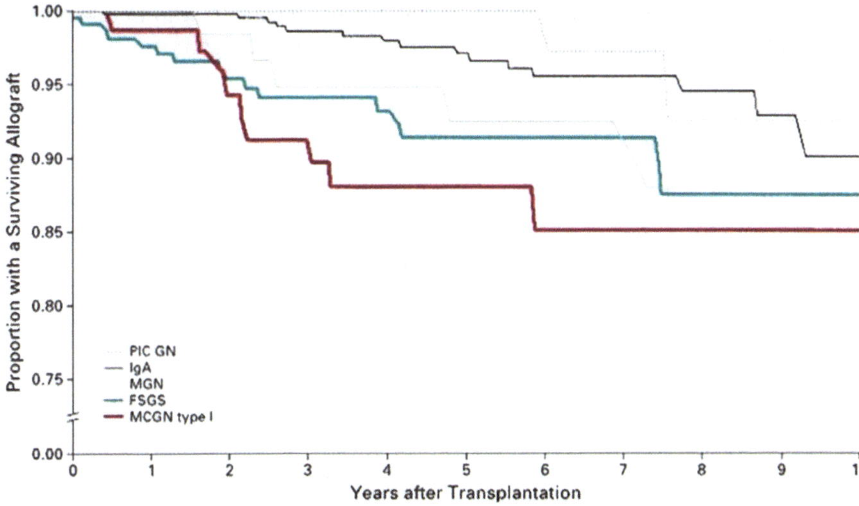

Fig. 7.5 Kaplan–Meier analysis of allograft loss due to recurrence of various forms of glomerulonephritis. *PIC GN* pauci-immune crescentic glomerulonephritis; *MGN* membranous glomerulonephropathy; *FSGS* focal segmental glomerulosclerosis; *MCGN* mesangiocapillary glomerulonephritis. Adapted from Briganti et al. [19]; used with permission

relevant studies are small and retrospective with variable follow-up periods. In one large study of patients transplanted after developing ESRD from glomerulonephritis, recurrence was the third most frequent cause of allograft loss at 10 years (after chronic rejection and death) [19].

BK Virus Infection

Even when viral infection has been controlled, there may be permanent and severe damage to the tubulo-interstium of the allograft. The management of BK virus infection has been discussed above.

Diabetic Nephropathy

Recurrence of diabetic nephropathy in the allograft has not been well studied. This reflects the poor long-term survival of diabetic transplant recipients; the duration of exposure to the diabetic milieu is often insufficient to allow development of severe diabetic nephropathy. Kim performed a case–control study of 78 transplanted patients with ESRD due to type I diabetes mellitus [20]. Overall allograft survival was poorer in the diabetic group. If death was excluded as a cause of allograft failure, however, allograft survival was little different. Six of 16 patients who were biopsied had histologic evidence of recurrence, but this resulted in allograft loss in only one case. New onset diabetes mellitus after transplant is a common problem. This can also lead to diabetic nephropathy; histological evidence of this may occur quite rapidly after transplant [21].

Management of Late Allograft Dysfunction

The history should be carefully reviewed especially with regard to the primary renal disease, early posttransplant course (severe DGF might indicate significant irreversible early allograft damage), episodes of acute rejection (if any), degree of hypertension, CNI levels, and compliance. Urinalysis is helpful as proteinuria suggests recurrence of primary disease or chronic AMR. Renal ultrasound should be performed to exclude an obstructive cause. If there is suspicion of renal artery stenosis or obstruction, testing can be performed as above. In most cases, however, intrinsic renal disease is the predominant cause of dysfunction: allograft biopsy is thus frequently performed. The aim of biopsy is to determine the predominant form of disease but sometimes this is difficult as multiple processes may be present. Ideally, staining for C4d and BK virus should be performed on all such biopsies. Despite improvements in our understanding of the causes of chronic dysfunction [17], treatment options for the various causes remain limited. In part this reflects that, whatever the cause, the nephron damage (as evidenced by the degree of interstitial fibrosis/tubular atrophy) is irreversible.

If there is histological evidence of a component of *acute* TCMR, pulse steroids are often used and baseline immunosuppression is increased. The management of chronic TCMR is less clear. At the very least, immunosuppression should not be reduced; if the allograft is not severely damaged (i.e., near "end-stage") then some centers slightly increase immunosuppression. If there is evidence of a component of *acute* AMR, then a plasmapheresis/IVIg protocol may be employed. The management of chronic AMR is not clear. Interventions such as rituximab and IVIg are under investigation; at this time a reasonable strategy is to switch to or continue a maintenance protocol of MMF + tacrolimus + steroids.

In cases where CNI toxicity appears to be an important cause of the allograft injury *and* there is no evidence of active rejection, reduction in CNI dosage is a reasonable strategy. Alternative agents such as MMF or sirolimus can be substituted but patients should be watched closely for late acute rejection. There is evidence that reduction or cessation of CNIs in this setting – with addition of MMF or sirolimus – does improve or stabilize GFR [22]. Sirolimus should probably be avoided in those with proteinuria or GFR <40 mL/min, because of a high risk of adverse effects [23].

Although there are no randomized controlled trials showing that treatment of hypertension in renal transplant recipients leads to improvement in renal and nonrenal outcomes, it seems reasonable to apply the Joint National Committee guidelines for patients with chronic kidney disease (CKD) and thus to rigorously control hypertension [24]. There are no randomized controlled trials of ACE-I/angiotensin receptor blocker therapy in renal transplantation but in practice these drugs are commonly used, especially when proteinuria is prominent.

The MDRD equation is increasingly used to estimate GFR in recipients with chronic dysfunction but its accuracy for an individual patient may be limited [25]. As GFR deteriorates, preparations should be made for a return to dialysis. Erythropoietin, vitamin D therapy, and other supportive measures may be required before dialysis resumes. The "CKD management" of the patient with the failing transplant can be difficult as the immunosuppressive medications may exacerbate hypertension, hyperlipidemia, anemia, and bone disease. Furthermore, resuming dialysis can be psychologically very traumatic for some patients. Patients may elect to go back on the transplant waiting list but they should be made aware that sensitization makes allograft matching more difficult and increases the risk of rejection.

Prevention of chronic allograft dysfunction is a major focus of current research. Strategies under investigation include CNI minimization, adequate "dosing" of functioning nephrons (including dual kidney transplantation), minimizing ischemia–reperfusion injury, further reduction in the incidence of acute rejection, aggressive treatment of hyperlipidemia and hypertension, and interruption of pathways leading to fibrosis. Protocol biopsies to identify early allograft damage have been advocated by some but outside the setting of high-risk recipients, their use remains controversial.

References

1. USRDS. USRDS 2008 Annual data report, Vol. 2009. NIH and NIDDK, Bethesda; 2009.
2. Johnston O, O'Kelly P, Spencer S, et al. Reduced graft function (with or without dialysis) vs immediate graft function – a comparison of long-term renal allograft survival. Nephrol Dial Transplant. 2006;21:2270–4.
3. Perico N, Cattaneo D, Sayegh MH, et al. Delayed graft function in kidney transplantation. Lancet. 2004;364:1814–27.
4. Moers C, Smits JM, Maathuis MH, et al. Machine perfusion or cold storage in deceased-donor kidney transplantation. N Engl J Med. 2009;360:7–19.
5. Ekberg H, Tedesco-Silva H, Demirbas A, et al. Reduced exposure to calcineurin inhibitors in renal transplantation. N Engl J Med. 2007;357:2562–75.
6. Meier-Kriesche HU, Schold JD, Srinivas TR, et al. Lack of improvement in renal allograft survival despite a marked decrease in acute rejection rates over the most recent era. Am J Transplant. 2004;4:378–83.
7. Solez K, Colvin RB, Racusen LC, et al. Banff 07 classification of renal allograft pathology: updates and future directions. Am J Transplant. 2008;8:753–60.
8. Chiurchiu C, Ruggenenti P, Remuzzi G. Thrombotic microangiopathy in renal transplantation. Ann Transplant. 2002;7:28–33.
9. Baid S, Pascual M, Williams Jr WW, et al. Renal thrombotic microangiopathy associated with anticardiolipin antibodies in hepatitis C-positive renal allograft recipients. J Am Soc Nephrol. 1999;10:146–53.
10. Vincenti F, Ghiggeri GM. New insights into the pathogenesis and the therapy of recurrent focal glomerulosclerosis. Am J Transplant. 2005;5:1179–85.

11. Saland JM, Shneider BL, Bromberg JS, et al. Successful split liver-kidney transplant for factor H associated hemolytic uremic syndrome. Clin J Am Soc Nephrol. 2009;4:201–6.
12. Vlaminck H, Maes B, Evers G, et al. Prospective study on late consequences of subclinical non-compliance with immunosuppressive therapy in renal transplant patients. Am J Transplant. 2004;4:1509–13.
13. Bruno S, Remuzzi G, Ruggenenti P. Transplant renal artery stenosis. J Am Soc Nephrol. 2004;15:134–41.
14. Hirsch HH, Brennan DC, Drachenberg CB, et al. Polyomavirus-associated nephropathy in renal transplantation: interdisciplinary analyses and recommendations. Transplantation. 2005;79:1277–86.
15. Drachenberg CB, Papadimitriou JC. Polyomavirus-associated nephropathy: update in diagnosis. Transpl Infect Dis. 2006;8:68–75.
16. Solez K, Colvin RB, Racusen LC, et al. Banff '05 Meeting Report: differential diagnosis of chronic allograft injury and elimination of chronic allograft nephropathy ('CAN'). Am J Transplant. 2007;7:518–26.
17. Gloor J, Cosio F, Lager DJ, et al. The spectrum of antibody-mediated renal allograft injury: implications for treatment. Am J Transplant. 2008;8:1367–73.
18. Lehtonen SR, Taskinen EI, Isoniemi HM. Histological alterations in implant and one-year protocol biopsy specimens of renal allografts. Transplantation. 2001;72:1138–44.
19. Briganti EM, Russ GR, McNeil JJ, et al. Risk of renal allograft loss from recurrent glomerulonephritis. N Engl J Med. 2002;347:103–9.
20. Kim H, Cheigh JS. Kidney transplantation in patients with type 1 diabetes mellitus: long- term prognosis for patients and grafts. Korean J Intern Med. 2001;16:98–104.
21. Wojciechowski D, Onozato ML, Gonin J. Rapid onset of diabetic nephropathy in three renal allografts despite normoglycemia. Clin Nephrol. 2009;71:719–24.
22. Birnbaum LM, Lipman M, Paraskevas S, et al. Management of chronic allograft nephropathy: a systematic review. Clin J Am Soc Nephrol. 2009;4:860–5.
23. Schena FP, Pascoe MD, Alberu J, et al. Conversion from calcineurin inhibitors to sirolimus maintenance therapy in renal allograft recipients: 24-month efficacy and safety results from the CONVERT trial. Transplantation. 2009;87:233–42.
24. Chobanian AV, Bakris GL, Black HR, et al. The Seventh Report of the Joint National Committee on Prevention, Detection, Evaluation, and Treatment of High Blood Pressure: the JNC 7 report. JAMA. 2003;289:2560–72.
25. Poggio ED, Batty DS, Flechner SM. Evaluation of renal function in transplantation. Transplantation. 2007;84:131–6.

Chapter 8
Approach to Medical Complications After Kidney Transplantation

John Vella

Abstract It is generally accepted that transplantation is the treatment of choice for selected patients with end-stage kidney disease as patient survival is improved when compared with dialysis. Transplant recipients experience an improvement in quality of life as well as reduced long-term health care costs. Unfortunately, for most individuals, the success of transplantation is based on an absolute requirement for immunotherapy from which most complications derive. Much of the medical care of the transplant patient involves assessing the risks of over- and under-immunosuppression, striving to minimize immunosuppression while avoiding the risks of rejection. Complications range from those that are minor in severity to those that are graft or life threatening. All complications need to be evaluated and managed appropriately in order to minimize nonadherence with medications, premature graft failure, and death.

Keywords Cardiovascular disease • Hypertension • Dyslipidemia • Diabetes mellitus • lymphoproliferative diseases

Introduction

It is generally accepted that transplantation is the treatment of choice for selected patients with end-stage kidney disease as patient survival is improved when compared with dialysis [1]. Transplant recipients experience an improvement in quality of life as well as reduced long-term health care costs. Unfortunately, for most individuals, the success of transplantation is based on an absolute requirement for

J. Vella MD, FRCP, FACP, FASN (✉)
Department of Medicine/Nephrology and Transplantation, Maine Medical Center, Portland, ME 04102, USA
e-mail: vellajp@mmc.org

A. Chandraker et al. (eds.), *Core Concepts in Renal Transplantation*,

DOI 10.1007/978-1-4614-0008-0_8,

Table 8.1 Noninfectious complications after kidney transplantation

• Cardiovascular
• Cancer
• Musculoskeletal
• Hematologic
• Cosmetic
• Neuropsychiatric
• Gastrointestinal

immunotherapy from which most complications derive. Such complications range from those that are minor in severity to those that are graft or life threatening (Table 8.1). All complications need to be evaluated and managed appropriately in order to minimize nonadherence with medications, premature graft failure, and death.

Posttransplant Cardiovascular Disease

Cardiovascular disease (CVD) is extremely prevalent in the transplant population and is the leading cause of death [2]. Patients with kidney disease are exposed to both traditional and nontraditional risk factors over a prolonged period of time (see Fig. 8.1 and Table 8.2). Many individuals come to transplantation with an established burden of atherosclerotic disease. The known survival benefit of transplantation is most likely derived from the elimination of uremia-related risk factors. In a study of almost 30,000 transplant patients reported to the United States Renal Data System (USRDS) between 1996 and 2000, the association between glomerular filtration rate (GFR) and hospitalization for treatment of acute coronary syndromes or congestive heart failure was examined. Reduced GFR at the end of the first year posttransplantation was significantly and independently associated with increased risks of both acute coronary syndromes and congestive heart failure [3].

"Nontraditional" Cardiovascular Risk Factors

What is it about transplantation that provides a cardiovascular benefit in spite of the fact that immunotherapy adversely impacts established CVD risk factors such as dyslipidemia, hypertension, anemia, and diabetes? In other words, how does improved GFR protect against CVD? Attention has focused on "nontraditional" risk factors that are prevalent in patients with chronic kidney disease (CKD) that are not effectively controlled by dialysis such as inflammation and oxidative stress. For example, our group has evaluated time-dependent changes in biomarkers of oxidative stress before and after living donor transplantation [4]. Blood levels of the pro-inflammatory proteins, IL-6, tumor necrosis factor alpha (TNF-α) and

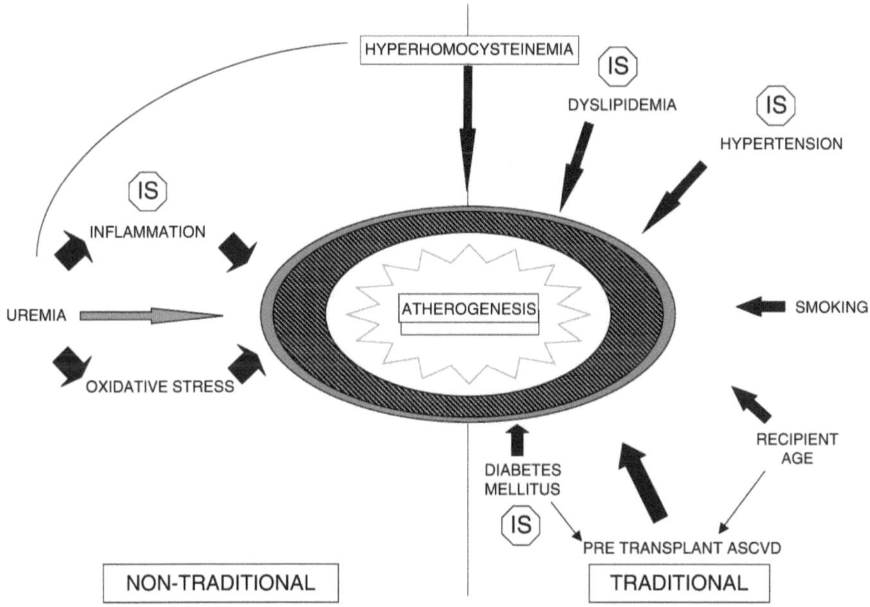

Fig. 8.1 Risk factors for cardiovascular disease after transplantation

Table 8.2 Cardiovascular complications

Complication	Relationship
Hypertension	Pretransplant hypertension
	Calcineurin inhibitor therapy
	Cyclosporine > tacrolimus
	Corticosteroids
Dyslipidemia	Pretransplant dyslipidemia
	Sirolimus > cyclosporine > tacrolimus
	Corticosteroids
Diabetes	Pretransplant diabetes mellitus
	New onset diabetes after transplantation
	Tacrolimus > cyclosporine
	Underlying disease
	Hepatitis C
	ADPKD
	Obesity
Nontraditional risk factors	Inflammation
	Allograft dysfunction
	Oxidative stress
	Hyperhomocysteinemia

C-reactive protein, as well as the oxidative stress markers plasma protein carbonyls and F_2-isoprostanes, were significantly elevated in CKD patients compared to healthy control subjects. However, a rapid and sustained decline in all of these biomarkers after transplant was observed.

Hypertension

Hypertension has long been associated with the development of CVD in both the general and CKD populations. Implicated factors include hypervolemia, hyperreninemia, and arterial calcification. Immunotherapy with corticosteroids and calcineurin inhibitors after transplantation may exacerbate preexisting hypertension. Hypertension early posttransplantation may increase rejection and delayed graft function rates. GFR posttransplantation impacts hypertension as well as both patient and allograft survival. Indeed, systolic blood pressure has been shown to drop significantly leading to improvements in left ventricular hypertrophy (LVH), left ventricular dilatation, and systolic dysfunction after transplantation. In addition, an inverse relationship between GFR and the average number of antihypertensive medications required by kidney transplant recipients has been demonstrated.

It has long been known that the calcineurin inhibitors induce hypertension. For example, cyclosporine activates the sympathetic nervous system, upregulates endothelin and inhibits inducible nitric oxide, the end result of which is potent vasoconstriction and systemic hypertension [5]. However, it is now generally accepted that tacrolimus is less likely to exacerbate hypertension compared with cyclosporine. It should be noted, however, that sirolimus if combined with tacrolimus may exacerbate hypertension as compared with a combination of tacrolimus/mycophenolate (MMF).

Another approach to dealing with hypertension is steroid minimization or withdrawal. While the transplant community seems to have gathered into opposing camps on this topic, it is perhaps more important to realize that steroid-sparing and withdrawal strategies showed benefits in reducing antihypertensive drug need, serum cholesterol, antihyperlipidemic drug need, new-onset diabetes after transplantation, and cataracts at the expense of increasing rejection risk [6]. Either way, such strategies neither increase nor decrease mortality or graft loss despite the increase in acute rejection. A European best practice guideline group made the following recommendations pertaining to the management of hypertension after transplantation that largely mirrors JNC-7 [7]:

- Careful monitoring and treatment of high blood pressure
- Blood pressure control goals
  - <130/85 mmHg for kidney transplant recipients without proteinuria
  - <125/75 mmHg for proteinuric patients

Long-term antihypertensive treatment is obligatory for most transplant patients in order to reduce cardiovascular risk and to protect allograft function. The use of angiotensin-converting enzyme (ACE) inhibitors in the antihypertensive treatment of kidney transplant recipients may be associated with hyperkalemia and anemia and may exacerbate prerenal azotemia. Calcium channel blockers have been widely regarded as the antihypertensive drugs of choice early after transplantation due to their ability to mitigate calcineurin inhibitor-mediated vasoconstriction although the impact of such therapy on long-term outcomes has been questioned. In a prospective double-blind study, 154 patients were randomized to receive either nifedipine or lisinopril and kidney function was assessed [8]. GFRs were significantly higher in the nifedipine group than in the lisinopril group (56 mL/min vs. 44 mL/min). In a prospective randomized study, the long-term effect of quinapril on blood pressure, kidney function, and proteinuria was compared with atenolol in 96 hypertensive kidney transplant recipients. After a 5-year observation period both agents, atenolol and quinapril, decreased systolic and diastolic blood pressure (SBP, DBP) as well as mean arterial pressure (MAP) and pulse pressure (PP) to a similar extent. Neither serum creatinine levels nor Cockcroft–Gault clearance had changed significantly and urinary protein excretion remained stable among the quinapril-treated patients, although a significant increase was observed in the atenolol group [9]. It has been demonstrated that losartan lowers macroproteinuria in diabetic or nondiabetic kidney transplant recipients similar to ACE inhibitors. Both losartan and candesartan have been studied in transplant recipients and have been shown to lower both systemic blood pressure and reduce microalbumenuria.

Posttransplant Dyslipidemia

Dyslipidemia occurs in approximately 60% of transplant recipients. It is known that pretransplant dyslipidemia as well as posttransplant immunosuppression impact lipid levels in the transplant recipient. The Assessment of Lescol in Kidney Transplantation study (ALERT) showed that treatment of kidney transplant recipients with fluvastatin over a period of 5–6 years significantly and safely reduced levels of low-density lipoprotein (LDL) cholesterol. Although the initial report indicated a nonstatistically significant reduction in the incidence of major adverse cardiac events at 5 years, further analysis of the data from this trial revealed a benefit of early initiation of fluvastatin on outcome at 7 years with a 29% reduction in death and myocardial infarction (MI) [10]. For patients commenced on therapy within the first 4 years of transplant, there was a risk reduction of 64% compared to 19% for patients commenced on therapy after 10 years. These observations are consistent with the development of CVD with the passage of time and the accumulation of multiple risk factors. The authors comment that the earlier the initiation of therapy with fluvastatin the greater was the reduction in cardiac events and that the "lipid-lowering and cardiovascular benefits of fluvastatin are comparable to those of statins in other patient groups, and support use of fluvastatin in kidney transplant recipients" [10].

In order to direct attention to the specific issues relating to the management of dyslipidemia in kidney transplant recipients, a workgroup of the National Kidney Foundation (NKF) has published clinical practice guidelines as part of the kidney Disease Outcome Quality Initiative (K/DOQI) that have been updated and summarized in the Kidney Disease: Improving Global Outcomes (KDIGO) guidelines [11]. The original NKF Task Force on CVD concluded that patients with CKD and kidney transplant recipients should be considered in the highest risk category. The guidelines recommend that all adult and adolescent kidney transplant recipient be evaluated for dyslipidemia with a complete lipid profile at the time of presentation; at 2–3 months after a change in treatment or other conditions known to cause dyslipidemia; and at least annually thereafter. Whenever possible the lipid profile should be measured after an overnight fast and if a dyslipidemia is recognized a potentially remediable secondary cause should be considered. In addition to the presumption that the recognition and treatment of dyslipidemias in transplant patients would reduce the incidence of atherosclerotic disease, the possibility was considered that preservation of kidney function would result, though evidence for such a benefit is limited. Evidence that the use of statins would reduce the incidence of acute rejection was regarded as unconvincing.

Readers are referred to the guidelines for precise treatment recommendations, which generally mirror those made in the general population, and require therapeutic lifestyle change (TLC) before drug therapy. In the event that an underlying cause cannot be corrected, the guidelines recommend treatment of adult patients with a fasting:

- Triglycerides of ≥500 mg/dL
- LDL of ≥100 mg/dL

The guidelines emphasize the effectiveness of statins while focusing attention on the impact of impaired GFR, cyclosporine administration, and other interacting agents on blood levels. Wiesbaur and colleagues have added to this literature by performing an analysis of statin use with patient and graft survival in a cohort of 2,041 first-time recipients of renal allografts between 1990 and 2003 [12]. Statin use was independently and significantly associated with lower mortality rates. Twelve-year survival rates were 73% for statin users and 64% for nonusers. The adjusted hazard ratio for all-cause mortality associated with statin use was 0.6 and graft survival rates during the same time period were 76% for statin users and 70% for nonusers. The adjusted hazard ratio for graft survival associated with statin use was 0.7. Statins can be used safely with cyclosporine if the statin dose is reduced, generally to approximately 50% of the standard dose. No specific statin drug was recommended. A baseline creatine phosphokinase (CK) level may help in the interpretation of subsequent muscle tenderness and elevated CK levels. The guidelines recommend against the combined administration of fibrates and statins, and bile acid sequestrants must be used with great care because of their potential impact on the intestinal absorption of immunosuppressive medications. It was felt that ezitimibe should probably not be used until its safety was established in the transplant population.

New-Onset Diabetes After Transplantation

New-onset diabetes mellitus (NODAT) is a known, serious, long-term complication of transplantation and a number of clinical studies have shown that it is associated with reduced patient and graft survival. The incidence of NODAT is, to some extent, definition-dependent. Older studies that defined this condition by the need for long-term insulin therapy underestimated the extent of the problem. A recent study reported that all patients with and 87% without pretransplantation diabetes had evidence of hyperglycemia (bedside glucose >200 mg/dL or physician-instituted insulin therapy) during the initial hospitalization after transplantation [13]. All patients with and 66% without pretransplantation diabetes required insulin at hospital discharge. Various studies indicate that NODAT persists in up to 20% of patients through the end of the first year posttransplant. Factors associated with the development of NODAT include recipient age, deceased kidney donor, hepatitis C, polycystic kidney disease (ADPKD), episodes of rejection, and the use of tacrolimus rather than cyclosporine. Steroid withdrawal or avoidance and statin therapy are associated with a reduced incidence of NODAT [6].

Coronary Artery and Vascular Calcification

Coronary artery calcification (CAC) is highly prevalent in the dialysis population, particularly in patients who are older, diabetic, obese, osteoporotic, and those with evidence of inflammation. CAC as measured by electron beam computerized tomography (EBCT) has been studied as a noninvasive technique to diagnose coronary artery disease and as a surrogate marker of coronary plaque load. The prevalence of CAC in the dialysis population is, not surprisingly, also reflected in the transplant population. Sixty-five percent of transplant recipients have CAC with higher scores found in diabetics, older patients, and those with hypercholesterolemia, and were lower in transplant recipients who had not been dialyzed [14].

Posttransplant Malignancy

Improvements in patient and graft survival rates in renal transplantation remain overshadowed by the long-term risk of malignancy. The relationship between the nature and intensity of immunotherapy and subsequent malignancy is well defined and has been reviewed extensively [15, 16]. It remains clear that the incidence of all types of cancer is higher for transplant recipients than the general population and is the second most common cause of death after CVD. The increase in cancer risk after transplantation is consequent on the interplay of numerous factors that include the cumulative exposure to immunotherapy leading to disruption of both antitumor and antiviral immunosurveillance (Table 8.3). Additionally, some drugs may impact carcinogenesis by mechanisms independent of their immunosuppressive effects.

Table 8.3 Cancer after transplantation

Complication	Relationship
Skin cancer (SCC > BCC)	Immunotherapy
	Human papillomavirus
	Sun exposure
Viral-mediated	Posttransplant lymphoproliferative disease: Epstein–Barr virus
	Kaposi sarcoma: human herpes virus 8
Renal cell carcinoma	Atrophic kidneys

Viral infections (including herpes and hepatitis viruses) are clearly linked to some malignancies and chronic antigen stimulation from the transplanted organ, repeated infections, and transfusions of blood products have also been implicated.

Impact of Immunosuppression

It has been suggested that the use of antilymphocyte antibody therapy and tacrolimus increase the risk of PTLD. Hardinger et al. recently reported the 10-year follow-up of a randomized trial of thymoglobulin or Atgam induction [17]. Event-free survival was significantly higher with thymoglobulin compared with Atgam (48 vs. 29%). At 10 years, patient and graft survival rates were similar, whereas acute rejection remained lower (11 vs. 42%) in the thymoglobulin group. The incidence of all types of cancer was numerically although not significantly lower with thymoglobulin compared with Atgam (8 vs. 21%). There were no posttransplant lymphoproliferative disorder in the thymoglobulin group and there were two cases in the Atgam group. Kidney function and measures of quality of life were found to be higher in the thymoglobulin compared with the Atgam group. The use of IL-2-receptor antagonists as induction therapy significantly reduced the cancer risk of transplant recipients. With the exception of mammalian target of rapamycin (mTOR) inhibitors (sirolimus and everolimus), tumor risk between immunosuppressive drugs typically used for maintenance immunosuppression was not significantly different. However, mTOR inhibitor-based immunosuppressive protocols showed a clear tendency for lower malignancy rates. Given the potential anticancer actions of the mTOR inhibitors demonstrated in clinical studies, de Fijter et al. analyzed the effect of conversion from calcineurin inhibitors in 53 renal transplant recipients developing nonmelanoma skin cancer after transplantation [18]. Remission was observed in 37 patients and therapy was generally well tolerated with minimal adverse events reported. Fifteen patients developed new lesions following conversion. Drug levels did not seem to affect the outcomes of conversion.

Reports continue to accumulate indicating that Kaposi Sarcoma (KS) after transplantation is exquisitely sensitive to conversion from calcineurin inhibitor to mTOR inhibitor therapy. As an example, Campestol et al. reported that conversion to either everolimus or sirolimus led to regression of KS lesions in 11 out of 12 patients [19]. Conversion was generally well tolerated, stable kidney function was maintained in most patients and there was no rejection. Patients with KS showed markedly increased basal P70 (S6K) activation and depressed phosphorylation of AKT. Long-term treatment with sirolimus was associated with marked inhibition of phosphorylation of both AKT and P70 (S6K), in parallel with regression of the dermal neoplasm.

It is certainly true that the mTOR inhibitors have failed to gain traction within the United States due to the high incidence of adverse effects that include increased risk of infection, wound problems, edema, and proteinuria. Clinical trials have indicated that up to 20% of patients randomized to sirolimus are withdrawn from therapy because of the nature and severity of adverse events. Nevertheless, for those recipients suffering from cancer after transplantation, such agents may be useful.

Posttransplant Lymphoproliferative Disease

Transplant recipients are at the greatest risk of developing PTLD within the first year after transplantation. Most cases of PTLD are induced by Epstein–Barr virus (EBV) infection causing uncontrolled proliferation of B cells. The incidence is higher in EBV seronegative children who receive seropositive grafts from adult donors. Heart-lung transplants showed the highest relative risk among different types of organ transplants. The use of tacrolimus and induction or rescue therapy with OKT3 or ATG is known to increase the risk of PTLD. The diagnosis of PTLD is generally suggested by clinical symptoms (organ involvement and/or fever) and imaging study results. Traditionally, computed tomography (CT) scanning with oral and intravenous contrast has been the test of choice for defining the presence and extent of PTLD.

Treatment of PTLD

The current approach to the treatment of PTLD involves a number of therapeutic options that include:

- Reduction of basal immunosuppression
- Antiviral treatment in the case of EBV-positive B-cell lymphoma
- Rituximab in the case of CD20-positive lymphomas
- Combination chemotherapy (cytoxan, adriamycin, vincristine and prednisone: CHOP) alone or in combination with rituximab for diffuse lymphoma or incomplete response to previous treatment

Swinnen et al. reported the results of a prospective, multicenter study that examined the efficacy of a PTLD treatment algorithm that started with a defined course of reduced immunotherapy and escalated to interferon-α (IFN-α), and finally to chemotherapy [20]. Intravenous acyclovir was given to all patients. The calcineurin inhibitor was reduced by 50% for 2 weeks and then by another 50% unless the patient was in complete remission. Sixteen patients with biopsy-proven PTLD (median age 47) were eligible to participate in the study of whom 13 had received heart transplants and three kidney transplants. Reduced immunotherapy resulted in only 1 of 16 partial responses and no complete remissions. Progressive disease developed in half and 40% experienced rejection. Only 1 of 13 patients achieved durable remission with IFN. Five of seven patients who received chemotherapy achieved remission. The applicability of such a study to kidney transplantation remains uncertain, as most patients in the above quoted study were heart transplant recipients. The authors concluded, "A strong case can be made for adding rituximab to reduced immunosuppression as initial therapy" [20]. Trappe and colleagues performed a retrospective analysis to determine the efficacy and safety of salvage therapy in recipients of solid organ transplants with progression of PTLD after rituximab first-line therapy [21]. Eleven patients who had received reduced immunotherapy and single-agent rituximab were analyzed. Of these, ten had received CHOP. This cohort seems to have been quite different from usual PTLD cohort in that most of these patients had late disease (median onset of disease 145 months posttransplant), had monomorphic histology and only 36% were associated with EBV. CHOP therapy achieved complete remission in 50% of patients at 44 months posttreatment and partial remission 20% patients. The median overall survival was 46.5 months.

Hematologic Complications of Transplantation

The hematologic complications of transplantation are mostly related to drug therapy or infection and are summarized in Table 8.4. A number of interrelated factors that include allograft dysfunction, myelosuppressive immuno- and antiviral drug therapies, thrombotic micro-angiopathy, inhibitors of the renin–angiotensin system and infection cause postkidney transplant anemia. In addition, transplant patients have a

Table 8.4 Hematologic complications of transplantation

Complication	Relationship
Anemia	Antibody induction therapy
	Antimetabolite immunosuppression
	ACE/ARB
Posttransplant erythrocytosis	Endogenous erythropoietin excess
Leucopenia	Polyclonal antibody induction
	Anti-metabolite immunosuppression
	Antiviral antibiotics
	CMV
	Bactrim
Thrombotic microangiopathy	Calcineurin inhibitors

higher incidence of enteric disease that may lead to gastrointestinal bleeding and many patients are iron deficient or have marrow fibrosis as sequelae of ESRD and dialysis. Indeed, iron deficiency anemia after kidney transplantation occurs in up to 40% of transplant recipients [22]. Allograft dysfunction after kidney transplantation often leads to anemia in the recipient.

In a retrospective, cohort study of the prevalence of anemia among 240 patients who underwent kidney transplantation at a single center, the mean hematocrit rose from 33% at 1 month after transplantation to 40% at 12 months after transplantation. The proportion of patients with hematocrits less than 36% was 76% at transplantation and 21% at 1 year and 36% at 4 years posttransplantation. Women had a significantly higher risk of anemia than men. Posttransplant anemia is often inadequately evaluated and treated. In the above quoted study, only 36% of patients with hematocrit readings of less than 30% had iron studies performed, 46% received iron supplementation, and 40% received recombinant human erythropoietin. A European study, the Transplant European Survey on Anemia Management (TRESAM), documented the prevalence and management of anemia in kidney transplant recipients. Data from 4,263 patients derived from 72 transplant centers in 16 countries were obtained. At enrollment, 38.6% of patients were found to be anemic. Of the 8.5% of patients who were considered severely anemic, only 17.8% were treated with erythropoietin. There was a strong association between hemoglobin and graft function; of the 904 patients with serum creatinine >2 mg/dL, 60.1% were anemic, vs. 29.0% of those with serum creatinine ≤2 mg/dL ($p<0.01$). Therapy with ACE inhibitors, angiotensin II receptor antagonists, mycophenolate mofetil (MMF), or azathioprine was also associated with a higher likelihood of anemia. In a single center retrospective study of 374 kidney transplant recipients, the prevalence of PTA was 28.6% [23]. Ten percent of all patients were on erythropoietin therapy, but only 41.6% of patients whose HCT was <30 received this treatment. Female gender and lower kidney function were associated with lower HCT by multivariate analysis. Patients on ACEI had significantly lower HCT compared with patients without such treatment. In addition, a significant curvilinear dose–response relationship was found between ACEI dose and HCT. Among the immunosuppressant drugs, MMF and tacrolimus were associated with a lower HCT. In a fourth study of 128 patients, 30% of patients were anemic at some time during the posttransplant period. In this longer-term study, the prevalence of PTA increased over time such that by 5 years posttransplant, 26% of the patients were anemic. Anemia occurred in 62.5% of patients converted from azathioprine to MMF. A multivariate logistic regression model demonstrated a significant correlation between anemia and serum total CO_2, BUN, and creatinine at 1 year posttransplant. At 5 years posttransplant, only serum total CO_2 correlated with anemia. Thus, diminished kidney excretory function and metabolic acidosis appear to be important correlates of late PTA. These four studies when taken together indicate that posttransplant anemia is prevalent, increases in frequency with time posttransplant and is often inadequately investigated and treated.

Parvovirus B19 virus infection has been reported in organ transplant recipients with persistent anemia. Diagnosis can be established by documenting seroconversion, however, detection of B19 virus DNA in serum is the best direct marker of active infection. In a study that evaluated the incidence and clinical role of active B19 virus infection in kidney transplant recipients presenting with anemia, 48 such recipients were investigated by PCR on serum samples. The controls were 21 recipients without anemia. Parvovirus DNA was demonstrated in serum from 23% of anemic patients, vs. only 5% of the controls. Seventy-three percent of these patients had DNA evidence of concomitant CMV infection; 27% recovered spontaneously from anemia whereas 73% needed therapy.

Hemophagocytic syndrome is a rare cause of anemia posttransplant, the clinical components of which include fever, hepatosplenomegaly, pancytopenia, hypofibrinogenemia, and liver dysfunction. The syndrome is defined by bone marrow and organ infiltration by activated, nonmalignant macrophages that phagocytoze red blood cells and is often caused by an infectious or neoplastic disease. A retrospective analysis of 17 cases of HPS after kidney transplantation revealed a median time between transplantation and hemophagocytosis of 52 days [24]. Sixty-four percent had received antilymphocyte globulins during the 3 months before presentation. Fever was present in all patients, and hepatosplenomegaly was present in 9 of 17 patients. Laboratory tests revealed anemia, thrombocytopenia, and leucopenia. Elevated liver enzymes were present in 12 of 17 patients, and cholestasis was present in 10 of 17 patients. HPS was related to viral infection in nine patients (cytomegalovirus, EBV, human herpes virus 6, and human herpes virus 8), bacterial infection in three patients (tuberculosis and Bartonella henselae), and other infections in two patients (toxoplasmosis and Pneumocystis carinii pneumoniae). PTLD was present in two patients. Despite broad-spectrum anti-infectious treatment and dramatic tapering of immunosuppression, death occurred in eight patients (47%). Graft nephrectomy was performed in four of the nine surviving patients [24].

It has been suggested that anemia posttransplantation may impact CVD. In a single-center population of 404 type 1 diabetic patients who underwent either cadaveric kidney transplantation alone or simultaneous pancreas-kidney transplantation, the effect of increasing hematocrit on the risk for cardiovascular was examined over time. More than 60% of the individuals in the study cohort had a hematocrit of less than or equal to 30% at least once during the first 30 days posttransplant. Forty-two individuals (10.4% of the study population) had at least one 30-day hematocrit less than or equal to 30% and a CV event (MI, CV death, angina, or congestive heart failure) during the first 26 weeks of the posttransplant course. In a retrospective study of 638 transplant recipients, age, diabetes, gender, hypertension, and anemia were identified as independent risk factors for de novo CHF. In another study, the same investigators identified anemia and hypertension as being independent risk factors for LVH posttransplantation [25].

Posttransplant Erythrocytosis

Posttransplant erythrocytosis (PTE) is defined as a persistently elevated hematocrit to a level greater than 51% after kidney transplantation [26]. It occurs in 10–15% of graft recipients and usually develops 8–24 months after engraftment. The cause remains incompletely understood although in some patients may be related to the production of inappropriately high levels of erythropoietin. In addition, an increase in angiotensin type I receptor density has been reported in erythroid precursors of some transplant patients with PTE compared to those without PTE and normal volunteers, and the level of AT1R expression in PTE correlated significantly with the hematocrit [27]. The cause of this upregulation is unknown although interestingly, both ACE inhibitors and ARBs can effectively manage PTE [28]. Approximately 60% of patients with PTE experience malaise, headache, plethora, lethargy, and dizziness. Thromboembolic events occur in 10–30% of the cases and 1–2% eventually die of associated complications [26]. The goal of therapy is to reduce the hematocrit to less than 50%. Most patients respond well to either ACEI or ARB although some still require periodic therapeutic phlebotomy.

Leucopenia

Myelosuppression after transplantation is a frequent sequela of both immuno- and antiviral therapy and is associated with an increased incidence of infections [29]. The antimetabolite immunotherapeutic agents are the greatest offenders in this regard although azathioprine has a greater tendency to cause leucopenia as compared with MMF [30]. Because of the pharmacokinetic interaction between azathioprine and allopurinol that causes profound leucopenia, this combination is best avoided or used with extreme caution. Ganciclovir is known to cause leucopenia and its more bioavailable analog, valganciclovir is especially prone to causing myelosuppression especially when used in combination with MMF [31].

Musculoskeletal Complications of Transplantation

The risk of fracture after kidney transplantation is about 2–3% per patient per year (Table 8.5). Immunotherapy and secondary hyperparathyroidism are considered to be the more important pathogenic factors. Other implicated causes include preexisting uremic osteodystrophy (with or without poor allograft function), adynamic bone disease, and vitamin D deficiency (± Vit D receptor polymorphisms). Vitamin D insufficiency has been reported in 29% of those who were less than 1 year posttransplant and 43% in those who were more than 1 year posttransplant. Severe deficiency was detected in 12 and 5%, respectively. An inverse correlation was found between PTH and vitamin D levels in the long term but not in recently transplanted patients. No correlation was found between vitamin D levels and bone mineral densitometry. Hypercalcemia was present in 40% of the recent and 25% of the long-term transplant recipients. Hypercalcemia after kidney transplantation is generally considered to result from PTH-induced osteoclast activation and bone resorption. Borchhardt recently reported a series of bone biopsies after tetracycline labeling obtained from

Table 8.5 Musculoskeletal complications of transplantation

Complication	Relationship
Osteoporosis	Pretransplant osteoporosis
	Cyclosporine
	Steroids
Osteitis	Residual hyperparathyroidism
Adynamic bone disease	Over-treatment of osteodystrophy
Tendonitis	Quinolone antibiotics (high dose)

17 such patients [32]. Interestingly, high-turnover renal osteodystrophy was present in nine and low turnover in eight patients. Regardless of the precise cause, the dominant clinical bone adverse events after transplantation include bone loss, fractures, osteonecrosis, and bone pain.

Bone mineral densitometry screening (dual-energy X-ray absorptiometry-DEXA) is currently recommended for all women over the age of 65 and postmenopausal women under age 65 who have one or more additional risk factors for osteoporosis. Bone mineral densitometry testing is recommended for transplant recipients based on the assumption that data from the general population are pertinent to this cohort [15, 16]. Akaberi investigated whether DEXA is of value for predicting fractures in transplant patients [33]. A total of 238 patients were studied between 1995 and 2007. During this time period, 46 patients had 53 fractures (19%). The risk of fracture for those with osteoporosis and osteopenia were 3.5 and 2.7 times, respectively, compared with those with normal BMD supporting the utility of DEXA for identifying at-risk patients.

Therapy

Therapeutic options for posttransplant bone disease have been focused on vitamin D analogs, calcium supplementation, bisphosphonates and to a lesser extent, calcitonin. It has recently been suggested that recombinant parathyroid hormone may be a promising therapeutic option. However as mentioned above, hyperparathyroidism is prevalent in the transplant population and theoretically, administration of such a drug might exacerbate bone disease. Nevertheless, Cejka reported the results of a 6-month trial in which 26 kidney transplant recipients were randomized to daily subcutaneous injections of teriparatide or placebo. Femoral neck BMD remained stable in the teriparatide group, although decreased significantly in the placebo group. Lumbar spine and radial BMD, histomorphometric bone volume and bone matrix mineralization status remained unchanged in both groups. Serologic bone markers were similarly reduced in both groups throughout the study. The authors concluded that teriparatide did not improve BMD early after kidney transplantation.

For those with persistent hyperparathyroidism, treatment options have included activated vitamin D analogs, cinacalcet, or surgery. Cinacalcet is a calcimimetic drug licensed for treatment of secondary hyperparathyroidism in patients with ESRD that has been shown to lower serum calcium and PTH levels in transplant recipients. Initial reports indicated that the effectiveness of therapy was short-lived [15]. More recently, Kruse et al. indicated that cessation of therapy after 12 months was associated with a sustained improvement in parameters such as calcium and PTH [34]. The impact of parathyroidectomy on the long-term risks for hip and other fractures has been unclear even though such procedures are often advised as a prelude to transplantation for those with refractory disease to mitigate bone disease and prevent nephrolithiasis. Rudser et al. compared long-term fracture rates among hemodialysis patients from the USRDS who underwent parathyroidectomy with a matched control group [35]. After adjustment, parathyroidectomy was associated with a 31% lower risk for fracture compared with the control group. Although this analysis excluded transplant recipients, another report by Chou et al. demonstrated that parathyroidectomy after kidney transplantation is indeed associated with a significant improvement in bone mineral density in as soon as a year [36].

Bone Pain

Osteoarticular pain soon after transplantation occurs in between 5 and 10% of patients and typically affects the lower extremities. This complication has been described in patients taking both cyclosporine and tacrolimus. The term "post-transplant distal limb syndrome" was recently coined to describe this benign but sometimes disabling complication [37]. The clinical evaluation is unremarkable and the described radiologic features include patchy epiphyseal osteoporosis by X-ray, increased focal or diffuse uptake of the tracer at bone scintigraphy and areas of low-signal intensity at T1-weighted images on MRI, consistent with areas of medullary edema. Clinical recovery is the rule and usually occurs within several weeks.

Tendonitis

Achilles tendonitis with ruptures was initially described in patients taking high-dose quinolone antibiotics more than a decade ago. More recently, a case–control study reported a fourfold overall increased risk for tendonitis and ruptures in patients taking steroids [38]. In this study, the sixfold increase in odds risk was observed in patients aged 60–79 years and 20-fold increase in odds risk in patients aged 80 years or older. In persons aged 60 years and older, the OR was 28 for current exposure to ofloxacin. Approximately 2–6% of all Achilles tendon ruptures in people older than 60 years can be attributed to quinolones. It has been suggested that high-dose quinolones be used with caution in older patients on steroids for this reason.

Neuropsychiatric Complications of Transplantation

The development of end-stage kidney disease combined with the realization that life may no longer be possible without medical intervention may lead to anxiety, depression, nonadherence, sexual dysfunction, and suicide (Table 8.6). Immunotherapy has also been implicated in inducing or exacerbating psychiatric disorders that include euphoria, delirium, generalized anxiety disorder, and occasionally, hallucinations [39]. Such disorders often require intervention with psychopharmacologic agents. However, psychotropic drug administration may be hazardous because of pharmacokinetic interactions with immunosuppressive drugs [40]. The neuropsychiatric issues that pertain to transplant recipients are summarized in Table 8.6.

Depression

End-stage kidney disease and transplantation are associated with depression, which impacts adversely upon compliance and may be associated with decreased longevity. In the kidney transplant population, depression occurs early after transplantation and has been associated with rejection. Depression is common in recipients also for up to 45% of other organ transplants. Factors that increase a transplant recipient's risk for depression and anxiety-related disorders include pretransplant psychiatric history, poor social support, the use of avoidance coping strategies for managing health problems and low self-esteem. Other implicated factors that may lead to depression include the disfiguring effects of immunosuppressive medication, such as high-dose corticosteroid therapy, and antihypertensive treatment with β blockers.

Table 8.6 Neuropsychiatric complications of transplantation

Complication	Relationship
Tremor	Tacrolimus > cyclosporine
Depression	Corticosteroids
Mania	β(beta)-blockers
Anxiety	
Delirium	Polypharmacy
	Infection
Nonadherence	Medication adverse effects
	Psychiatric disease
	Education
	Recipient age
Visual changes	Cataracts
	Diabetes
	Steroid-induced retinopathy
	Infection

In one study, the suicide rate in kidney transplant recipients was 24 per 100,000 patient-years, a finding that was 84% higher than the general population [41]. In multivariate models, age greater than 75 years, male gender, white or Asian race, geographic region, alcohol or drug dependence, and recent hospitalization with mental illness were significant independent predictors of death as a result of suicide.

Nonadherence

Nonadherence with diet and medication is a significant problem among some transplant recipients. With organ transplantation, nonadherence is a major risk factor for graft rejection episodes and is responsible for up to 25% of deaths after the initial recovery period [42]. In one study, the risk of acute graft rejection was 4.2 times greater among recipients who were not compliant with medications. The numerous factors implicated include psychiatric disturbances, adverse effects of medications, lack of knowledge concerning the need for medications, and financial concerns. This problem is particularly prevalent in adolescents and young adults. Characteristics linked to noncompliance include younger and older age, marital status (single), anxiety, denial, personality disorders and mental retardation and substance abuse.

Psychopharmacology

Previous therapeutic options for depression were hampered by the adverse effects associated with traditional agents. By comparison, newer antidepressant medications are more effective and safer in both the general population and medically ill patients. This diverse group of compounds possesses distinct pharmacokinetic properties that are unrelated to either the tricyclic/tetracyclic antidepressants or the monoamine oxidase inhibitors. Such newer agents include selective serotonin reuptake inhibitors (SSRIs), such as fluoxetine, paroxetine, sertraline, trazodone, and fluvoxamine. Agents with serotonin reuptake activity that also prevent the uptake of other neurotransmitters (such as norepinephrine and dopamine) include nefazodone, bupropion, and venlafaxine.

A problem associated with the use of these agents may be drug interactions resulting in elevated immunosuppressive drug levels due to alterations in the cytochrome CYP3A4 isoenzyme system. Among the newer antidepressant medications, fluvoxamine and nefazodone have the strongest inhibitory action on the CYP3A4 isoenzyme. In fact, we have previously reported interactions between cyclosporine and nefazodone or fluvoxamine that led to severe cyclosporine toxicity, allograft dysfunction, and uncontrolled hypertension [40]. The corollary of such observations is that agents with minimal inhibitory effects on the CYP3A4 isoenzyme, such as paroxetine and sertraline, would not be expected to cause a pharamacokinetic interaction. Although fluoxetine has moderate inhibitory potency, it has not been implicated in causing such interactions. Information is lacking for trazodone, venlafaxine, and bupropion. Caution dictates that levels of affected drugs should be carefully monitored in any transplant patient who requires treatment for major affective disorders. Appropriate dosage adjustments should be performed as necessary to circumvent toxicity. For patients who require antidepressant medications, fluoxetine or bupropion are often used as first-line therapy since these agents have not been shown to have significant interactions with calcineurin inhibitors.

Neurologic Complications

Tremors after transplantation are extremely common and are generally related to calcineurin inhibitor therapy. Cyclosporine has long been known to activate the sympathetic nervous system and increase circulating catechol levels and it is now understood that tacrolimus has an even greater effect in this regard. Most often, such tremors are related to the higher levels that are required early posttransplantation in order to prevent allograft rejection. In general terms, tremors abate over time as the levels are allowed to run at a lower range. A new onset tremor in a transplant recipient may be due to calcineurin inhibitor toxicity and should prompt a measurement of the drug level. Sirolimus and the antimetabolite immunosuppressive agents are not generally associated with this adverse event.

Visual Disturbances After Transplantation

Ocular complications after transplantation are frequently encountered and range in severity from blurred vision from poorly controlled hyperglycemia to sight-threatening steroid-induced retinopathy. Cataracts develop in approximately 40% of transplant patients and lead to surgery in many of those afflicted. Risk factors include diabetes mellitus, older age, and the use of corticosteroids. Diabetic retinopathy is often "burned out" by the time a diabetic comes to transplantation. However, for type I diabetics undergoing pancreas transplantation, active retinopathy may regress. Ocular infections consequent on immunotherapy such as CMV or toxoplasmosis are fortunately rare in the organ transplant population. There have been recent reports of uveitis induced by cidofovir, an antiviral antibiotic approved for the treatment of CMV retinitis in HIV patients that is sometimes used off label as rescue therapy for refractory polyoma virus allograft nephropathy. As visual disturbances after solid organ transplantation may be sight threatening, any new symptoms are most appropriately evaluated by ophthalmology. Routine ophthalmologic examinations are currently recommended for high-risk patients on an annual basis.

Gastrointestinal Complications of Transplantation

Gastrointestinal complications commonly occur after transplantation and are summarized in Table 8.7. The commonest GI adverse events after transplantation are related to the use of either MMF or mycophenolic acid (MPA). Mycophenolate causes nausea or diarrhea in up to 40% of patients. The incidence of gastrointestinal (GI) symptoms is greater when individuals take higher doses. Altering the drug dose or frequency often ameliorates symptoms although there has been concern of late that under-dosing or discontinuing MMF may increase the relative risk of allograft rejection by a factor of 2.3–2.7 [43]. Although it has been suggested that the incidence of GI adverse effects may be lower when using MPA, the Physician Desk Reference indicates that there is no difference in the reported incidence of GI symptoms (constipation 38 vs. 39%, nausea 29 vs. 27%, diarrhea 23 vs. 24%, vomiting 23 vs. 20%).

Sirolimus is a potent inhibitor of cellular proliferation that binds to the mTOR and in so doing, inhibits response to cytokine signaling. It has been approved for the prevention of kidney allograft rejection by the U.S. Food and Drug Administration (FDA). The reported adverse GI effects include abdominal pain (28–36%), nausea (25–36%), vomiting (19–25%), and diarrhea (25–42%). The incidence of diarrhea seems to be higher when sirolimus is used in the context of calcineurin inhibitor withdrawal or as adjunctive therapy with MMF. Stomatitis and mouth ulcers (similar in appearance to aphthous ulcers) occur in approximately 30% of patients treated with sirolimus. The precise etiology remains uncertain, although an earlier theory that stomatitis may be related to viral infection seems to have been abandoned. A dose reduction may allow such ulcers to heal although symptoms often persist and on occasion, one has little choice other than to discontinue the medication.

Table 8.7 Gastrointestinal complications of transplantation

Complication	Relationship
Gastritis/PUD	Stress
	Corticosteroids
	CMV
Hepatitis	Noninfectious
	Hepatitis B/hepatitis C virus
	Statin therapy
	Amlodipine
	Azathioprine
Diarrhea	Mycophenolate
	Sirolimus
	Proton pump inhibitors
Stomatitis	Noninfective – Sirolimus
	Candida

Hepatitis

Reactivation of viral hepatitis is dealt with in Chap. 9. Noninfective hepatitis occurs with some regularity in transplant recipients most often as an adverse consequence of drug therapy. Historically, azathioprine was occasionally associated with hepatotoxicity, jaundice, and rarely hepatic veno-occlusive disease. This was especially prevalent in patients with underlying chronic viral hepatitis. However, the latter drug is rarely used in de novo transplant recipients since it was replaced by MMF in the 1990s. Currently, asymptomatic transaminitis is seen on occasion related to either statin therapy for dyslipidemia or rarely, amlodipine for hypertension and typically resolves promptly on discontinuation of the offending agent. Hepatotoxicity has also been associated with the use of calcineurin inhibitors therapy, often although not always, associated with toxic blood levels.

Peptic Ulcer Disease After Transplantation

Peptic ulcer disease is a common complication after transplantation and is related to stress, immunotherapy, and, to a lesser extent, helicobacter infection. The incidence has been reported to be as high as 40% in a single center study of 465 kidney recipients over a decade [44]. In this report, the most frequent types of peptic ulcer disease were gastritis, gastric ulcer, duodenal ulcer, esophagitis, duodenitis, and esophageal ulcer. By multivariate analysis, the use of methylprednisolone pulse therapy and history of pretransplant peptic ulcer disease were independent risk factors for posttransplant peptic ulcer disease. The provision of prophylaxis against peptic ulceration has been the standard of care for more than two decades based on clinical acumen in the absence of clinical trial data.

Cosmetic Complications of Transplantation

This chapter concludes with a collection of relatively minor complications (summarized in Table 8.8) that can still impact on patient wellbeing and in some circumstances can lead to noncompliance and rejection. The term "cosmetic complication" is not intended to diminish the symptoms that are experienced by our patients. Indeed, in a prospective cohort study, 80% of surveyed patients reported immunosuppression-induced hirsutism, gingival hyperplasia, acne, alopecia, or Cushingoid facies [45]. Interestingly, the patient-reported incidence of physical changes significantly exceeded observations by health care professionals for every condition. However, 85% of affected patients reported feeling "happy to endure" changes "for the sake of having a transplant." Patients also reported emotional and social effects due to physical changes, an outcome underestimated by transplant

Table 8.8 Cosmetic complications of transplantation

Complication	Relationship
Edema	Drugs
	Dihydropyridine calcium channel blockers
	Sirolimus
	Thiazolidinediones
	Allograft dysfunction
	Proteinuria
	Allograft dysfunction
	Lymphocele
Hypertrichosis	Cyclosporine
Alopecia	Tacrolimus
Gingival hyperplasia	Dihydropyridine calcium channel blockers
	Cyclosporine
Weight gain/Cushingoid appearance	Corticosteroids
Acne	Corticosteroids
	Sirolimus

professionals. Although most physicians believed changes could be addressed, doctors recommended treatment for less than half of the affected patients. When recommended therapy changes were pursued, treatments were effective in the majority of cases.

Mucocutaneous Complications of Transplantation

In addition to the skin cancers previously described, a variety of other skin problems have been described after transplantation. Acne vulgaris is commonly seen after transplantation and previously was attributed to the widespread use of corticosteroids. Newer evidence indicates that cyclosporine is more likely to be associated with acne as compared with tacrolimus. Sirolimus has also been implicated as a cause of a variety of cutaneous problems that include: acne-like eruptions (46%), scalp folliculitis (26%), and hidradenitis suppurativa (12%); mucous membrane disorders, including aphthous ulceration (60%), epistaxis (60%), chronic gingivitis (20%), and chronic fissure of the lips (11%); and last, nail disorders including chronic onychopathy (74%) and periungual infections (16%). Such symptoms were of sufficient severity in 7% of the patients that sirolimus was discontinued. Changes in hair growth have been associated with the use of both calcineurin inhibitors although with diametrically opposite results. For example, one of the most common side effects of treatment with cyclosporine is hirsutism. Conversely, up to 30% of women who receive tacrolimus develop alopecia. Gingival hyperplasia has long been associated with use of cyclosporine although not tacrolimus. Specific risk factors include the dose and serum levels of cyclosporine as well as the use of cyclosporine microemulsion. Nifedipine, gingivitis, and plaque have also been implicated as cofactors. Treatment options include antibiotics and withdrawal of cyclosporine under cover of sirolimus. As tacrolimus has become the principal calcineurin inhibitor used, gingival hyperplasia is rarely seen currently.

References

1. Wolfe RA, Ashby VB, Milford EL, Ojo AO, Ettenger RE, Agodoa LY, et al. Comparison of mortality in all patients on dialysis, patients on dialysis awaiting transplantation, and recipients of a first cadaveric transplant. N Engl J Med. 1999;341(23):1725–30.
2. Kasiske BL. Risk factors for accelerated atherosclerosis in renal transplant recipients. Am J Med. 1988;84(6):985–92.
3. Abbott KC, Yuan CM, Taylor AJ, Cruess DF, Agodoa LY. Early renal insufficiency and hospitalized heart disease after renal transplantation in the era of modern immunosuppression. J Am Soc Nephrol. 2003;14(9):2358–65.
4. Simmons EM, Langone A, Sezer MT, Vella JP, Recupero P, Morrow JD, et al. Effect of renal transplantation on biomarkers of inflammation and oxidative stress in end-stage renal disease patients. Transplantation. 2005;79(8):914–9.
5. Vella JP, Cohen DJ. Transplantation NephSAP J Am Soc Nephrol. 2009;8(6):424–503.
6. Pascual J, Zamora J, Galeano C, Royuela A, Quereda C. Steroid avoidance or withdrawal for kidney transplant recipients. Cochrane Database Syst Rev. 2009;(1):CD005632.
7. EBPG Expert Group on Renal Transplantation. European best practice guidelines for renal transplantation. Section IV: Long-term management of the transplant recipient. IV.5.2. Cardiovascular risks. Arterial hypertension. Nephrol Dial Transplant. 2002;17(Suppl 4):25–6.
8. Midtvedt K, Hartmann A, Foss A, Fauchald P, Nordal KP, Rootwelt K, et al. Sustained improvement of renal graft function for two years in hypertensive renal transplant recipients treated with nifedipine as compared to lisinopril. Transplantation. 2001;72(11):1787–92.
9. Suwelack B, Kobelt V, Erfmann M, Hausberg M, Gerhardt U, Rahn KH, et al. Long-term follow-up of ACE-inhibitor versus beta-blocker treatment and their effects on blood pressure and kidney function in renal transplant recipients. Transpl Int. 2003;16(5):313–20.
10. Holdaas H, Fellstrom B, Cole E, Nyberg G, Olsson AG, Pedersen TR, et al. Long-term cardiac outcomes in renal transplant recipients receiving fluvastatin: the ALERT extension study. Am J Transplant. 2005;5(12):2929–36.
11. Kasiske BL, Zeier MG, Chapman JR, Craig JC, Ekberg H, Garvey CA, et al. KDIGO clinical practice guideline for the care of kidney transplant recipients: a summary. Kidney Int. 2010;77(4):299–311.
12. Wiesbauer F, Heinze G, Mitterbauer C, Harnoncourt F, Horl WH, Oberbauer R. Statin use is associated with prolonged survival of renal transplant recipients. J Am Soc Nephrol. 2008;19(11):2211–8.
13. Chakkera HA, Weil EJ, Castro J, Heilman RL, Reddy KS, Mazur MJ, et al. Hyperglycemia during the immediate period after kidney transplantation. Clin J Am Soc Nephrol. 2009;4(4):853–9.
14. Rosas SE, Mensah K, Weinstein RB, Bellamy SL, Rader DJ. Coronary artery calcification in renal transplant recipients. Am J Transplant. 2005;5(8):1942–7.
15. Vella JP, Danovitch GD. Transplantation NephSAP. J Am Soc Nephrol. 2008;7(1):6–62.
16. Vella JP, Danovitch GM. Transplantation NephSAP. J Am Soc Nephrol. 2006;5(4):201–75.
17. Hardinger KL, Rhee S, Buchanan P, Koch M, Miller B, Enkvetchakul D, et al. A prospective, randomized, double-blinded comparison of thymoglobulin versus Atgam for induction immunosuppressive therapy: 10-year results. Transplantation. 2008;86(7):947–52.
18. de Fijter JW. Use of proliferation signal inhibitors in non-melanoma skin cancer following renal transplantation. Nephrol Dial Transplant. 2007;22 Suppl 1:i23–6.

19. Campistol JM, Schena FP. Kaposi's sarcoma in renal transplant recipients – the impact of proliferation signal inhibitors. Nephrol Dial Transplant. 2007;22 Suppl 1:i17–22.
20. Swinnen LJ, LeBlanc M, Grogan TM, Gordon LI, Stiff PJ, Miller AM, et al. Prospective study of sequential reduction in immunosuppression, interferon alpha-2B, and chemotherapy for posttransplantation lymphoproliferative disorder. Transplantation. 2008;86(2):215–22.
21. Trappe R, Riess H, Babel N, Hummel M, Lehmkuhl H, Jonas S, et al. Salvage chemotherapy for refractory and relapsed posttransplant lymphoproliferative disorders (PTLD) after treatment with single-agent rituximab. Transplantation. 2007;83(7):912–8.
22. Lorenz M, Kletzmayr J, Perschl A, Furrer A, Horl WH, Sunder-Plassmann G. Anemia and iron deficiencies among long-term renal transplant recipients. J Am Soc Nephrol. 2002;13(3): 794–7.
23. Winkelmayer WC, Kewalramani R, Rutstein M, Gabardi S, Vonvisger T, Chandraker A. Pharmacoepidemiology of anemia in kidney transplant recipients. J Am Soc Nephrol. 2004;15(5):1347–52.
24. Karras A, Thervet E, Legendre C. Hemophagocytic syndrome in renal transplant recipients: report of 17 cases and review of literature. Transplantation. 2004;77(2):238–43.
25. Rigatto C, Foley R, Jeffery J, Negrijn C, Tribula C, Parfrey P. Electrocardiographic left ventricular hypertrophy in renal transplant recipients: prognostic value and impact of blood pressure and anemia. J Am Soc Nephrol. 2003;14(2):462–8.
26. Vlahakos DV, Marathias KP, Agroyannis B, Madias NE. Posttransplant erythrocytosis. Kidney Int. 2003;63(4):1187–94.
27. Gupta M, Miller BA, Ahsan N, Ulsh PJ, Zhang MY, Cheung JY, et al. Expression of angiotensin II type I receptor on erythroid progenitors of patients with post transplant erythrocytosis. Transplantation. 2000;70(8):1188–94.
28. Yildiz A, Cine N, Akkaya V, Sahin S, Ismailoglu V, Turk S, et al. Comparison of the effects of enalapril and losartan on posttransplantation erythrocytosis in renal transplant recipients: prospective randomized study. Transplantation. 2001;72(3):542–4.
29. EBPG Expert Group on Renal Transplantation. European best practice guidelines for renal transplantation. Section IV: Long-term management of the transplant recipient. IV.9.2. Haematological complications. Leukopenia. Nephrol Dial Transplant. 2002;17(Suppl 4):49.
30. Halloran P, Mathew T, Tomlanovich S, Groth C, Hooftman L, Barker C. Mycophenolate mofetil in renal allograft recipients: a pooled efficacy analysis of three randomized, double-blind, clinical studies in prevention of rejection. The International Mycophenolate Mofetil Renal Transplant Study Groups [erratum appears in Transplantation. 1997;63(4):618]. Transplantation. 1997;63(1):39–47.
31. Rerolle JP, Szelag JC, Le Meur Y. Unexpected rate of severe leucopenia with the association of mycophenolate mofetil and valganciclovir in kidney transplant recipients. Nephrol Dial Transplant. 2007;22(2):671–2.
32. Borchhardt K, Sulzbacher I, Benesch T, Fodinger M, Sunder-Plassmann G, Haas M. Low-turnover bone disease in hypercalcemic hyperparathyroidism after kidney transplantation. Am J Transplant. 2007;7(11):2515–21.
33. Akaberi S, Simonsen O, Lindergard B, Nyberg G. Can DXA predict fractures in renal transplant patients? Am J Transplant. 2008;8(12):2647–51.
34. Kruse AE, Eisenberger U, Frey FJ, Mohaupt MG. Effect of cinacalcet cessation in renal transplant recipients with persistent hyperparathyroidism. Nephrol Dial Transplant. 2007;22(8):2362–5.
35. Rudser KD, de Boer IH, Dooley A, Young B, Kestenbaum B. Fracture risk after parathyroidectomy among chronic hemodialysis patients. J Am Soc Nephrol. 2007;18(8):2401–7.
36. Chou FF, Hsieh KC, Chen YT, Lee CT. Parathyroidectomy followed by kidney transplantation can improve bone mineral density in patients with secondary hyperparathyroidism. Transplantation. 2008;86(4):554–7.
37. Tillmann FP, Jager M, Blondin D, Oels M, Rump LC, Grabensee B, et al. Post-transplant distal limb syndrome: clinical diagnosis and long-term outcome in 37 renal transplant recipients. Transpl Int. 2008;21(6):547–53.

38. van der Linden PD, Sturkenboom MC, Herings RM, Leufkens HM, Rowlands S, Stricker BH. Increased risk of achilles tendon rupture with quinolone antibacterial use, especially in elderly patients taking oral corticosteroids. Arch Intern Med. 2003;163(15):1801–7.
39. Jowsey SG, Taylor ML, Schneekloth TD, Clark MM. Psychosocial challenges in transplantation. J Psychiatr Pract. 2001;7(6):404–14.
40. Vella JP, Sayegh MH. Interactions between cyclosporine and newer antidepressant medications. Am J Kidney Dis. 1998;31(2):320–3.
41. Kurella M, Kimmel PL, Young BS, Chertow GM. Suicide in the United States end-stage renal disease program. J Am Soc Nephrol. 2005;16(3):774–81.
42. Bunzel B, Laederach-Hofmann K. Solid organ transplantation: are there predictors for post-transplant noncompliance? A literature overview. Transplantation. 2000;70(5):711–6.
43. Bunnapradist S, Lentine KL, Burroughs TE, Pinsky BW, Hardinger KL, Brennan DC, et al. Mycophenolate mofetil dose reductions and discontinuations after gastrointestinal complications are associated with renal transplant graft failure. Transplantation. 2006;82(1):102–7.
44. Chen KJ, Chen CH, Cheng CH, Wu MJ, Shu KH. Risk factors for peptic ulcer disease in renal transplant patients – 11 years of experience from a single center. Clin Nephrol. 2004;62(1):14–20.
45. Peters TG, Spinola KN, West JC, Aeder MI, Danovitch GM, Klintmalm GB, et al. Differences in patient and transplant professional perceptions of immunosuppression-induced cosmetic side effects. Transplantation. 2004;78(4):537–43.

Chapter 9
Infectious Complications in Renal Transplant Recipients

Erik R. Dubberke and Daniel C. Brennan

Abstract Despite improved outcomes in kidney transplant patients over the years, infectious complications remain a significant cause of morbidity and mortality in this population. Infection is now more common than acute rejection and associated with poor graft and patient outcomes. Several studies have shown that allograft and patient survival were reduced at 1 and 3 years after transplantation in recipients with infection and febrile episodes, and even in the current era infection remains the third largest cause of death in renal transplant recipients. Approximately two-thirds of renal transplant recipients will experience an infectious-related complication in the first year after transplantation and approximately 20% eventually will die from infection. These alarming rates reflect the overall or "net state" of immunosuppression associated with end-stage renal disease (ESRD) and transplantation as well as donor and environmental exposures. In addition, the robustness of a recipient's immune system depends on several factors including age, nutrition, and comorbid conditions.

Keywords Polyoma virus BK • Cytomegalovirus • Hepatitis C • Fungal infections • Mycobacterium

Introduction

Despite improved outcomes in kidney transplant patients over the years, infectious complications remain a significant cause of morbidity and mortality in this population. Infection is now more common than acute rejection and associated with poor graft

---

E.R. Dubberke, MD, MSPH
Department of Medicine, Washington University School of Medicine, St. Louis, MO, USA

D.C. Brennan, MD (✉)
Department of Internal Medicine, Renal Division, Washington University in St. Louis, 660 S. Euclid Avenue, St. Louis, MO 63110, USA
e-mail: Brenan@wdosis.wustl.edu

A. Chandraker et al. (eds.), *Core Concepts in Renal Transplantation*,
DOI 10.1007/978-1-4614-0008-0_9, © Springer Science+Business Media, LLC 2012

and patient outcomes [1]. Approximately two-thirds of renal transplant recipients will experience an infectious-related complication in the first year after transplantation, and approximately 20% eventually will die from infection [2]. These alarming rates reflect the overall or "net state" of immunosuppression associated with end-stage renal disease (ESRD) and transplantation as well as donor and environmental exposures [3]. In addition, the robustness of a recipient's immune system depends on several factors including age, nutrition, and comorbid conditions.

Increasing age, diabetes, malnourishment from ESRD, uremia, and the dialysis procedure itself are all immunosuppressive [4]. Thus, the immunosuppressed state begins pre-transplantation. Renal transplant recipients may develop infections due to immunomodulatory infectious agents such as cytomegalovirus (CMV) and hepatitis C virus (HCV) which can cause disease and predispose to other opportunistic infections. The intensity of the immunosuppressive regimen contributes significantly to the net state of immunosuppression. Finally, all individuals are exposed constantly to infection in the community and increasingly more resistant organisms in the hospital environment.

Pre-Transplant Evaluation

The pre-transplant evaluation begins with a detailed history and physical examination. The goal is to assess for conditions or exposures that predispose the candidate to future complications, particularly infections, which require treatment or prophylaxis. The evaluation process is a comprehensive overview to uncover past exposures, including childhood illnesses with attention to viral infections and mononucleosis, endemic infections like coccidioidomycosis or histoplasmosis, and sexually transmitted infections such as hepatitis B (HBV), human immunodeficiency virus (HIV), human papillomavirus (HPV), syphilis, and herpes. Occupational and pet exposures as well as consumption of well water are also queried. The medical history also includes an extensive review of systems to determine the presence of any active infectious disease or predisposing risk factors. These include a history of dental caries, sinusitis, chronic obstructive pulmonary disease (COPD), tuberculosis (TB) or a positive purified protein derivative (PPD), valvular heart disease, diverticulosis, hepatitis, urinary tract infections (UTI), prostatitis, diabetes mellitus (diabetes), blood transfusions, and alcohol or drug abuse. Pre-transplant screening studies for occult and latent infections are listed in Table 9.1, and appropriate evaluation and treatment of positive studies are necessary prior to transplantation.

Patients on immunosuppressive medications as treatment for their primary renal disease will be predisposed to infectious complications and recurrence of their disease post-transplantation. Pre-transplant nephrectomy may be necessary for infected nephrolithiasis, polycystic kidney disease, or reflux nephropathy.

An immunization history is obtained and pre-transplant vaccinations should include tetanus, diphtheria, pertussis, inactivated polio, influenza, pneumococcus [5], HBV, hepatitis A, and *Hemophilus influenza* type b [6]. Live vaccines for measles and varicella should be given several months prior to transplantation. The varicella vaccine is safe and effective in pediatric transplant patients [7] and should be

Table 9.1 Pre-transplant screening

Serologies
Cytomegalovirus
Epstein-Barr virus
Varicella-zoster virus
Herpes simplex 1 and 2 viruses
Hepatitis A, B, and C viruses
Human immunodeficiency virus
Rapid plasma reagin
Endemic fungi
Tuberculin skin test
Urinalysis with culture
Pelvic or prostate exam
Chest radiogram
Dental evaluation
Tests to consider
Endemic fungi
Trypabosoma cruzi
Toxoplasma serology
Human T-cell leukemia virus
Gallbladder ultrasound
Stool culture
Stool ova and parasite

considered for adults without a history of chickenpox or who have a negative varicella zoster virus (VZV) titer prior to transplant. Currently there is insufficient data on whether the zoster vaccine is safe and effective in solid organ transplant recipients.

Donor-Related Infectious Disease

Plausible reports of organ transmission through kidney transplants of infectious organisms have been described for a number of agents, including HIV, CMV, herpes simplex virus (HSV), rabies virus, HBV, the delta agent (HDV), HCV, adenovirus, West Nile virus (WNV), polyoma viruses BK and JC, rabies, lymphocytic choriomeningitis virus (LCMV), bacteria, fungi (histoplasma, *Cryptococcus*, *Candida*), monosporium, mycobacteria (TB and atypical mycobacteria), malaria, toxoplasma, trypanosoma, and strongyloides [8]. All donors require screening for HIV 1 and 2, human T-cell leukemia (HTLV), hepatitis A, B, and C, CMV, Epstein-Barr virus (EBV), HSV, VZV, syphilis, and *Toxoplasma gondii* which can be transmitted from donor to recipient. Donors should have screening urinalysis and urine cultures. Cadaveric donors should have screening blood cultures especially when there has been a prolonged hospitalization prior to donation. Screening of living donors should occur as close to time of transplant as reasonably possible. If an extended period of time has passed from when the donor screening originally occurred, screening should be repeated for pathogens for which the donor was originally negative.

Viral infections transmitted from donor to recipient may cause primary infection, disseminated disease, and viral associated cancer such as post-transplantation

Table 9.2 Human herpes viruses and associated diseases

Virus	Disease
HHV-1: Herpes simplex 1 (HSV 1)	Herpes labialis
HHV-2: Herpes simplex 2 (HSV 2)	Herpes genitalis
HHV-3: Varicella zoster virus (VZV)	Chicken pox
	Shingles
HHV-4: Epstein-Barr virus	Mononucleosis
	Burkitt's lymphoma
	Nasopharyngeal carcinoma
	Post-transplant lymphoproliferative disorder (PTLD)
	Oral hairy leukoplakia
HHV-5: Cytomegalovirus (CMV)	Cytomegalovirus disease
	Salivary gland virus disease
HHV-6: Human herpes virus 6	Roseola subitum
HHV-7: Human herpes virus 7	Roseola subitum
	Pityriasis rosea
HHV-8: Human herpes virus 8	Kaposi's sarcoma
	Effusion lymphoma
	Multifocal Castleman's disease

lymphoproliferative disease (PTLD) from EBV or Kaposi's sarcoma (KS) from human herpes virus (HHV) 8 (Table 9.2). HIV remains a contraindication to organ donation. Similarly, donor seropositivity for HBV as evidenced by HBV surface antigen (HBsAg) positivity is a contraindication to organ donation. The risk of transmission of HBV to kidney recipients from donors with evidence of prior HBV infection with core antibody positive but surface antigen negative (HBcAb+, HBsAg–) is low and is only a relative contraindication to transplantation, however, recipients who are HBcAb+, HBsAb– are at risk for reactivation [9]. Transplantation of HCV donor seropositive (D+) kidneys into recipients who are HCV seronegative (R–) has been associated with post-transplant liver disease and increased mortality and is generally avoided. Transplantation of HCV D+ into recipients who are seropositive (R+) is controversial but does not appear to effect short-term graft survival or mortality [10]. In general, donor seropositivity for HSV, VZV, EBV, HHV 8, or CMV is not a contraindication to donation even when the recipient is seronegative.

Cadaveric donors typically receive a cephalosporin antibiotic during the procurement operation and recipients often receive peri-operative antibiotic prophylaxis [11]. Systemic bacterial infection of a donor is considered a contraindication to transplantation. Other infections such as syphilis, TB, fungal, and other viral infections should be evaluated on a case-by-case basis.

Timing of Post-Transplant Infections

Infections occurring post-transplant can be divided into three time frames: the first month, the second through sixth month, and beyond 6 months (Table 9.3). Recipients are susceptible to certain infections in each period because of the different levels of

Table 9.3 Timetable of infections after renal transplantation

Time after transplantation	Infection
0–1 month	Wound infections
	Line sepsis
	Urinary tract infections
	Pneumonia
	Herpesviruses
	Oral Candidiasis
1–6 months	Polyoma virus
	Cytomegalovirus
	Pneumocystis carinii
	Aspergillus fumigatus
	Candida species
	Nocardia species
	Toxoplasma gondii
	Listeria monocytogenes
	Hepatitis B and C
	Histoplasmosis
	Coccidioidomycosis
Beyond 6 months	Community infections
	Cytomegalovirus retinitis
	Cryptococcus
	Polyoma virus
	Mycobacteria

Table 9.4 Prophylaxis in transplant patients

Infection	Prophylaxis
Wound infections	Perioperative antibiotics
Oral candidiasis	Clotrimazole or nystatin
Cytomegalovirus	Ganciclovir or valganciclovir
Herpes simplex viruses	Acyclovir
Pneumocystis carinii	TMP-SMX,[a] dapsone, pentamidine
Urinary tract infections	TMP-SMX,[a] ciprofloxacin
Varicella zoster virus	Zoster immune globulin, acyclovir

[a]Trimethoprim-sulfamethoxazole

immunosuppression and environmental exposures. However, some infectious agents may shift out of their typical time frame with a change in antirejection medications or preemptive and prophylactic antimicrobials (Table 9.4).

The infectious risk during the first month is primarily nosocomial and related to the surgical procedure and the initial hospitalization, and only occasionally due to occult infections present in the recipient prior to transplantation. Reduction in post-surgical risk of infection relies on the technical skill of the surgical team and early removal of foreign bodies such as endotracheal tubes, vascular access lines, drainage tubes, and catheters. Reverse isolation or the use of gowns, gloves, and masks for those having contact with the patient is also not warranted even when the patient is neutropenic [12].

The classical mnemonic (the 5W's) for evaluation of fever in any surgical patient: wind, wound, water, walking, wonder drugs, is germane for the kidney transplant recipient. These patients are at risk for conventional bacterial pneumonia from atelectasis; bacterial and candidal wound infection – particularly when fat necrosis occurs or when hematomas, seromas, urinomas, or lymphoceles are present; and UTIs associated with indwelling urinary catheters. Good pulmonary toilet and early ambulation reduce the risk of pneumonia. The prophylactic use of double-strength trimethoprim/sulfamethoxazole (TMP-SMX 320/1,600 mg) orally (PO) regardless of the serum creatinine while the bladder catheter remains in place has reduced the risk of bacterial UTI to <10% and the risk of blood stream infections by tenfold [13]. The optimal duration and dose of continued prophylaxis are unknown. Because of its protection against multiple opportunistic infections (see below), we continue TMP-SMX prophylaxis for life in non-allergic patients, although many centers only continue such prophylactic therapy for the first 6–12 months post-transplant year.

HSV 1 and 2, and HHV-6 may be reactivated in the first month. Less commonly VZV, EBV, and CMV in the recipient also may reactivate early. New or primary viral infection from the donor generally does not become symptomatic until after the first month. Oral ganciclovir and valganciclovir are highly effective for preventing most herpes virus infections including HSV 1 and 2, VZV, EBV, CMV, and possibly HHV-6 but not HHV-7 [14, 15].

The second to the sixth-month post-transplantation is the period when transplant-related opportunistic infections are most likely to arise. These infections include CMV, *Pneumocystis jieroveci* (formerly *carinii*), *Aspergillus* species, *Candida* species, *Cryptococcus neoformans*, *Nocardia* species, *T. gondii*, and *Listeria monocytogenes*. Reactivation of quiescent donor and recipient infections also occur such as CMV, HBV, HCV, HHV 8, polyoma virus (BK), mycobacterium, histoplasmosis, and coccidioidomycosis.

By 6 months most transplant programs have significantly tapered immunosuppression to a relatively low basal state, and the profound immunosuppressive effects of antilymphocyte induction therapy are less as well. Thus, historically after 6 months most patients suffer from the same infections seen in the general community including recurrent cold sores, influenza, UTIs, diarrhea, and pneumococcal pneumonia. There are a few exceptions to this general rule. CMV retinitis tends to occur late and may occur contemporaneously with reactivation of other herpes infections including EBV, HSV, and VZV [16]. The presence of herpes or zosteriform lesions may be sentinel lesions for CMV [16]. Another exception to this general rule is that some patients develop acquired immunoglobulin deficiencies post-transplantation. These may develop from immunosuppression, CMV infection, or vitamin B12 deficiency and especially predispose the patients to recurrent infections with encapsulated organisms [17]. Finally, the time course of infections described above reflects the state of transplantation from approximately 1985–1995.

Beyond the sixth month, there is increased risk of opportunistic infections in patients with poor allograft function and those with repeated episodes of acute rejection requiring increased immunosuppressive therapy. In these patients, the recovery of the immune system from the antilymphocyte agents over the first 3–6 months does not occur. Instead, it may be replaced by a continuous and prolonged increase in the net state of immunosuppression from the combination and higher levels of these immunosuppressive medications. The combination of tacrolimus and MMF being more immunosuppressive, than previous immunosuppressive regimens. Finally, episodes of acute rejection and chronic rejection are treated by increasing the net state of immunosuppression further predisposing patients to opportunistic infections.

Evaluation of Fever in the Renal Transplant Recipient

The presence of fever in the transplant recipient may represent a broad range of conditions including infection and rejection. Fever early after transplantation along with an acute decline in kidney function and graft tenderness suggests rejection rather than infection [18]. The presenting signs and symptoms of infection may be unusual because of the use of immunosuppression. An aggressive approach to diagnosis is appropriate because of the differences in treatment and potential morbidity. Cultures of urine and blood and a chest radiograph (CXR) are obtained. A blood specimen is sent for detection of CMV by polymerase chain reaction (PCR) for those patients at risk. Clues from the history, physical, and environmental exposures help direct the investigation. Empirical broad-spectrum antimicrobial therapy is initiated early, prior to the determination of a specific etiology. A more aggressive evaluation is pursued when there is an inadequate response to treatment or failure to identify an etiologic agent. The likelihood of *P. jieroveci* (formally *P. carinii*) pneumonia (PCP) is low in patients without a recent history of CMV or in patients compliant with TMP-SMX prophylaxis; so bronchoscopy with lavage and biopsy are not usually necessary.

For outpatient therapy, a fluoroquinolone can be used. The dose should be reduced for those fluoroquinolones that are renally excreted since the glomerular filtration rate (GFR) for most transplant patients does not exceed 50 mL/min. Alternatively, oral azithromycin 500 mg PO on day 1 followed by 250 mg PO daily for 4 days can be initiated. Ciprofloxacin has mild effects on cyclosporine and tacrolimus metabolism that can usually be monitored. Achilles tendonitis and tendon ruptures have been reported in renal transplant patients taking fluoroquinolone antibiotics [19]. Although azithromycin is a macrolide antibiotic, it does not inhibit the cytochrome P450 IIIa enzyme system and does not increase cyclosporine and tacrolimus levels like other macrolide antibiotics such as erythromycin and clarithromycin. For patients who require hospitalization, we typically use vancomycin and ceftazidime or cefepime for the first 48–72 h pending the identification of a specific infectious agent.

Bacterial Infections

Over 50% of renal transplant recipients will experience a bacterial infection within the first year. The major sites of infection include the urinary tract, blood stream, and lungs, as well as surgical site infections in the first month after transplant. Renal transplant recipients are also at increased risk for bacterial infections that otherwise occur in non-immunosuppressed patients and bacterial infections rarely seen in non-immunosuppressed patient.

Urinary Tract Infections

The incidence of UTI in patients who are not receiving antimicrobial prophylaxis has been reported to vary from 35 to 79% [20]. Beyond 3 months after transplantation, the incidence of UTI decreases progressively. Risk factors include pre-transplantation UTI, a prolonged period of postoperative hemodialysis, polycystic kidney disease, diabetes, prolonged postoperative bladder catheterization, immunosuppression, allograft trauma, and technical complications associated with ureteral anastomosis [20] and being a female recipient. Typical pathogens include *Klebsiella*, *Escherichia coli*, *Proteus*, *Enterococci*, *Enterobacter*, *Staphylococci*, *Pseudomonas*, and rarely *Corynebacterium*. Recurrent infections should be investigated with ultrasound or computed tomography to rule out abscess or other nidus of infection.

Prophylactic antimicrobial therapy is now universally used and is maintained for a minimum of 6–12 months following kidney transplantation with either ciprofloxacin and TMP-SMX, TMP-SMX offering the additional advantage of preventing PCP pneumonia.

Septicemia

The urinary tract is the most common source of septicemia, followed by the lungs, the wound site, and the abdomen [21]. Most cases occur within the first 6 months after transplantation. Poor prognostic factors for survival included persistent septicemia beyond 7 days, pulmonary portal of entry, leucopenia (WBC ≤ 3,000), metastatic abscesses, acute respiratory failure, and shock. There is an increased incidence of hospitalizations for septicemia in patients with diabetes, urologic disease, female gender, delayed graft function, rejection, and pre-transplantation dialysis.

Wound Infections

Early reports of surgical wound infections (SWI) described a rate of 14–34% with a subsequent decline to 3–4% [22]. The declining incidence of postoperative wound infections over the years is likely multifactorial. Intraoperative antibiotic bladder irrigation, perioperative antibiotics, and meticulous surgical techniques avoiding hematoma, seroma, and urinoma are important preventative measures. The most significant risk factors for wound infections are obesity, urine leak, reoperation through the transplant incision, diabetes, and use of MMF as opposed to AZA.

Legionellosis

Legionella pneumophilia is the most common *Legionella* species causing infection in renal transplant recipients. It usually presents as pneumonia with a peripheral patchy infiltrate on CXR that may progress to consolidation. *Legionella* is frequently associated with epidemics and has been linked to drinking water, contaminated respiratory equipment, and heating and air conditioning ventilation systems. In patients hospitalized with pneumonia at risk for legionellosis, the first tests are a urine *Legionella* antigen and culture with selective media. Direct fluorescent antibody (DFA) testing of sputum or broncheoalveolar lavage specimens is rapid and specific but technically difficult [23]. Azithromycin is the antibiotic of choice for *Legionella* because it does not interfere with cyclosporine or tacrolimus metabolism. Doxycycline, TMP-SMX, and rifampin (RIF) also have activity against *Legionella* but RIF increases cytochrome P450 activity and drastically reduces cyclosporine and tacrolimus levels.

Nocardiosis

Nocardia species are ubiquitous in the environment. Pulmonary infections are most commonly caused by *N. asteroids*, and *N. brasiliensis* is the most common cause of progressive cutaneous or lymphoreticular (sporotricoid) disease. Pulmonary disease is the most common presentation. The infection typically begins in the lungs and then may disseminate in up to 50% of patients usually to the central nervous system (CNS) or subcutaneous tissue. The most common presentation is pulmonary nodules on CXR that may cavitate or form abscesses. CNS involvement is common and all patients with a diagnosis of *Nocardia* require that CNS involvement be excluded [24]. Diagnosis is presumptive with the find of long, narrow, branching, Gram-positive filamentous organisms on Gram stain and confirmed with culture. The treatment of choice is TMP-SMX to prevent relapses; a long duration of therapy is necessary with recommendations that vary up to 1 year.

Listeriosis

L. monocytogenes is found naturally in soil and water and may contaminate raw foods including dairy products, vegetables, and meats. Infections historically have been most common during the first 2 months post-transplantation and most commonly during the months of July to October. The portal of entry is the gastrointestinal tract (GI) and patients may present with gastroenteritis or CNS infection. Listerial meningitis has been associated with a 33% fatality rate [25]. Examination of the cerebrospinal fluid (CSF) shows a predominance of monocytes with a relatively low glucose content and Gram-positive bacilli. The absence of bacteria in the CSF is actually more common and the exam should be repeated in 1–2 days. Intravenous (IV) ampicillin is the treatment of choice, but TMP-SMX is also effective for treatment.

Viral Infections

Infections with the herpes virus group followed by hepatitic infections are the most common and most concerning viral infections encountered in renal transplantation. Other viruses of concern include adenoviruses, respiratory syncytial virus (RSV), influenza virus, and polyoma viruses.

Herpes Virus Infections

There are currently eight HHV identified. All are fairly ubiquitous and characterized by development of a latent state that may be reactivated with stress or immunosuppression.

Herpes Simplex Virus

Human simplex virus (HSV) occurs as types 1 and 2. Type 1 is commonly associated with herpes labialis and type 2 is more often associated with herpes genitalis. However, both types may be cultured from either location. Up to 66% of adults have evidence of prior infection with HSV. After acute infection the virus remains latent in the sensory nerve ganglia. Reactivation may occur within the first month after transplantation and most commonly presents as mild ulcer-like mucocutaneous lesions but may cause zosteriform lesions or other skin lesions. HSV esophagitis may cause dysphagia and mimic candidiasis. Less commonly HSV can cause pneumonitis, hepatitis, encephalitis, nephritis, and rarely disseminated disease. Diagnosis is made by demonstration of multinucleated giant cells on a Tzanck test, culture, PCR for HSV DNA, or DFA. PCR for HSV DNA in the CSF is the preferred test for CNS infection. The standard therapy for mucocutaneous lesions is acyclovir 200 mg PO 4–5 times/day. Valacyclovir and famciclovir are alternatives with less frequent dosing schedules. More serious cases may require treatment with IV acyclovir 5–15 mg/kg every 8 h adjusted for renal function as needed. Patients who do not respond to treatment after 1 week or who develop new lesions while on therapy require the virus be isolated for antibiotic susceptibilities. Immunosuppressed patients are about 10 times more likely to have resistant HSV that requires treatment with foscarnet or cidofovir [26].

Varicella-Zoster Virus

Over 90% of adults have prior evidence of infection with VZV. Reactivation causes shingles or zoster in a dermatomal distribution. However, dermatomal pain without cutaneous manifestations occurs. The appearance of dermatomal vesicular lesions is usually enough to make the diagnosis and it can be confirmed with the finding of multinucleated giant cells on Tzanck smear, PCR, and DFA. The cutaneous lesions may act as a portal of entry for secondary bacterial or fungal infections. Primary infection in the remaining 10% may present as skin lesions, pneumonia, encephalitis, pancreatitis, hepatitis, or disseminated intravascular coagulation and has a high mortality rate.

Treatment for zoster is a 7-day course of either acyclovir 800 mg PO 5 times/day, famciclovir 500 mg PO 3 times daily, or valacyclovir 1,000 mg PO 3 times daily. Renal transplant recipients with primary VZV or disseminated zoster should receive acyclovir 10 mg/kg every 8 h for 7 days. These patients must be placed in negative pressure isolation until all lesions crust over to prevent spread to non-immune patients and healthcare providers. For seronegative patients with exposure to chicken pox or VZV, varicella immunoglobulin should be administered within 72 h (where available) and acyclovir 200 mg PO 5 times/day begun. A minority of patients will develop post-herpetic neuralgia, although immunosuppression is not a risk factor [27]. Multiple agents, including gabapentin, tricyclic antidepressants such as amitriptyline, narcotics, pregabalin, tramadol, topical lidocaine, and topical capsaicin, are moderately effective for reducing symptoms [28].

Epstein-Barr Virus

Approximately 95% of the adult population has serologic evidence of previous infection with EBV, and the majority of seronegative recipients seroconvert within the first year after transplantation. EBV may cause a mononucleosis-like syndrome, chronic fatigue, or fever of unknown origin (FUO), but has also been associated with Burkitt's lymphoma, nasopharyngeal carcinoma and in transplant recipients, PTLD. PTLD represent a heterogeneous group of abnormal lymphoid proliferations that occur in the setting of ineffective T-cell function because of pharmacologic immunosuppression after organ transplantation. The majority of PTLD are of B-cell origin and are associated with EBV infection. T-cell PTLD are comparatively rare and less frequently associated with EBV [29]. Increasing immunosuppression augments the rate of EBV reactivation [30]. Levels of EBV by semiquantitative DNA PCR in blood higher than 500 EBV DNA copies/75,000 peripheral blood mononuclear cells were found in all patients with PTLD but in only 7.5% of RTR without that complication [31]. PTLD can be potentially fatal.

Cytomegalovirus

CMV is the most important infectious agent affecting renal transplant recipients and is a significant cause of increased morbidity and mortality in this population.

CMV infection occurs in up to 80% of all renal transplant recipients [32], while disease occurs in only 8–32% [33]. The wide range in the incidence of infection and disease results from varying intensities of immunosuppression used and the frequency and methods used to monitor CMV infection. Infections can occur as primary infections in a seronegative patient or as reactivation of a latent virus or re-infection in a seropositive patient. New infections can be acquired from the community, CMV positive blood products, or a CMV positive donor kidney. Infection may progress to disease with a wide variety of end organ involvement. Symptomatic disease can present as a CMV syndrome of fever, leukopenia, thrombocytopenia, and elevated liver enzymes. Severe disease can involve the lungs, liver, GI, pancreas, kidneys, lower urinary tract, heart, eyes, and skin. CMV has been implicated as a cause of acute and chronic graft dysfunction as well as long-term graft loss. CMV has been associated with atherosclerosis including coronary artery restenosis and renal artery stenosis. Finally, CMV is able to suppress the immune response and predisposes to co-infections with other viruses, bacteria, and fungi. Risk factors for CMV disease include antilymphocyte therapy for induction or rejection treatment, active infection with other herpesviruses, high-dose steroids, high-dose mycophenolate mofetil, and CMV sero-mismatch.

The incidence and severity of CMV disease has been most strongly associated with the CMV serostatus of the kidney donor and recipient. Concern has mainly focused on avoiding CMV infection in the CMV D+/R– group because this group has historically been at greatest risk for severe primary infection during the first 3 months post-transplant. Although the incidence of infection is similar between D+/R– and D+/R+, the D+/R+ patients only experience about half the number of symptomatic infections. Rapid and accurate diagnosis of CMV is important because of its increased morbidity. Newer techniques include shell vial, pp65 antigenemia, and nucleic acid detection assays including PCR of RNA and DNA, hybrid capture assay, branched DNA assay, and nucleic acid sequence-based amplification. In addition to a rapid result, these assays provide a quantitative measure of viral burden that allows for diagnosis, therapeutic monitoring, and assessment of new medications and treatment protocols. Molecular tests for diagnosis of CMV are considered most appropriate as they are rapid, quantitative, and can be performed on stored samples [34].

Multiple strategies have been used to reduce the morbidity and mortality of CMV infection and its associated costs. Universal prophylaxis refers to giving prophylactic therapy to all renal transplant patients regardless of their CMV serostatus. Selected prophylaxis refers to giving prophylaxis to patients at high risk for CMV, namely the D+/R– category. The preemptive approach treats asymptomatic CMV infection in an effort to prevent CMV disease, and the deferred approach treats active CMV disease. Each approach has its advantages and disadvantages and there is no consensus on the best approach to use.

Prophylactic therapy is very effective in reducing CMV disease in high-risk patients such as D+/R– patients receiving antilymphocyte therapy [35]. The evidence for benefit in low-risk patients and in patients not receiving antilymphocyte therapy is established but not as strong [14, 36]. Although CMV hyperimmune globulin, acyclovir, valacyclovir, ganciclovir, and valganciclovir have all been found to be effective at preventing CMV disease, ganciclovir and valganciclovir are superior [35, 37]. A concern with the prophylactic strategy is 20–30% of high-risk patients go on to develop late onset CMV disease after the prophylaxis is stopped, and the incidence of ganciclovir-resistance may be higher in those who receive prophylaxis. Since CMV infection occurs in 66–88% of D+/R– patients, critics of the universal prophylactic approach claim that it exposes a significant proportion of patients who would never have developed disease to a prolonged course of antiviral therapy that may have side effects, encourage viral resistance, is costly, and may be only delaying the disease [14, 38–40].

A number of studies have shown that prophylactic treatment of CMV with ganciclovir delays the onset of CMV infections, reduces CMV infections, reduces severity of CMV disease, decreases acute rejection episodes, improves graft survival, and reduces steroid-resistant rejection [35, 37, 41, 42]. It further suggests that prolonged prophylaxis for 6 months to 1 year may be necessary when the donor is seropositive.

Valganciclovir is a valyl-ester prodrug of oral ganciclovir, and has a bioavailability of nearly 70% (compared to 7% for oral ganciclovir) and at doses of 450–900 mg produces ganciclovir levels that are similar to IV administration of ganciclovir at 2.5–5 mg/kg [43, 44]. In one study 372 CMV D+/R– solid organ transplant recipients were randomized 2:1 to receive oral valganciclovir 900 mg/day or oral ganciclovir 1,000 mg 3 times/day with dose adjustments for renal insufficiency for 100 days as prophylaxis for CMV [43]. During prophylaxis only 0.8 and 1.6% of the patients developed CMV disease. Thus, this study did not show a significant difference between valganciclovir compared to oral ganciclovir.

Preemptive therapy of CMV infection involves serial monitoring for CMV viremia and starting treatment before the development of signs or symptoms of disease. This method avoids complications and cost of drug therapy in low-risk patients and initiates treatment early to lessen symptomatic disease in high-risk patients. The preemptive approach appears to be equivalent to the prophylactic approach for preventing CMV disease, but the preemptive approach may be associated with a decrease in the development of late CMV disease [45, 46]. The major limitation of the preemptive approach is the need to perform frequent determinations of CMV viremia, and this may not always be feasible or cost-effective [45, 46].

Deferred therapy involves waiting for the development of symptomatic CMV disease before starting anti-CMV medication. During CMV disease, MMF or azathioprine doses should be reduced or discontinued. Therapeutic treatment of established CMV disease is primarily with the anti-viral agent ganciclovir given intravenously. There is accumulating data that valganciclovir, which is approved for prophylaxis of CMV may also be effective for treatment and may be given orally. Typical treatment is ganciclovir 5 mg/kg IV every 12 h or valganciclovir 900 mg orally twice daily for 2–3 weeks although longer courses may be necessary. Dose and duration adjustments are necessary because of its renal excretion. The addition of hyperimmune globulin may be beneficial for patients with organ involvement.

Foscarnet and cidofovir may also be used, however, their use is limited by nephrotoxicity. DNA PCR can be used to evaluate response to treatment [47]. When using a quantitative CMV DNA assay, predictors of CMV relapse were higher median pretreatment viral loads and persistent detectable viral DNA after treatment with IV ganciclovir [48]. Inadequate response could indicate ganciclovir resistance necessitating further evaluation and foscarnet therapy. In addition, co-infections with CMV are not uncommon and should be considered.

Ganciclovir Resistance

Ganciclovir resistance is relatively uncommon in kidney transplant recipients. It is postulated that persistent high subclinical CMV levels in the presence of relatively low serum concentrations of oral ganciclovir for a long period of time may lead to the emergence of resistance [38]. It tends to occur after prolonged exposure to ganciclovir, and may lead to serious complications such as allograft loss, progressive allograft dysfunction, rejection, or CMV retinitis. The most common mechanism of resistance is a mutation in the UL97 gene encoding the viral protein kinase. A UL97 mutation confers resistance to ganciclovir, but foscarnet and cidofovir remain active. Isolates with mutations in the UL54 gene that encodes the DNA polymerase can exhibit resistance to ganciclovir, foscarnet, and cidofovir depending on where the mutation is located in the gene [49].

Leflunomide, an immunosuppressant used in the treatment of rheumatoid arthritis, has activity against CMV independent of the actions of the UL97 and UL 54 genes. The exact mechanism of action is not known, but it appears to interfere with virion assembly and has activity against ganciclovir-resistant strains.

Maribavir, a benzimidazole riboside, is a novel antiviral with activity against CMV and EBV that was found to be ineffective as CMV prophylaxis in stem cell and liver transplant recipients. Maribavir is a direct inhibitor of the UL97 kinase and acts independently from the UL54 DNA polymerase. Although maribavir inhibits this kinase, its activity does not appear to be decreased against CMV strains with mutations in the UL97 gene. Maribavir interferes with ganciclovir but may be useful in the treatment of ganciclovir-resistant CMV disease [50].

Human Herpesvirus 6–8

HHV-6 is a beta herpes virus like CMV and causes roseola infantum, or exanthema subitum in children. Most HHV-6 infections are minor, self-limited, febrile illnesses, often followed by a rash. By 2 years of age, 90% of children are infected. However, it remains latent in lymphocytes and is usually benign. In renal transplant recipients, reactivation of HHV-6 is frequent and ranges from 4 to 66%, but this variability is confounded by different diagnostic techniques and population seroprevalence [51]. HHV-6 reactivation is associated with primary and reactivated CMV infections and symptomatic CMV infections Also, HHV-6 infection can present as a CMV-like illness without CMV reactivation. It has been reported to cause hepatitis, encephalitis, and a hemophagocytic syndrome in a renal transplant recipient [52]. Reports of therapy against HHV-6 are limited, but ganciclovir, foscarnet, and cidofovir are potentially effective [53].

HHV-7 is also a beta herpesvirus like CMV and HHV-6. It is ubiquitous and seroprevalence ranges from 60% to over 90%. HHV-7 has been associated with roseola and pityriasis rosea in children. Reactivation in renal transplant patients is common and has been associated with progression to CMV disease and rejection [54]. In general, ganciclovir has minimal in vitro activity against HHV-7 [55] and is ineffective as prophylaxis and of the available agents, cidofovir is the most likely to be effective [55].

Human Herpesvirus 8

HHV-8, a recently discovered herpesvirus, is the cause of KS, multifocal Castleman's disease, and primary effusion lymphoma. Unlike HHV-6 and HHV-7, the seroprevalence in the US is <3% and shows marked geographic variation with seroprevalence >25% in Italy and regions of Africa [56]. Seroconversion of HHV-8 negative patients post-transplantation likewise is variable with rates as high as 12% [57]. HHV-8 is primarily transmitted via sexual contact but also can be acquired from the donated kidney [58]. The development of transplant-associated KS occurs both in patients seropositive prior to transplantation and in patients who seroconverted [57]. It has been suggested that KS develops as a result of reactivation in endemic regions and from donor transmission otherwise [57]. The incidence of KS in transplant recipients is 0.1–5% and varies by regional seroprevalence [59]. The disease tends to occur within the first 3 years after transplantation and often is aggressive. Reduction in immunosuppression may lead to regression of the tumor but predisposes to rejection and loss of the graft. Traditional therapies include radiation and cytotoxic regimens. In HIV-infected patients, foscarnet has been shown to slow progression of KS lesions [60] and ganciclovir reduced the incidence of KS [61]. Prophylaxis of CMV with ganciclovir may reduce the incidence of KS in renal transplant patients as well.

Hepatitis Viruses

Chronic liver disease affects about 15% of the renal allograft recipients [62]. Renal transplant recipients with chronic viral hepatitis have a significant increase in mortality from hepatic failure and concomitant sepsis [63]. There is an increased risk of infection attributed to infection with HCV namely an increased risk of bloodstream, pulmonary and CNS infections, and Gram-negative bacterial infections [62]. This may be explained by the immunomodulatory effects of the hepatitis viruses.

In addition to infecting hepatocytes, the hepatitis viruses infect the peripheral blood mononuclear cells [64]. Through their suppressive effect on the host immune response, the hepatitis viruses may contribute to improved survival by reducing the incidence of allograft rejection, but at the same time, they increase the overall risk of infection [62].

HBV is a DNA virus commonly seen in dialysis and transplant patients that may remain latent, progress to cirrhosis, or cause fulminant hepatitis. It can occur in transplant patients as a result of primary infection, reactivation, or donor transmission. Controversy exists regarding the impact of HBV serostatus of the donor and recipient on transplantation as well as patient and graft survival. The role of HBV in renal transplantation has been reviewed [65]. Concern for reactivation of HBV during immunosuppression exists as HBsAg– but HBsAb+ and HBcAb+ patients have developed reactivation and hepatitis [66]. Likewise, recipients from HBsAg– but HBcAb+ donors have seroconverted but without evidence of active infection. The risk of progression to active infection is higher if HBsAg+ is noted in the donor or recipient prior to transplantation. The effect of HBsAg+ status on mortality in transplant patients is controversial, but HBsAg– serostatus likely imparts a long-term survival advantage [67]. This difference may be secondary to pre-existing liver disease prior to transplantation, emphasizing the need for pre-transplant liver biopsy. The use of lamivudine as preemptive, prophylactic, and salvage treatment improves survival but long-term studies are needed as prolonged therapy is associated with increasing lamivudine resistance [68]. Other antivirals with activity against HBV are adefovir, tenofovir, entecavir, and emtricitabine. The use of HBcAb+ donor kidneys has been evaluated and is considered safe in vaccinated patients and those with evidence of prior HVB infection [9].

HCV is a single-stranded RNA virus and is the major cause of liver disease after renal transplant. The prevalence of HCV varies by geographic region and center from 10 to 41%, which is about 10 times that of the general population [69]. The majority of anti-HCV antibody-positive patients are also HCV RNA positive, and patients may be HCV RNA positive but lack an antibody response because of the humoral immune suppression. The virus is transmitted parenterally and in most cases acquired from hemodialysis. Seroconversion after transplantation of a HCV RNA-positive donor kidney is nearly universal. Whereas, anti-HCV antibody-positive but HCV RNA-negative kidneys rarely cause infection. Because of the shortage of donor organs, these anti-HCV antibody-positive kidneys are considered for HCV RNA-positive recipients. Over 60% of HCV-infected renal transplant patients will develop chronic hepatitis [70]. Mathurin et al. [67] showed after 10 years patient and graft survival of 65 and 49%, respectively, for HCV-positive recipients compared to 80 and 63% HCV-negative recipients. Besides progression to liver cirrhosis, other potential complications of HCV include fibrosing cholestatic hepatitis, hepatocellular carcinoma, cryoglobulinemia, membranoproliferative glomerulonephritis, membranous glomerulonephritis, and thrombotic microangiopathy. Treatments for HCV include interferon alpha, ribavirin, and amantidine. However, none of these treatments is both safe and effective after transplantation. Therefore, in renal transplant candidates, pre-transplant evaluation for HCV, liver biopsy, genotyping, RNA quantification, and pre-transplant treatment for HCV-positive individuals is recommended.

Influenza

Influenza is a major cause of acute respiratory illness and affects immunocompromised individuals more severely than immunocompetent individuals. In addition to the typical viral prodrome of fever, headache, myalgias, and dry cough, influenza has been associated with viral pneumonia, secondary bacterial pneumonia, rhabdomyolysis, and multiple neurological complications including encephalitis, and hemolytic-uremic syndrome [71]. It is recommended that transplant patients, their family, and transplant personnel receive yearly vaccinations for influenza. However, for non-vaccinated patients, those with egg allergies, and vaccine failures, two classes of drugs are available for prophylaxis and treatment: M2 blockers including amantadine and rimantadine and viral neuraminidase inhibitors including zanamivir (Relenza) and oseltamivir (Tamiflu). The M2 blockers are only active against influenza A, the neuraminidase inhibitors have activity against both influenza A and B. In general, it is not recommended to treat with antivirals if symptoms have been present for >2–3 days. A concern with M2 blockers is rapid resistance can develop on treatment. Care should be taken in patients with decreased renal function since all four drugs are cleared through the kidneys.

Human Immunodeficiency Virus

Infection with the HIV has been considered a contra-indication to renal transplantation until recently. Prior to the use of highly active anti-retroviral therapy (HAART), the concern of unchecked viral replication from immunosuppressive regimens and accelerated progression of a fatal disease led to a general consensus to reserve a limited supply of donor kidneys to those most like to benefit, non-HIV-infected patients. Since the use of HAART, HIV patients survive longer and suffer less opportunistic complications. Now they face other challenges including ESRD from HIV-associated nephropathy. The number of HIV patients on hemodialysis for ESRD is increasing and hemodialysis increases mortality in HIV patients. With a wider array of immunosuppressive medications, antibiotics, infectious disease detection methods, and prophylactic strategies, HIV patients will likely see a mortality and morbidity benefit from kidney transplantation compared to hemodialysis. Many complexities will arise as transplantation into HIV-positive recipients becomes more common including pre-transplant screening for appropriate level of viral suppression and estimating risk of progression to AIDS, polypharmacy with medication interactions, possible recurrence of HIV-associated nephropathy, and infection surveillance and management with a doubly compromised immune system.

Polyoma Viruses

The polyoma viruses (simian virus 40, JC, BK) are double-stranded non-enveloped DNA viruses that can lead to nephropathy and graft failure. BK virus (BKV) remains dormant in the urinary tract and circulating leukocytes after the primary childhood infection and becomes reactivated during immunosuppression. Adult seroprevalence rates for BKV range from 65 to 90% and BKV reactivation can come from the recipient or the donor [72, 73]. BKV viremia occurs in 13% and BKV nephropathy in 8% of kidney transplant recipients [74]. Analysis of risk factors for reactivation has underscored the central role played by serologic status of the donor, immunosuppressive regimens, injury to the uroepithelial tissue, and acute rejection [75]. Distinction of BKV infection from allograft rejection is of particular importance, although these processes may coexist in some cases [74].

Among renal transplant recipients who are receiving immunosuppressive therapy, 10–60% have reactivation of BKV accompanied by shedding of urothelial cells, and this shedding is inconsistently associated with allograft dysfunction [76]. Once the virus has reactivated, an ascending infection via cell-to-cell spread occurs. Early retrospective studies identified tacrolimus and mycophenolate mofetil, as risk factors for BKV nephropathy, however, subsequent studies indicate the overall state of immunosuppression is likely more important than the specific immunosuppressants used. Viral replication begins early after transplantation and progresses through detectable stages – viruria then viremia then nephropathy [74, 75]. Viruria can be detected by PCR for BKV DNA, reverse transcription (RT)-PCR for BKV RNA, cytology for BKV inclusion bearing epithelial cells termed "decoy cells," or electron microscopy for viral particles [74, 75]. Viruria is not specific for nephropathy, but viremia may be a better indicator of nephropathy [75, 77]. Although higher levels of viremia correlate with the risk of developing nephropathy, there are no established thresholds of viremia to indicate nephropathy. Therefore, the gold standard for establishing BKV nephropathy remains biopsy.

Currently no established antiviral treatment is available, and control of viral infection is tentatively obtained by means of reduction of immunosuppression [75, 77]. Treatment attempts have included immunoglobulins without proof of efficacy [78]. Immunoglobulins can have a dual effect, treating polyoma infection and allograft rejection. Retinoic acid, 5-bromo-2-deoxyuridine, cidofovir, leflunomide, fluoroquinolones, and gyrase inhibitors have antiviral activity in vitro but have not been tested in patients in a systematic fashion. Cidofovir use is limited by its nephrotoxicity. Retransplantation remains an option if other therapies fail [51].

It has been recommended that screening for BKV should be performed every 3 months for the first 2 years after transplantation then annually through the fifth year, when allograft dysfunction occurs, and when a transplant kidney biopsy is performed [79]. Screening should be based on a urinary assay for decoy cells, BKV DNA, or BKV RNA. A positive screening test should be confirmed within 4 weeks along with a quantitative assay. Recipients with persistent high viral levels for more than 3 weeks should undergo biopsy and intervention. Monitoring should continue every 2–4 weeks until the viral level falls below threshold values and preferably to undetectable levels.

Fungal Infections

Systemic fungal infections occur in 2–14% of renal transplant recipients [80, 81]. Although systemic mycoses encompass a broad range of diseases, about two-thirds of renal transplant recipients with fungal infections die [81, 82]. Risk factors for development of systemic fungal infections include age, prolonged hospitalization, medications like broad spectrum antibiotic and corticosteroids, comorbid conditions such as diabetes, liver disease, and CMV disease, and breaches in the innate defenses such as indwelling catheters, disruption of intestinal mucosa, and tissue ischemia [81–83]. The clinical manifestations of these infections are often non-specific. Therefore, a high index of suspicion and an aggressive approach to diagnosis are important. Therapy includes specific antifungal agents and risk factor reduction, such as removing IV catheters and decreasing immunosuppression (Table 9.5).

Several new antifungals, including new antifungal classes, have become available in the last 10 years or so. These include the triazoles voriconazole and posaconazole and the echinocandins caspofungin, micafungin, and anidulafungin. When selecting an empiric antifungal in a patient with a suspected fungal infection it is important to keep in mind these medications may have potentially important differences in antifungal coverage as well as risk for drug–drug interactions with immunosuppressants. Even with the increase in the number of antifungals available, amphotericin B formulations are often still considered the drug of choice in critically ill and immunocompromised patients with fungal infections, particularly with increasing use of non-amphotericin B prophylactic antifungals.

Voriconazole and posaconazole are broad spectrum triazole antifungals with activity against a wide variety of yeasts, including many fluconazole resistant *Candida* spp., and moulds [84]. The major difference in antifungal coverage between voriconazole and posaconazole is posaconazole covers *Zygomycetes*. Both will increase cyclosporine and tacrolimus levels and levels need to be monitored closely. Currently there is no IV formulation available for posaconazole It is also important to keep in mind posaconazole levels are increased when it is taken with food and decreased by proton pump inhibitors. Caution should be used with posaconazole if the patient has poor oral intake or is on a proton pump inhibitor. In contrast to the new triazoles, echinocandins are relatively narrow spectrum with activity limited generally to *Candida* spp. and *Aspergillus* [85]. In regards to in vitro and in vivo activity, there is little that distinguishes one echinocandin from another. All three echinocandins are well tolerated and are rarely associated with significant adverse events. Caspofungin is hepatically metabolized and when co-administered with cyclosporine, cyclosporine will increase caspofungin levels. Caspofungin will decrease cyclosporine and tacrolimus levels. Neither micafungin nor anidulafungin will interfere with cyclosporine or tacrolimus levels.

Candidiasis

Candidiasis is the most common fungal infection effecting renal transplant patients. *Candida albicans* is the usual causative pathogen, however, the incidence

Table 9.5 Fungal Infections Complicating Transplantation

Fungus	Common clinical syndromes	Diagnosis	Treatment options: Primary[a]	Treatment options: Secondary[a]
Aspergillus	Pneumonia/pulmonary cavity Sinusitis CNS mass Disseminated	Culture of suspected site of infection Histopathology Serum galactomannan[c]	Voriconazole	Echinocandin[a] Itraconazole Amphotericin Posaconazole
Candida	Urinary tract infection Fungemia Surgical site infection	Culture of suspected site of infection	*Severely ill or at risk for infection with azole resistant strain*: amphotericin,[b] echinocandin[d] *Mildly ill*: Fluconazole	Itraconazole Posaconazole Voriconazole
Coccidioides	Pneumonia/pulmonary cavity Meningitis Disseminated[e]	Culture of suspected site of infection Histopathology Serology: compliment fixation	*Severely ill or meningitis*: Amphotericin[b] followed by itraconazole suppression *Mild or moderately ill*: Itraconazole	Posaconazole Voriconazole Fluconazole
Cryptococcus	Fungemia Meningitis Pneumonia Cellulitis	Culture of suspected site of infection Serum cryptococcal antigen CSF cryptococcal antigen Histopathology (mucicarmine stain)	*Meningitis*: Amphotericin[b] plus flucytosine followed by fluconazole suppression *No Meningitis*: amphotericin[b] followed by fluconazole suppression	Fluconazole Itraconazole Posaconazole Voriconazole

Histoplasma	Pneumonia/pulmonary cavity Disseminated[f]	Culture of suspected site of infection (including bone marrow) Histopathology Isolator blood cultures Urine or serum histoplasma antigen Serology: compliment fixation and immunodiffusion	*Severely ill*: amphotericin[b] followed by itraconazole suppression *Mild or moderately ill*: itraconazole	Fluconazole Posaconazole Voriconazole
Mucormycosis	Sinusitis Pneumonia/pulmonary cavity CNS mass Disseminated	Culture of suspected site of infection Histopathology	Amphotericin[b]	

CSF cerebral spinal fluid; *CNS* central nervous system

[a]If more than antifungal listed, antifungals listed alphabetically, not by order of preference

[b]Amphotericin B deoxycholate, amphotericin B lipid complex, liposomal amphotericin B, or amphotericin B colloidal dispersion

[c]Serum galactomannan testing has a sensitivity <50% in solid organ transplant recipients

[d]Caspofungin, micafungin, and anidulafungin demonstrate similar in vitro and in vivo activity against *Candida* and *Aspergillus* species. Of note, *Candida parapsilosis* has been associated with clinical failures

[e]Disseminated coccidioides has a predilection for skin, joints, and bones

[f]Disseminated histoplasma has a predilection for the lymphoreticular system

of non-albicans species causing disease has been increasing [86]. Other reported species include *C. (Torulopsis). glabrata, C. parapsilosis. C. tropicalis*, and *C. krusei*. Candidal infections are generally manifest as mucocutaneous overgrowth including thrush, intertrigo, onychomycosis, esophagitis, or vaginitis. Invasive candidiasis usually occurs when the mucocutaneous barrier is breached by bladder and IV catheters or surgical trauma. This may present as catheter-related sepsis. The risk of hematogenous dissemination is tenfold higher in immunosuppressed patients compared to normal hosts. Manifestations of disseminated (often metastatic) candidal infections are diverse, and include skin lesions, intra-abdominal abscesses, meningitis, brain abscess, endophthalmitis, endocarditis, aortitis, arthritis, osteomyelitis, pneumonitis, pyelonephritis, and urinary tract obstruction by fungus balls. Diagnosis of candidal infections in renal transplant recipients is made by performing fungal stains and cultures of appropriate specimens, usually tissue biopsies.

Treatment of candidal infections depends on the location, *Candida* species, and prior treatment therapies. In general, oral, vaginal, and cutaneous candidasis can be treated by topical therapy with either nystatin or clotrimazole. Oral fluconazole is generally effective for esophagitis, UTI, or topical therapy failure. Asymptomatic candiduria should be treated in post-transplant patients after removal of the bladder catheter because of the use of high-dose immunosuppressives, bladder dysfunction, and frequent underlying diabetes [87]. In addition, this finding may be the only evidence of disseminated disease. Invasive candidal infections require removal of foreign devices and prolonged IV antibiotic therapy. Therapy options and therapy duration depend on severity of illness of the patient, site of infection, likelihood of azole resistance, and the presence of any infectious complications [88].

Cryptococcosis

C. neoformans is the most common cause of CNS fungal infection in kidney transplant patients. *C. neoformans* is present in soil contaminated with bird excreta. Infections are acquired by inhalation and occur in 0.3–4% of renal transplant recipients [89, 90]. In the immunocompromised host, the fungus quickly can disseminate from the lungs. The most common sites of isolated infection are the CNS (55%), skin (13%), and lungs (6%) [91]. The majority of cases of cryptococcal meningitis occur after 6 months following transplantation. The presentation is generally subacute or chronic, and symptoms include fever, headache, mental status changes, and focal neurologic deficits. Cutaneous involvement may be manifested as a cellulitis, nodular skin lesion, or an acneiform eruption. Cryptococcal pneumonia may be indistinguishable from other community-acquired pneumonia.

Treatment with amphotericin B and 5-flucytosine is most effective for acutely ill patients [92]. Less severe infections have been successfully managed with fluconazole.

Aspergillosis

The most common cause of aspergillosis is *Aspergillus fumigatus*. However, other species, including *A. flavus* and *A. niger*, can cause disease. The fungus is ubiquitous in the environment and is readily aerosolized. Inhalation of spores results in infections of the respiratory tract and a means of dissemination. Infection is rare except in immunocompromised patients but occurs in up to 3% of renal transplant recipients [81, 82]. Infections usually occur during the first 3 months following transplantation but nosocomial outbreaks have been associated with hospital construction and renovation. Characteristic presenting symptoms include fever, cough, hemoptysis, and pleuritic chest pain. Disseminated aspergillosis most often involves the CNS and is manifest as meningitis, encephalitis, brain abscesses, or granulomas. Symptoms are non-specific and include headache, altered mental status, seizures, and evolving stroke. Other organs that may be affected include the GI, kidneys, liver, thyroid, heart, pericardium, spleen, bones, and joints. Risk factors for invasive aspergillosis include renal failure, immunosuppression (high-dose corticosteroids and antilymphocyte antibody), neutropenia, and CMV infection [93].

The key to diagnosis is clinical suspicion and demonstration of *Aspergillus* in tissue biopsy or aspirate and growth in culture. Detection of *Aspergillus* in the respiratory tract (sputum, nasal swab, and bronchoalveolar lavage) is very suggestive of disease in immunocompromised patients [94]. Also, the characteristic radiographic findings of wedge-shaped pleural-based densities or cavities on CXR and the "halo sign" on CT may aid in early invasive diagnosis and treatment.

Disseminated aspergillosis has a poor prognosis and a crude mortality approaching 100%. Voriconazole is considered the treatment of choice or aspergillosis. A randomized controlled trial demonstrated superior treatment response and survival among patients who received voriconazole compared to amphotherICn. Amphotericin B has been the standard therapy, often requiring high dosing regimens for long periods. However, lipid soluble formulations of amphotericin B have comparable efficacy but reduced renal side effects [95]. Survival with fewer severe side effects compared to amphotericin B deoxycholate [96]. Caspofungin has been approved as salvage therapy for invasive aspergillosis. Posaconazole is approved for the salvage treatment of aspergillosis in Europe. In addition to medical therapy, surgery may be required to remove necrotic tissue and localized infections.

Mucormycosis

Infections with fungi of the class *Zygomycetes* cause mucormycosis. This class includes *Rhizopus* species, *Mucor* species, *Absidia* species, *Rhizomucor* species, and *Cunninghamella* species. These fungi are ubiquitous found in food, air, and soil. Infection is uncommon although occurs with a prevalence of 0–1.2% in renal transplant recipients. Risk factors include uncontrolled diabetic mellitus, chelation therapy with deferoxamine, corticosteroids, and hematologic malignancies. Similar to *Aspergillus*, fungal spores are inhaled into the respiratory tract, hyphae invade the small vessels causing hemorrhage and infarction, and then the fungus can disseminate. Clinical manifestations include rhinocerebral, pulmonary, cutaneous, CNS, and GI involvement. Signs and symptoms of infections are non-specific and can present as fever, orbital cellulitis, ophthalmoplegia, hemoptysis, cough, chest pain, headache, mental status changes, and GI bleeding. Diagnosis is made by tissue biopsy and histologic examination. Treatment consists of aggressive surgical debridement of necrotic tissue, minimizing risk factors, and antifungal therapy with amphotericin B. Posaconazole is approved for salvage therapy of mucormycosis in Europe. Rapid diagnosis and treatment of patient at risk are critical because of the high morbidity and mortality (80%) associated with mucormycosis.

Endemic Mycoses

These infections can occur at any time following transplantation. Histoplasmosis and coccidioidomycosis are more common in transplant patients and are caused by *Histoplasma capsulatum* and *Coccidioides immitis*, respectively. The clinical presentation of these mycoses is varied and dissemination is common.

Histoplasmosis

Histoplasmosis is endemic in the central United States and is acquired by inhalation. Infection with *H. capsulatum* occurs in 0.4–2.1% of renal transplant recipients [97, 98]. Most cases represent primary exogenous infection. Histoplasmosis can be transmitted from the organ donor, and reactivation of latent foci can occur. Disseminated disease is common and clinical presentation may be nonspecific. Disseminated histoplasmosis has manifested as cellulitis, allograft involvement, necrotizing myofasciitis, and CNS disease. In reported cases of disseminated histoplasmosis in renal transplants, patients had received antilymphocyte therapy and IV pulse steroids in the 3 months prior to the onset of infection [99]. Diagnosis relies on serology, fungal stains, culturing the organism from specific foci or the bone marrow in cases of disseminated disease, or identification of the histoplasma antigen in the serum or urine. The antigen can be detected in the urine of 90% of patients with disseminated infection and 75% of patients with diffuse acute pulmonary histoplasmosis. Treatment with amphotericin B and alternatively with itraconazole for milder cases is very effective.

Coccidioidomycosis

Coccidioidomycosis is endemic in the southwestern United States, northern Mexico, and regions of Latin America. Patients who have lived in or traveled to these areas are at increased risk of infection with *C. immitis*. The majority of cases can be attributed to reactivation of old foci of infection, and occur within the first year post-transplant. However, coccidioidomycosis can result from a primary infection and may occur at any time in an immunosuppressed host [100].

Transplant recipients infected with *C. immitis* usually develop progressive disseminated disease associated with a high mortality. Risk factors include male sex and blood group B [101]. Organ-systems most commonly involved are the lungs, CNS, skin, joints, and kidney. The radiographic manifestations are highly variable and extrathoracic infection without evidence of pulmonary disease occurs not infrequently. Diagnosis of coccidioidomycosis is made by histologic examination of tissue specimens, culture, and serology. Treatment options include amphotericin B, fluconazole, and itraconazole. Treatment is with amphotericin B for severe disseminated disease. This should be followed by long-term suppressive therapy with itraconazole.

Pneumocystosis

Pneumocystis jiroveci (previously known as *Pneumocystis carinii*) is an extracellular organism resembling both fungi and a protozoan parasites. In solid organ transplants not receiving prophylaxis for pneumocystis (PCP), 6–20% develop PCP within the first year after transplantation [102]. The clinical presentation of PCP is usually subacute with symptoms of fever, non-productive cough, dyspnea and interstitial infiltrates with or without cysts, and variable degrees of hypoxemia. Patients with PCP may also have an elevated serum lactate dehydrogenase (LDH) level. Pneumocystis infection is often associated with CMV infection, and may carry a high mortality rate. Diagnosis relies on identification of the organisms using silver stains or immunofluorescent monoclonal antibody on deep respiratory specimens. Pneumocystis infection can be prevented by using prophylaxis with TMP-SMX or alternatively with dapsone or aerosolized pentamidine for 6–12 months post-transplantation. The treatment of choice is TMP-SMX in addition to steroids in severe cases. Alternative choices for treatment include a combination of primaquine and clindamycin, dapsone, or atovaquone.

Mycobacterium Tuberculosis

Approximately 1–15% of renal transplant recipients develop active *Mycobacterium tuberculosis* infection (TB) and prevalence varies by geography and endemicity [103]. The lowest incidence is in North America and the highest in India. The majority of TB occurs within the first year post-transplant, although it can occur at any time following transplantation [104]. Immunosuppressed patients are at increased risk for both primary infection and reactivation. Transmission of *M. tuberculosis* from the renal allograft has been reported. TB can involve almost any organ system, but it most commonly presents either as pulmonary disease or as disseminated disease. The GI tract is the most common extra-pulmonary site. Clinical manifestations include fever, weight loss, pulmonary disease with focal infiltrates (40%) or a miliary pattern (22%) on CXR [104], GI involvement most commonly in the ileocecal region, osteomyelitis, septic arthritis, cutaneous lesions, meningitis, nephropathy, and lymphadenitis. Risk factors for active TB include non-Caucasian race, aging, malnutrition, diabetes, CMV, renal failure, liver disease, co-existing infections, upper gastrointestinal surgery, a history of inadequately treated disease, and immunosuppressive therapy. Mortality in renal transplant patients is 30% overall and is greatest in disseminated TB.

Evaluation for *M. tuberculosis* infection in kidney transplant patients should begin pre-transplant. Risk factors should be queried including high-risk exposures, prior positive PPD, and prior treatment. A positive PPD in patients with chronic renal failure is >10 mm. A PPD >5 mm is considered positive with CXR evidence of prior TB infection or close contacts of TB cases. These patients require further evaluation for evidence of active disease. Patients with latent disease should undergo treatment prior to transplant to prevent reactivation and medication interactions. After transplantation, a positive PPD is >5 mm [105]. Use of the QuantiFERON-TB test for diagnosis of latent or active TB is not recommended in the pre- or post-transplant setting [106]. Patients suspected of having active TB should be isolated to avoid transmission to other susceptible hosts. Three induced sputum specimens should be obtained in the early morning and sent for acid-fast stain and culture. Bronchoalveolar lavage fluid and post-bronchoscopy sputum samples can also be sent for acid-fast stain and culture. In the case of extrapulmonary disease, other body fluids (pleural, ascitic, cerebrospinal, synovial, urine, or other) should be concentrated prior to staining. Histopathologic examination of biopsy tissue (acid-fast bacilli and granulomata) may also be useful if disease is suspected and body fluid analysis is non-diagnostic. Rapid assay kits are also available and utilize nucleic acid amplification techniques to detect the organism.

Patients with latent TB require treatment with isoniazid (INH) for 9 months. Alternative therapies including INH for 6 months and RIF for 4 months can be considered because of adverse effects, drug interactions, high cost, or poor compliance [105]. Because of the high prevalence of drug-resistant *M. tuberculosis*, active TB should be treated with directly observed therapy consisting of a 2-month initial phase of INH, RIF, pyrazinamide (PZA), and ethambutol (EMB). Alterations to this regimen are allowed if drug susceptibilities are known in advance and for certain underlying medical conditions. After 2 months, the regime can be tailored based on the drug sensitivities and continued for 4–7 months [107]. Renal transplant recipients receiving treatment for active or latent TB should be followed closely and liver enzymes should be checked because of the high prevalence of liver disease and possible drug interactions. The adverse effects and toxicity of anti-tuberculous agents are well described. One effect, of particular importance to patients receiving immunosuppression, is that INH and RIF induce hepatic cytochrome P450 enzymes and increase the metabolism of glucocorticoids, cyclosporine, tacrolimus, and sirolimus. This can lead to under-immunosuppression and rejection if blood levels of immunosuppressive drugs are not followed closely.

Conclusion

Approximately two-thirds of renal transplant recipients will experience an infectious related complication in the first year after transplantation. This reflects the overall, or net state, of immunosuppression associated with ESRD and transplantation as well as donor and environmental exposures. Renal transplant candidates often are immunosuppressed prior to transplantation from age, nutrition, comorbid conditions, and medications. After transplantation, immunosuppressive medications are used to maintain the donor kidney but further hinder the immune response. This difficult balance favors the reactivation and progression of infections. These infections may come from the donor kidney, transfused blood products, the environment, or occult and latent infections within the recipient. The intensity of the immunosuppressive regimen predisposes recipients to specific infections. As the intensity of therapy declines over the first year, the frequency of infections with specific agents changes as well. Understanding the degree of immunosuppression and the time course of infection aids in the diagnosis of infections, and the appropriate use of preemptive, prophylactic and treatment strategies.

References

1. Dharnidharka VR, Stablein DM, Harmon WE. Post-transplant infections now exceed acute rejection as cause for hospitalization: a report of the NAPRTCS. Am J Transplant. 2004;4(3):384–9.
2. Gill JS, Abichandani R, Kausz AT, Pereira BJ. Mortality after kidney transplant failure: the impact of non-immunologic factors. Kidney Int. 2002;62(5):1875–83.
3. Rubin RH. Infection in the organ transplant recipient. In: Rubin RH, Young LS, editors. Clinical approach to infection in the compromised host. New York: Plenum Medical Book Company; 1994. p. 629–705.
4. Vanholder R, Van Loo A, Dhondt AM, De Smet R, Ringoir S. Influence of uraemia and haemodialysis on host defence and infection. Nephrol Dial Transplant. 1996;11(4):593–8.
5. Kazancioglu R, Sever MS, Yuksel-Onel D, Eraksoy H, Yildiz A, Celik AV, et al. Immunization of renal transplant recipients with pneumococcal polysaccharide vaccine. Clin Transplant. 2000;14(1):61–5.
6. Huzly D, Neifer S, Reinke P, Schroder K, Schonfeld C, Hofmann T, et al. Routine immunizations in adult renal transplant recipients. Transplantation. 1997;63(6):839–45.
7. Furth SL, Fivush BA. Varicella vaccination in pediatric kidney transplant candidates. Pediatr Transplant. 2002;6(2):97–100.
8. Gottesdiener KM. Transplanted infections: donor-to-host transmission with the allograft. Ann Intern Med. 1989;110(12):1001–16.
9. Fong TL, Bunnapradist S, Jordan SC, Cho YW. Impact of hepatitis B core antibody status on outcomes of cadaveric renal transplantation: analysis of United network of organ sharing database between 1994 and 1999. Transplantation. 2002;73(1):85–9.
10. Batty Jr DS, Swanson SJ, Kirk AD, Ko CW, Agodoa LY, Abbott KC. Hepatitis C virus seropositivity at the time of renal transplantation in the United States: associated factors and patient survival. Am J Transplant. 2001;1(2):179–84.

11. Midtvedt K, Hartmann A, Midtvedt T, Brekke IB. Routine perioperative antibiotic prophylaxis in renal transplantation. Nephrol Dial Transplant. 1998;13(7):1637–41.
12. Nauseef WM, Maki DG. A study of the value of simple protective isolation in patients with granulocytopenia. N Engl J Med. 1981;304(8):448–53.
13. Fox BC, Sollinger HW, Belzer FO, Maki DG. A prospective, randomized, double-blind study of trimethoprim-sulfamethoxazole for prophylaxis of infection in renal transplantation: clinical efficacy, absorption of trimethoprim-sulfamethoxazole, effects on the microflora, and the cost-benefit of prophylaxis. Am J Med. 1990;89(3):255–74.
14. Brennan DC, Garlock KA, Singer GG, Schnitzler MA, Lippmann BJ, Buller RS, et al. Prophylactic oral ganciclovir compared with deferred therapy for control of cytomegalovirus in renal transplant recipients. Transplantation. 1997;64(12):1843–6.
15. Brennan DC, Storch GA, Singer GG, Lee L, Rueda J, Schnitzler MA. The prevalence of human herpesvirus-7 in renal transplant recipients is unaffected by oral or intravenous ganciclovir. J Infect Dis. 2000;181(5):1557–61.
16. Lippmann BJ, Brennan DC, Wong J, Lowell JA, Singer GG, Howard TK. Are varicella zoster and herpes simplex sentinel lesions for cytomegalovirus in renal transplant recipients? Lancet. 1995;346(8979):914–5.
17. Miller BW, Brennan DC, Korenblat PE, Goss JA, Flye MW. Common variable immunodeficiency in a renal transplant patient with severe recurrent bacterial infection: a case report and review of the literature. Am J Kidney Dis. 1995;25(6):947–51.
18. Toogood GJ, Roake JA, Morris PJ. The relationship between fever and acute rejection or infection following renal transplantation in the cyclosporin era. Clin Transplant. 1994;8(4):373–7.
19. Donck JB, Segaert MF, Vanrenterghem YF. Fluoroquinolones and Achilles tendinopathy in renal transplant recipients. Transplantation. 1994;58(6):736–7.
20. Tolkoff-Rubin NE, Rubin RH. Urinary tract infection in the immunocompromised host. Lessons from kidney transplantation and the AIDS epidemic. Infect Dis Clin North Am. 1997;11(3):707–17.
21. Wagener MM, Yu VL. Bacteremia in transplant recipients: a prospective study of demographics, etiologic agents, risk factors, and outcomes. Am J Infect Control. 1992;20(5): 239–47.
22. Koyle MA, Ward HJ, Twomey PA, Glassock RJ, Rajfer J. Declining incidence of wound infection in cadaveric renal transplant recipient. Urology. 1988;31(2):103–6.
23. Waterer GW, Baselski VS, Wunderink RG. Legionella and community-acquired pneumonia: a review of current diagnostic tests from a clinician's viewpoint. Am J Med. 2001;110(1):41–8.
24. Arduino RC, Johnson PC, Miranda AG. Nocardiosis in renal transplant recipients undergoing immunosuppression with cyclosporine. Clin Infect Dis. 1993;16(4):505–12.
25. Stamm AM, Dismukes WE, Simmons BP, Cobbs CG, Elliott A, Budrich P, et al. Listeriosis in renal transplant recipients: report of an outbreak and review of 102 cases. Rev Infect Dis. 1982;4(3):665–82.
26. Bacon TH, Levin MJ, Leary JJ, Sarisky RT, Sutton D. Herpes simplex virus resistance to acyclovir and penciclovir after two decades of antiviral therapy. Clin Microbiol Rev. 2003;16(1):114–28.
27. Balfour Jr HH. Varicella zoster virus infections in immunocompromised hosts. A review of the natural history and management. Am J Med. 1988;85(2A):68–73.
28. Hempenstall K, Nurmikko TJ, Johnson RW, A'Hern RP, Rice AS. Analgesic therapy in postherpetic neuralgia: a quantitative systematic review. PLoS Med. 2005;2(7):e164.
29. Stadlmann S, Fend F, Moser P, Obrist P, Greil R, Dirnhofer S. Epstein-Barr virus-associated extranodal NK/T-cell lymphoma, nasal type of the hypopharynx, in a renal allograft recipient: case report and review of literature. Hum Pathol. 2001;32(11):1264–8.
30. Cheeseman SH, Henle W, Rubin RH, Tolkoff-Rubin NE, Cosimi B, Cantell K, et al. Epstein-Barr virus infection in renal transplant recipients. Effects of antithymocyte globulin and interferon. Ann Intern Med. 1980;93(1):39–42.

31. Frias C, Lauzurica R, Bayes B, Ausina V. Prospective follow-up of Epstein-Barr virus load in adult kidney transplant recipients by semiquantitative polymerase chain reaction in blood and saliva samples. Eur J Clin Microbiol Infect Dis. 2001;20(12):892–5.
32. Farrugia E, Schwab TR. Management and prevention of cytomegalovirus infection after renal transplantation. Mayo Clin Proc. 1992;67(9):879–90.
33. Sia IG, Patel R. New strategies for prevention and therapy of cytomegalovirus infection and disease in solid-organ transplant recipients. Clin Microbiol Rev. 2000;13(1):83–121.
34. Preiksaitis JK, Brennan DC, Fishman J, Allen U. Canadian society of transplantation consensus workshop on cytomegalovirus management in solid organ transplantation final report. Am J Transplant. 2005;5(2):218–27.
35. Hodson EM, Barclay PG, Craig JC, Jones C, Kable K, Strippoli GF, et al. Antiviral medications for preventing cytomegalovirus disease in solid organ transplant recipients. Cochrane Database Syst Rev. 2005;(4):CD003774.
36. Jassal SV, Roscoe JM, Zaltzman JS, Mazzulli T, Krajden M, Gadawski M, et al. Clinical practice guidelines: prevention of cytomegalovirus disease after renal transplantation. J Am Soc Nephrol. 1998;9(9):1697–708.
37. Snydman DR, Werner BG, Heinze-Lacey B, Berardi VP, Tilney NL, Kirkman RL, et al. Use of cytomegalovirus immune globulin to prevent cytomegalovirus disease in renal-transplant recipients. N Engl J Med. 1987;317(17):1049–54.
38. Limaye AP, Corey L, Koelle DM, Davis CL, Boeckh M. Emergence of ganciclovir-resistant cytomegalovirus disease among recipients of solid-organ transplants. Lancet. 2000;356(9230):645–9.
39. Geddes CC, Church CC, Collidge T, McCruden EA, Gillespie G, Matthews E, et al. Management of cytomegalovirus infection by weekly surveillance after renal transplant: analysis of cost, rejection and renal function. Nephrol Dial Transplant. 2003;18(9):1891–8.
40. Emery VC. Prophylaxis for CMV should not now replace pre-emptive therapy in solid organ transplantation. Rev Med Virol. 2001;11(2):83–6.
41. Rondeau E, Bourgeon B, Peraldi MN, Lang P, Buisson C, Schulte KM, et al. Effect of prophylactic ganciclovir on cytomegalovirus infection in renal transplant recipients. Nephrol Dial Transplant. 1993;8(9):858–62.
42. Sancho A, Gorriz JL, Crespo JF, Avila A, Alcaraz MJ, Garcia Ramos JL, et al. Prophylaxis of cytomegalovirus disease with intravenous ganciclovir in renal transplantation. Transplant Proc. 1999;31(6):2337–8.
43. Paya C, Humar A, Dominguez E, Washburn K, Blumberg E, Alexander B, et al. Efficacy and safety of valganciclovir vs. oral ganciclovir for prevention of cytomegalovirus disease in solid organ transplant recipients. Am J Transplant. 2004;4(4):611–20.
44. Pescovitz M, Rabkin J, Merion R, Paya C, Pirsch J, Freeman R, et al. Valganciclovir provides ganciclovir plasma exposure similar to IV ganciclovirin transplant recipients. Transplantation. 1999;67:S126.
45. Small LN, Lau J, Snydman DR. Preventing post-organ transplantation cytomegalovirus disease with ganciclovir: a meta-analysis comparing prophylactic and preemptive therapies. Clin Infect Dis. 2006;43(7):869–80.
46. Khoury JA, Storch GA, Bohl DL, Schuessler RM, Torrence SM, Lockwood M, et al. Prophylactic versus preemptive oral valganciclovir for the management of cytomegalovirus infection in adult renal transplant recipients. Am J Transplant. 2006;6(9):2134–43.
47. Roberts TC, Brennan DC, Buller RS, Gaudreault-Keener M, Schnitzler MA, Sternhell KE, et al. Quantitative polymerase chain reaction to predict occurrence of symptomatic cytomegalovirus infection and assess response to ganciclovir therapy in renal transplant recipients. J Infect Dis. 1998;178(3):626–35.
48. Sia IG, Wilson JA, Groettum CM, Espy MJ, Smith TF, Paya CV. Cytomegalovirus (CMV) DNA load predicts relapsing CMV infection after solid organ transplantation. J Infect Dis. 2000;181(2):717–20.

49. Baldanti F, Lurain N, Gerna G. Clinical and biologic aspects of human cytomegalovirus resistance to antiviral drugs. Hum Immunol. 2004;65(5):403–9.
50. Drew WL, Miner RC, Marousek GI, Chou S. Maribavir sensitivity of cytomegalovirus isolates resistant to ganciclovir, cidofovir or foscarnet. J Clin Virol. 2006;37(2):124–7.
51. Gabardi S, Waikar SS, Martin S, et al. Evaluation of fluoroquinolones for the prevention of BK viremia after renal transplantation. Clin J Am Soc Nephrol. 2010;5(7):1298–304.
52. Rossi C, Delforge ML, Jacobs F, Wissing M, Pradier O, Remmelink M, et al. Fatal primary infection due to human herpesvirus 6 variant A in a renal transplant recipient. Transplantation. 2001;71(2):288–92.
53. Yoshida M, Yamada M, Tsukazaki T, Chatterjee S, Lakeman FD, Nii S, et al. Comparison of antiviral compounds against human herpesvirus 6 and 7. Antiviral Res. 1998;40(1–2): 73–84.
54. Kidd IM, Clark DA, Sabin CA, Andrew D, Hassan-Walker AF, Sweny P, et al. Prospective study of human betaherpesviruses after renal transplantation: association of human herpesvirus 7 and cytomegalovirus co-infection with cytomegalovirus disease and increased rejection. Transplantation. 2000;69(11):2400–4.
55. Zhang Y, Schols D, De Clercq E. Selective activity of various antiviral compounds against HHV-7 infection. Antiviral Res. 1999;43(1):23–35.
56. Schulz TF. Epidemiology of Kaposi's sarcoma-associated herpesvirus/human herpesvirus 8. Adv Cancer Res. 1999;76:121–60.
57. Regamey N, Tamm M, Wernli M, Witschi A, Thiel G, Cathomas G, et al. Transmission of human herpesvirus 8 infection from renal-transplant donors to recipients. N Engl J Med. 1998;339(19):1358–63.
58. Luppi M, Barozzi P, Santagostino G, Trovato R, Schulz TF, Marasca R, et al. Molecular evidence of organ-related transmission of Kaposi sarcoma-associated herpesvirus or human herpesvirus-8 in transplant patients. Blood. 2000;96(9):3279–81.
59. Antman K, Chang Y. Kaposi's sarcoma. N Engl J Med. 2000;342(14):1027–38.
60. Robles R, Lugo D, Gee L, Jacobson MA. Effect of antiviral drugs used to treat cytomegalovirus end-organ disease on subsequent course of previously diagnosed Kaposi's sarcoma in patients with AIDS. J Acquir Immune Defic Syndr Hum Retrovirol. 1999;20(1):34–8.
61. Martin DF, Kuppermann BD, Wolitz RA, Palestine AG, Li H, Robinson CA. Oral ganciclovir for patients with cytomegalovirus retinitis treated with a ganciclovir implant. Roche Ganciclovir Study Group. N Engl J Med. 1999;340(14):1063–70.
62. Rao KV, Ma J. Chronic viral hepatitis enhances the risk of infection but not acute rejection in renal transplant recipients. Transplantation. 1996;62(12):1765–9.
63. Rao KV, Kasiske BL, Anderson WR. Variability in the morphological spectrum and clinical outcome of chronic liver disease in hepatitis B-positive and B-negative renal transplant recipients. Transplantation. 1991;51(2):391–6.
64. Feray C, Zignego AL, Samuel D, Bismuth A, Reynes M, Tiollais P, et al. Persistent hepatitis B virus infection of mononuclear blood cells without concomitant liver infection. The liver transplantation model. Transplantation. 1990;49(6):1155–8.
65. Gane E, Pilmore H. Management of chronic viral hepatitis before and after renal transplantation. Transplantation. 2002;74(4):427–37.
66. Roberts RC, Lane C, Hatfield P, Clutterbuck E, Atkins M, Brown A, et al. All anti-HBc-positive, HBsAg-negative dialysis patients on the transplant waiting list should be regarded as at risk of hepatitis B reactivation post-renal transplantation – report of three cases from a single centre. Nephrol Dial Transplant. 2006;21(11):3316–9.
67. Mathurin P, Mouquet C, Poynard T, Sylla C, Benalia H, Fretz C, et al. Impact of hepatitis B and C virus on kidney transplantation outcome. Hepatology. 1999;29(1):257–63.
68. Fabrizi F, Dulai G, Dixit V, Bunnapradist S, Martin P. Lamivudine for the treatment of hepatitis B virus-related liver disease after renal transplantation: meta-analysis of clinical trials. Transplantation. 2004;77(6):859–64.
69. Boletis JN. Epidemiology and mode of transmission of hepatitis C virus infection after renal transplantation. Nephrol Dial Transplant. 2000;15 Suppl 8:52–4.

70. Kallinowski B, Hergesell O, Zeier M. Clinical impact of hepatitis C virus infection in the renal transplant recipient. Nephron. 2002;91(4):541–6.
71. Asaka M, Ishikawa I, Nakazawa T, Tomosugi N, Yuri T, Suzuki K. Hemolytic uremic syndrome associated with influenza A virus infection in an adult renal allograft recipient: case report and review of the literature. Nephron. 2000;84(3):258–66.
72. Knowles WA. Discovery and epidemiology of the human polyomaviruses BK virus (BKV) and JC virus (JCV). Adv Exp Med Biol. 2006;577:19–45.
73. Bohl DL, Storch GA, Ryschkewitsch C, Gaudreault-Keener M, Schnitzler MA, Major EO, et al. Donor origin of BK virus in renal transplantation and role of HLA C7 in susceptibility to sustained BK viremia. Am J Transplant. 2005;5(9):2213–21.
74. Hirsch HH, Knowles W, Dickenmann M, Passweg J, Klimkait T, Mihatsch MJ, et al. Prospective study of polyomavirus type BK replication and nephropathy in renal-transplant recipients. N Engl J Med. 2002;347(7):488–96.
75. Brennan DC, Agha I, Bohl DL, Schnitzler MA, Hardinger KL, Lockwood M, et al. Incidence of BK with tacrolimus versus cyclosporine and impact of preemptive immunosuppression reduction. Am J Transplant. 2005;5(3):582–94.
76. Randhawa PS, Demetris AJ. Nephropathy due to polyomavirus type BK. N Engl J Med. 2000;342(18):1361–3.
77. Nickeleit V, Klimkait T, Binet IF, Dalquen P, Del Zenero V, Thiel G, et al. Testing for polyomavirus type BK DNA in plasma to identify renal-allograft recipients with viral nephropathy. N Engl J Med. 2000;342(18):1309–15.
78. Sener A, House AA, Jevnikar AM, Boudville N, McAlister VC, Muirhead N, et al. Intravenous immunoglobulin as a treatment for BK virus associated nephropathy: one-year follow-up of renal allograft recipients. Transplantation. 2006;81(1):117–20.
79. Hirsch HH, Brennan DC, Drachenberg CB, Ginevri F, Gordon J, Limaye AP, et al. Polyomavirus-associated nephropathy in renal transplantation: interdisciplinary analyses and recommendations. Transplantation. 2005;79(10):1277–86.
80. Tharayil John G, Shankar V, Talaulikar G, Mathews MS, Abraham Abraham M, Punnakuzhathil Thomas P, et al. Epidemiology of systemic mycoses among renal-transplant recipients in India. Transplantation. 2003;75(9):1544–51.
81. Bren A, Koselj M, Kandus A, Kovac D, Lindic J, Crnej A, et al. Severe fungal infections in kidney graft recipients. Transplant Proc. 2002;34(7):2999–3000.
82. Altiparmak MR, Apaydin S, Trablus S, Serdengecti K, Ataman R, Ozturk R, et al. Systemic fungal infections after renal transplantation. Scand J Infect Dis. 2002;34(4):284–8.
83. Howard RJ, Simmons RL, Najarian JS. Fungal infections in renal transplant recipients. Ann Surg. 1978;188(5):598–605.
84. Sabatelli F, Patel R, Mann PA, Mendrick CA, Norris CC, Hare R, et al. In vitro activities of posaconazole, fluconazole, itraconazole, voriconazole, and amphotericin B against a large collection of clinically important molds and yeasts. Antimicrob Agents Chemother. 2006;50(6):2009–15.
85. Cappelletty D, Eiselstein-McKitrick K. The echinocandins. Pharmacotherapy. 2007;27(3):369–88.
86. Pfaller MA, Diekema DJ. Epidemiology of invasive candidiasis: a persistent public health problem. Clin Microbiol Rev. 2007;20(1):133–63.
87. Edwards Jr JE, Bodey GP, Bowden RA, Buchner T, de Pauw BE, Filler SG, et al. International conference for the development of a consensus on the management and prevention of severe candidal infections. Clin Infect Dis. 1997;25(1):43–59.
88. Pappas PG, Rex JH, Sobel JD, Filler SG, Dismukes WE, Walsh TJ, et al. Guidelines for treatment of candidiasis. Clin Infect Dis. 2004;38(2):161–89.
89. Husain S, Wagener MM, Singh N. *Cryptococcus neoformans* infection in organ transplant recipients: variables influencing clinical characteristics and outcome. Emerg Infect Dis. 2001;7(3):375–81.
90. John GT, Mathew M, Snehalatha E, Anandi V, Date A, Jacob CK, et al. Cryptococcosis in renal allograft recipients. Transplantation. 1994;58(7):855–6.

91. Chugh KS, Sakhuja V, Jain S, Talwar P, Minz M, Joshi K, et al. High mortality in systemic fungal infections following renal transplantation in third-world countries. Nephrol Dial Transplant. 1993;8(2):168–72.
92. Saag MS, Graybill RJ, Larsen RA, Pappas PG, Perfect JR, Powderly WG, et al. Practice guidelines for the management of cryptococcal disease. Infectious Diseases Society of America. Clin Infect Dis. 2000;30(4):710–8.
93. Gustafson TL, Schaffner W, Lavely GB, Stratton CW, Johnson HK, Hutcheson Jr RH. Invasive aspergillosis in renal transplant recipients: correlation with corticosteroid therapy. J Infect Dis. 1983;148(2):230–8.
94. Perfect JR, Cox GM, Lee JY, Kauffman CA, de Repentigny L, Chapman SW, et al. The impact of culture isolation of Aspergillus species: a hospital-based survey of aspergillosis. Clin Infect Dis. 2001;33(11):1824–33.
95. Bowden R, Chandrasekar P, White MH, Li X, Pietrelli L, Gurwith M, et al. A double-blind, randomized, controlled trial of amphotericin B colloidal dispersion versus amphotericin B for treatment of invasive aspergillosis in immunocompromised patients. Clin Infect Dis. 2002;35(4):359–66.
96. Herbrecht R, Denning DW, Patterson TF, Bennett JE, Greene RE, Oestmann JW, et al. Voriconazole versus amphotericin B for primary therapy of invasive aspergillosis. N Engl J Med. 2002;347(6):408–15.
97. Wheat LJ, Smith EJ, Sathapatayavongs B, Batteiger B, Filo RS, Leapman SB, et al. Histoplasmosis in renal allograft recipients. Two large urban outbreaks. Arch Intern Med. 1983;143(4):703–7.
98. Davies SF, Sarosi GA, Peterson PK, Khan M, Howard RJ, Simmons RL, et al. Disseminated histoplasmosis in renal transplant recipients. Am J Surg. 1979;137(5):686–91.
99. Sridhar NR, Tchervenkov JI, Weiss MA, Hijazi YM, First MR. Disseminated histoplasmosis in a renal transplant patient: a cause of renal failure several years following transplantation. Am J Kidney Dis. 1991;17(6):719–21.
100. Blair JE, Logan JL. Coccidioidomycosis in solid organ transplantation. Clin Infect Dis. 2001;33(9):1536–44.
101. Cohen IM, Galgiani JN, Potter D, Ogden DA. Coccidioidomycosis in renal replacement therapy. Arch Intern Med. 1982;142(3):489–94.
102. Spieker C, Barenbrock M, Tepel M, Buchholz B, Rahn KH, Zidek W. Pentamidine inhalation as a prophylaxis against *Pneumocystis carinii* pneumonia after therapy of acute renal allograft rejection with orthoclone (OKT3). Transplant Proc. 1992;24(6):2602–3.
103. Higgins RM, Cahn AP, Porter D, Richardson AJ, Mitchell RG, Hopkin JM, et al. Mycobacterial infections after renal transplantation. Q J Med. 1991;78(286):145–53.
104. Singh N, Paterson DL. *Mycobacterium tuberculosis* infection in solid-organ transplant recipients: impact and implications for management. Clin Infect Dis. 1998;27(5):1266–77.
105. American Thoracic Society and CDC. Targeted tuberculin testing and treatment of latent tuberculosis infection. Am J Respir Crit Care Med. 2000;161(4 Pt 2):221–47.
106. Mazurek GH, Villarino ME. Guidelines for using the QuantiFERON-TB test for diagnosing latent *Mycobacterium tuberculosis* infection. Centers for Disease Control and Prevention. MMWR Recomm Rep. 2003;52(RR-2):15–8.
107. Blumberg HM, Burman WJ, Chaisson RE, Daley CL, Etkind SC, Friedman LN, et al. American Thoracic Society/Centers for Disease Control and Prevention/Infectious Diseases Society of America: treatment of tuberculosis. Am J Respir Crit Care Med. 2003;167(4):603–62.

Chapter 10
Recurrent and De Novo Glomerulonephritis After Kidney Transplantation

Austin Hunt and Mark D. Denton

Abstract Glomerulonephritis is the primary disease in over a third of patients undergoing renal transplantation. All forms of glomerulonephritis may recur histologically in the renal allograft, but the incidence and severity of clinical recurrence vary greatly according to the type of glomerular disease. Recurrence may be early post-transplant or may take many years. Glomerular diseases that recur late will increase in clinical significance as advances in immunosuppression reduce rejection-mediated graft loss and prolong transplant survival. Registry data shows that the risk of graft loss from recurrence increases with the number of follow-up years, from 0.6% at the first postoperative year to 8.4% at 10 years. Recurrence was the third most frequent cause of allograft loss at 10 years, after chronic allograft failure and death with a functioning allograft. Interestingly, the use of more potent maintenance immunosuppressive agents or more potent induction agents such as alemtuzumab do not appear to reduce recurrence rates. De novo glomerulonephritis may also occur in renal transplants. This chapter reviews the incidence, clinical features, treatment, and impact on renal transplant survival of the major forms of de novo and recurrent glomerular disease.

Keywords IgA nephropathy • Focal segmental glomerulonephritis • Systemic lupus erythematosus • Membranoproliferative glomerulonephritis • Membranous glomerulonephritis

A. Hunt, MBChB
Renal Unit, Derriford Hospital, Plymouth, England, UK

M.D. Denton, MD, PhD (✉)
Renal Unit, Beaumont Hospital, Beaumont Road, Dublin, Ireland
e-mail: Mark.Denton@beaumont.ie

A. Chandraker et al. (eds.), *Core Concepts in Renal Transplantation*,
DOI 10.1007/978-1-4614-0008-0_10, © Springer Science+Business Media, LLC 2012

Introduction

Glomerulonephritis is the primary disease in over a third of patients undergoing renal transplantation. All forms of glomerulonephritis may recur histologically in the renal allograft, but the incidence and severity of clinical recurrence vary greatly according to the type of glomerular disease. Recurrence may be early post-transplant or may take many years. Glomerular diseases that recur late will increase in clinical significance as advances in immunosuppression reduce rejection-mediated graft loss and prolong transplant survival. Registry data shows that the risk of graft loss from recurrence increases with the number of follow-up years, from 0.6% at the first postoperative year to 8.4% at 10 years [1, 2]. Recurrence was the third most frequent cause of allograft loss at 10 years, after chronic allograft failure and death with a functioning allograft [1, 2]. Interestingly, the use of more potent maintenance immunosuppressive agents or more potent induction agents such as alemtuzumab do not appear to reduce recurrence rates [3]. De novo glomerulonephritis may also occur in renal transplants. This chapter reviews the incidence, clinical features, treatment, and impact on renal transplant survival of the major forms of de novo and recurrent glomerular disease. There are several excellent reviews covering this subject [4, 5].

Interpreting the Literature on Recurrent Glomerular Disease

Due to the small number of cases within any single nephrology center, the literature on recurrent glomerular disease predominantly consists of anecdotal reports and retrospective case series. Results from such studies must be interpreted with caution particularly when subgroup analysis is performed. Retrospective data is subject to limitations of documentation, recall, and variations in local practice, and changes in practice over time. Registries capture data on large numbers of patients, but there is a limitation in the quality and accuracy of data due to incomplete or inaccurate identification, collection, and submission of data.

In order to correctly diagnose recurrent disease one needs an accurate histological diagnosis of both the native renal disease and the glomerular diseases in the transplant. However, many patients with chronic glomerulonephritis enter end-stage kidney disease (ESKD) without ever having had a renal biopsy. Furthermore, transplant patients with signs of glomerular disease such as mild proteinuria or slow deterioration in graft function are often not biopsied; when biopsies are performed immunostaining and electron microscopy are not always carried out. These factors lead to an under-estimation of the rate of recurrence.

The lack of specificity in the pathological features of some conditions may lead to errors in diagnosis; examples include the difficulty in differentiating primary from secondary focal segmental glomerulonephritis (FSGS) (a nonspecific feature of progressive renal disease), the similarity in light microscopic findings between transplant glomerulopathy (a feature of chronic humoral rejection), chronic thrombotic microangiopathy (TMA), and mesangiocapillary glomerulonephritis, and the common vascular changes observed in hemolytic uremic syndrome (HUS), malignant hypertension, scleroderma and cyclosporine toxicity. Also recurrence rates can be complicated by the existence of de novo disease such as de novo TMA, de novo membranous, and de novo mesangiocapillary glomerulonephritis. All the above factors may lead to an overestimation of recurrence rates.

Finally, caution must also be taken when estimating the incidence of graft loss from recurrence. Pathological features of acute and chronic rejection may coexist with glomerular pathology and it may be difficult to determine the exact cause of graft loss. A study of recurrent FSGS reported a high rate of acute cellular rejection in patients with recurrent disease. Furthermore, the primary disease may influence graft survival by mechanisms independent of disease recurrence; for example patients with IgA nephropathy have a higher than average graft survival despite frequent histological recurrence, whereas patients with systemic lupus erythematosus (SLE) may have poorer graft survival despite a negligible recurrence rate.

Primary Focal Segmental Glomerulonephritis

Primary FSGS is increasing in prevalence and is now the most common cause of nephrotic syndrome in children and adults and the most common primary glomerular disease leading to end-stage renal disease in the United States. The pathogenesis of primary FSGS is multifactorial but central to the pathogenesis is podocyte injury [6]. FSGS may be inherited and caused by mutations of genes encoding podocin or alpha-actinin-4 (familial FSGS) or acquired due to immunological, viral or toxin-induced injury to podocytes. These primary forms of FSGS are characterized by diffuse foot process fusion and segmental sclerosis. Secondary FSGS is a common histological finding in kidneys undergoing hyperfiltration injury following any renal injury but particularly reflux nephropathy. Secondary FSGS does not recur post-transplantation.

On the basis of glomerular morphology, D'Agati proposed a classification of primary FSGS variants known as the Columbia classification [7]. This classification distinguishes five variants of FSGS:

- The tip lesion variant, a lesion located near the origin of the proximal tubule
- The cellular variant characterized by endocapillary hypercellularity
- The collapsing variant, showing collapse of the glomerular tuft together with epithelial cell hypertrophy and hyperplasia
- The perihilar variant, a lesion predominantly located at the vascular pole
- FSGS not otherwise specified

If each variant represents a distinct pathogenic disease then it would be expected that morphology of recurrent disease would mimic the original native FSGS morphology. Ijpelaar et al. found that of 21 cases of FSGS recurrence, 81% recurred in the same pattern, supporting this hypothesis [8]. In fact, no transitions between the cellular and collapsing variant were seen, supporting the view that these are separate entities. The tip lesion variant of FSGS may be particularly prone to recurrence post-transplantation.

Overall the incidence of recurrence of primary FSGS is estimated at between 30 and 40%; approximately half of these grafts will fail due to recurrence [1, 9]. Thus recurrent FSGS is a major problem in the spectrum of recurrent glomerular disease and significantly impacts on graft survival. The coexistence of certain well-defined risk factors such as pediatric recipient, a rapid progression into ESKD, recurrence in a previous transplant, and mesangial hypercellularity on the native biopsy increases the likelihood of recurrence. Pediatric recipients with prior recurrence in a graft resulting in graft failure have an 85–100% risk of recurrence in future grafts.

Early reports suggested that recurrence of FSGS was more likely in live donor grafts compared with those of the deceased. Data from the North American Pediatric Renal Transplant Cooperative Study (NAPRTICS) database showed that there was a trend of increased graft failure from recurrence in live donor transplants compared with those of the deceased. However, overall survival of live donor grafts remained higher than that of the deceased. Similarly, examination of the United States Renal Data System (USRDS) database consisting of nearly 20,000 patients with FSGS showed that zero mismatch live donor kidney transplants had the best overall survival [10]. Some centers advocate not to use live donor kidneys in patients with previous graft loss from recurrence simply because of the high rate of expected graft loss. Live donation is contraindicated in patients with familial FSGS; recurrence has been described in recipients with homozygous podocin mutation who have received a kidney from a heterozygote parent.

Although primary FSGS in black patients generally takes a more aggressive course, several studies confirm that actual recurrence rates are less in the black population perhaps suggesting a distinct pathogenic mechanism of FSGS in these patients. Analysis of the NAPRTICS database revealed that native nephrectomy may be associated with a greater risk of recurrence; it is speculated that the presence of native kidneys provides a sponge for the circulating etiological factor.

Recurrence of FSGS in Patients with a Circulating Permeability Factor

Recurrent FSGS is most common in those forms of FSGS associated with a circulating factor responsible for inducing podocyte injury [11]. Indeed it was the rapidity of onset of recurrent FSGS that led to the hypothesis of a circulating permeability factor being a causative agent. Characterization of this permeability factor has revealed it to be anionic low-molecular-weight protein (30–50 kD) that binds galactose, can be removed by plasmapheresis and by absorption to a protein A column. The exact biochemical nature of this factor, however, remains to be elucidated. In vitro this factor rapidly affects glomerular permeability and induces altered phosphorylation of intracellular proteins and redistribution and loss of nephrin and podocin in podocytes.

Recurrence of FSGS in Patients with Familial FSGS

There have been exciting developments in understanding the genetic basis of inherited forms of FSGS [6]. Mutations of the gene NPHS2 (encoding for podocin) are the commonest cause of familial FSGS. Mutations of other genes encoding slit diaphragm proteins, e.g., NPHS1 (encoding nephrin) and α-actinin-4 are also associated with nephrotic syndrome. Sporadic mutations of any of these genes may account for cases of nephrotic syndrome in the absence of a family history. Indeed, homozygous/complex heterozygous NPHS2 mutations have been reported in 8% of sporadic FSGS causing nephrotic syndrome in early childhood [12]. Heterozygous carriers of NPHS2 mutations present variable clinical features with onset of proteinuria generally later in life.

In general, patients with homozygous/compound heterozygous NPHS2 mutations showed a low recurrence rate of less than 10%. When recurrence occurs it may be due to inadvertent transplantation of a kidney from a related heterozygous carrier. An alternative explanation for recurrence in patients with podocin mutations is the development of anti-podocin antibodies by the recipient (analogous to the development of anti-glomerular basement membrane antibodies(anti-GBMs) in patients with Alport's syndrome post-transplantation). In contrast, recurrent nephrotic syndrome is common after renal transplantation in patients with congenital nephritic syndrome of the Finnish type (due to the NPHS1 mutation encoding nephrin). Kuusniemi et al. reported the outcome of 19 transplants in patients with NPHS1 mutations. Recurrent nephrotic syndrome was observed in all transplants and was associated with the development of anti-nephrin antibodies [13]. It is hypothesized that transplantation results in the immune system being exposed to a previously "unseen" antigen resulting in anti-nephrin antibody production.

Clinical Presentation of Recurrent FSGS

The clinical severity of recurrent FSGS is highly variable, reflecting the heterogeneity of this condition. Classically, heavy proteinuria can occur immediately following vascular anastomosis, leading to frank nephrotic syndrome and rapid graft loss. In contrast some patients may develop low-grade proteinuria months after transplantation and exhibit a slow deterioration in graft function. The severity of recurrence usually mimics the severity of the primary involvement of native kidneys. Delayed graft function and acute tubular necrosis are more common post-transplant in patients who have immediate recurrence presumably because heavy proteinuria inhibits tubular recovery from ischemic injury. It has been reported that acute rejection is also more frequent in patients with recurrent FSGS. This may be due to changes in the antigenicity of the graft. Alternately it may be from reduced bioavailability of cyclosporine A due to hyperlipidemia associated with the nephrotic syndrome.

Treatment of Recurrent FSGS

Treatment regimens reported include plasmapheresis, double filtration plasmapheresis, immunoadsorption, high-dose calcineurin inhibitors (CNIs), cyclosphosphamide, rituximab, and anti-tumor necrosis factor (TNF) therapy alone or in combination. Most studies consist of case series in which results are compared to historical data. There are no randomized controlled trials.

Many studies have reported the efficacy of plasmapheresis for the treatment of recurrent FSGS [9]. Plasmapheresis can reduce proteinuria, often to negligible levels associated with coexistent loss of the circulating permeability factor in the serum and improvement of the histological lesion of podocyte effacement. Plasmapheresis is also effective in patients with congenital nephrotic syndrome who have recurrence associated with the development of anti-nephrin antibodies. Unfortunately in a large proportion of patients, nephrotic syndrome returns with a cessation of treatment. Patients who relapse after stopping plasmapheresis may often require further treatments extending over months to years. Plasmapheresis typically involves a 3.5 L exchange daily for 3–4 exchanges followed by alternate day and later weekly exchanges. The replacement solution is usually 5% human albumin solution and saline. However recent data demonstrating the ability of plasma to inhibit the activity of the FSGS-associated circulating permeability factor suggests that fresh frozen plasma may be the more appropriate replacement solution [11]. Additional reports have claimed success when combining plasmapheresis with high-dose cyclosporine, cyclophosphamide or mycophenolate mofetil. Canaud et al. reported the outcome of ten adult kidney transplant recipients with FSGS recurrence treated with high-dose steroids, intravenous cyclosporine for 14 days followed by oral cyclosporine therapy, and an intensive and prolonged course of plasma exchanges [14]. Complete remission was achieved in 90% of patients and maintained after stopping plasmapheresis at 9 months.

In general, long-term remission may be seen in 50–70% of patients with recurrent FSGS treated with plasmapheresis. Children may have a more favorable response than adults. Complete remission appears to be more likely if treatment is initiated early after recurrence develops. Patients therefore need to be monitored frequently by urine protein/creatinine ratio assessments post-transplantation. It is important that patients with FSGS have minimal proteinuria at the time of transplantation in order to best detect recurrence. Some advocate either "medical nephrectomy" (use of angiotensin II blockade and non-steroidal anti-inflammatory agents) or nephrectomy to remove any native proteinuria prior to transplantation.

In patients with a high risk of recurrence, some advocate prophylactic plasmapheresis pre- and post-transplantation. Using serum taken from patients pre-transplant, Savin et al. have developed an in vitro permeability assay using isolated glomeruli to successfully identify those patients who recur post-transplant [11]. This assay may be used to determine which patients may benefit from prophylactic plasmapheresis. Gohh et al. used a combination of pre- and post-operative plasmapheresis in high-risk adult patients (defined by either previous recurrence or rapid progression to ESKD) [15]. Simply performing eight sessions of plasmapheresis in the perioperative period reduced the rate of recurrence by 50%.

Other groups have examined the efficacy of high-dose CNIs. Raafat achieved complete remission in 11 of 16 cases of recurrence by increasing the cyclosporine dose to 24 mg/kg/day [16]. Remission was achieved between 14 days and 19 months. High-dose CNIs certainly reduce proteinuria but this may simply be due to a hemodynamic effect of these agents rather than a disease modulatory effect.

There are anecdotal reports of pediatric patients with post-transplant lymphoproliferative disorder (PTLD) and recurrent FSGS who have had remission of proteinuria after treatment with rituximab. This prompted the speculation that rituximab may inhibit production of a circulatory permeability factor. Dello Strologo et al. reported effect of rituximab in seven children or young adults with recurrent FSGS who did not respond to intensive plasmapheresis [17]. The majority had complete or partial remission. A randomized controlled trial of rituximab is needed in this setting.

IgA Nephropathy

Globally, IgA nephropathy is the commonest type of glomerulonephritis leading to ESKD. Histological recurrence of IgA nephropathy in renal allografts is common and may occur early. Most studies report a 50–60% rate of histological recurrence within 6 months post-transplantation [18]. When protocol biopsies are performed, mesangial IgA deposition may be seen within weeks post-transplantation. Diagnosis of recurrence may be complicated by the fact that IgA deposits may be a component of donor disease. Clinical recurrence may be associated with hematuria, proteinuria, and/or graft dysfunction. In general, the clinical course of recurrent IgA nephropathy in transplanted kidneys is relatively indolent; with 10–20% reaching ESKD after 10 years. Therefore, the clinical impact of recurrent disease reported by studies is very dependent on the duration of follow-up of the study. Early studies report that the clinical manifestations of recurrence are mild and that graft loss secondary to recurrent disease is rare. More recent reports involving longer follow-up have noted significant graft dysfunction and high rates of graft loss. Kessler reported on the outcome of 71 patients with a mean follow-up of 5 years post-transplant [19]. Clinically significant recurrence was seen in 15% of patients.

Some reports suggest that recurrence is more common following live donor transplantation and in human leukocyte antigen (HLA) identical grafts. Andresdottir et al. reported the outcome post-transplant of 79 patients with IgA nephropathy. Clinical recurrence occurred in 20% of patients with a living related donor graft vs. 4% in patients receiving a cadaveric kidney [20]. Analysis of the Australia and New Zealand database showed that of 1,354 transplants performed in patients with IgA nephropathy, those who received zero-HLA mismatched live donor kidneys had more than double the recurrence rate compared with those receiving a cadaveric or less well-matched live donor kidney. The impact of recurrence on graft survival however was counterbalanced by the survival advantage associated due to reduced rejection with receiving a zero-mismatched kidney.

Prolonged time on dialysis prior to transplantation is not associated with a reduced rate of recurrence suggesting that "burn out" of the disease process does not occur following ESKD. No difference in recurrence rates has been reported with more potent maintenance immunosuppressive regimens. Interestingly Berthoux et al. examined the effect of anti-thymocyte globulin (ATG) induction on recurrence [21]. They reported on 116 patients with IgA nephropathy who were transplanted. The 10-year cumulative recurrence rate was only 9% after ATG induction compared with 41% in patients who did not receive ATG induction.

Despite the high rate of recurrence, overall graft survival in patients with IgA nephropathy is good. Indeed several studies have shown higher graft survival in this transplant population compared with those transplanted for ESKD due to other forms of renal disease. Andresdottir reported that 5-year graft survival for cadaveric kidneys was 86% in patients with IgA nephropathy vs. 67 and 60% in patients with polycystic kidney disease and non-IgA glomerular disease, respectively [20]. Closer observation shows that the benefit in graft survival occurs within 3 months post-transplantation, perhaps due to less severe acute rejection. It has been proposed that immunological changes such as high pre-transplant levels of IgA antibodies to HLA class I molecules in patients with IgA nephropathy favor allograft acceptance.

In those patients with established recurrence, risk factors for the progression of recurrent disease are similar to those for primary IgA nephropathy, namely heavy proteinuria, hypertension, mesangial proliferation, and glomerulosclerosis on biopsy. Patients with crescentic IgA nephropathy in native kidneys and those with a rapid course to ESKD are more likely to have clinically significant recurrence often with recurrent crescentic disease. A retrospective analysis showed that patients with recurrent IgA nephropathy had improved graft survival if they were treated with renin–angiotensin–aldosterone system (RAAS) blockade. RAAS blockade is therefore recommended with recurrence. There is only anecdotal evidence for fish oil therapy and corticosteroids in recurrent IgA nephropathy. Several Japanese groups describe the benefit of tonsillectomy on reducing proteinuria in patients with recurrent IgA nephropathy. Kennoki et al. report on 28 established cases of recurrent IgA nephropathy [22]. Sixteen patients underwent tonsillectomy with a reduction in mean proteinuria from 800 to 200 mg/day compared with no reduction in proteinuria in the 12 cases who did not undergo tonsillectomy. Best results were achieved in patients with mild mesangial changes on biopsy.

Membranoproliferative Glomerulonephritis

Membranoproliferative glomerulonephritis (MPGN) is a common histological response to a several distinct etiologies. The light microscopic changes of MPGN (lobulated glomeruli with mesangial hypercellularity and glomerular basement membrane splitting) are shared with transplant glomerulopathy, chronic TMA (either from CNIs or familial HUS), paraprotein deposition disorders and classic immune complex associated MPGN [23]. Distinguishing the underlying cause of MPGN requires ultrastructural assessment of the glomerulus using electron microscopy together with immunofluorescent studies. Chronic TMA and transplant glomerulopathy are characterized by a lack of immune complex deposition, and paraprotein deposition disorders can usually be distinguished by unique electron microscopic changes. MPGN associated with immune complex deposition can be further divided into MPGN Type 1 associated with chronic hepatitis C (HCV) infection, SLE, and lymphoma and MPGN type 2 also known as dense deposit disease (DDD). DDD arises from over activity of the alternative complement pathway either due to an autoantibody to C3 convertase (C3 nephritic factor) or from factor H mutations. Early studies have not satisfactorily separated out the underlying causes of MPGN and therefore have limited value in determining recurrence rates post-transplantation. Recurrence rates are likely to vary depending on the specific etiology. This section focuses on recurrence of non-HVC-related MPGN Type 1, DDD, and HCV-associated de novo MPGN.

Non-HCV-Associated MPGN Type 1

Lorenz reported the transplant outcome of 29 patients with ESKD secondary to type 1 MPGN [24]. Post-transplant protocol biopsies were performed in this center. During an average follow-up of 53 months, 41% had recurrent disease diagnosed 1 week to 14 months post-transplant. The majority had subclinical disease at biopsy. Five patients lost their grafts. Low complement levels predicted recurrence. The presence of serum monoclonal proteins predicted a poor outcome. The recurrence rate quoted in this study is similar to earlier reports. Recurrence usually manifests with significant proteinuria and reduced graft survival. Treatment options include plasmapheresis and cyclophosphamide, but their effectiveness is not established.

Dense Deposit Disease

DDD, or MPGN type 2, has a high recurrence rate post-transplantation; histological recurrence is observed in 50–80%. Braun et al. performed an analysis of the NAPRTICS database and identified 75 patients with DDD who were transplanted [25]. Recurrent disease occurred in 75% and 5-year graft survival was 50% compared with 75% for the database as a whole. Other groups confirm high recurrence rates and poor graft survival. The C3 nephritic factor and C3 levels do not always correlate with severity of recurrence. Optimal management of recurrence depends on the nature of the complement dysregulation. If C3 nephritic factor is present then regular plasmapheresis to remove and rituximab to inhibit production of this factor is warranted. In contrast if there is a factor H deficiency then plasma infusion is warranted. A therapeutic role for sulindoxide in recurrent DDD is under investigation.

HCV-Associated MPGN Type 1

HCV infection may result in de novo MPGN type 1 in renal transplant patients [26]. This is of concern given the high incidence of HCV infection in some dialysis populations. In a cohort of 98 HCV-infected transplant patients, eight patients developed nephrotic syndrome (2 months to 10 years post-transplant) of whom five patients had biopsy proven MPGN [27]. Other groups show a higher incidence of glomerular disease and indeed graft loss and recommend transplant biopsy of HCV-positive recipients even in the presence of mild clinical or laboratory findings compatible with glomerular disease. In order to prevent de novo glomerular disease in this patient population, patients with HCV infection awaiting transplantation should receive anti-viral treatment with interferon-α and ribavirin prior to transplantation. Unfortunately approximately 50% do not respond. Preliminary reports suggest that HCV infection may be eradicated and both cryoglobulinemia and associated glomerular disease improved with interferon-α and ribavirin treatment post-transplant. Several reports suggests that rituximab, by depleting peripheral B cells, may reduce HCV associated cryoglobulins and improve glomerular inflammation and reduce proteinuria without enhancing HCV replication.

Recurrent Membranous Glomerulopathy

Dabade et al. performed surveillance biopsies in 19 transplant patients with ESKD secondary to membranous nephropathy (MN) and found that histological recurrence was seen in 42% with a median follow-up of 4 months [28]. The majority of these patients had very subtle changes on light microscopy and were only diagnosed with the aid of immunofluorescence and electron microscopy. At the time of diagnosis most patients had minimal proteinuria. Longer-term follow-up of these patients showed that some went on to develop nephrotic syndrome. Similar findings were reported recently by El-Zoghby et al. [29]. The incidence of recurrent MN was 41% and median time of diagnosis was 4 months. Although clinical disease was mild at diagnosis, the majority of patients with recurrent MN had progressive increases in proteinuria. Briganti reported the outcome of 81 patients who had membranous glomerulopathy as a primary renal disease. After 10 years 12.5% of this group lost their grafts due to recurrent disease [1].

Clinical presentation of recurrence is with increasing proteinuria; the mean time to development of nephrotic range proteinuria is 10 months post-transplant. Recurrence in successive transplants has also been reported. Unlike native disease, spontaneous remission of membranous glomerulopathy in transplants is rare. There are only anecdotal reports on treatment. Secondary causes for membranous glomerulopathy such as drugs and hepatitis viruses should be excluded. The beneficial effects of steroids combined with cyclophosphamide or chlorambucil have not been validated. Several groups have reported a rapid reversal of the nephrotic syndrome with rituximab. The rationale for using this agent comes from preliminary data showing a beneficial effect in primary MN. El-Zoghby et al. treated eight patients with nephritic range proteinuria with rituximab. Seventy-five percent of treated patients underwent complete or partial remission [29].

De Novo Membranous Glomerulopathy

De novo membranous glomerulopathy is one of the most common forms of glomerular disease seen in the renal allograft, occurring in 1–2% of all transplants. Only transplant glomerulopathy is responsible for more cases of nephrotic syndrome in transplant recipients. The glomerular changes are identical to recurrent membranous glomerulopathy, and differentiation between the two requires an accurate knowledge of primary renal disease pre-transplantation. The incidence appears to increase with time post-transplant reaching 5% at 10 years. In general de novo membranous is reported to occur later and have a more severe clinical course than recurrent membranous glomerulopathy. In a retrospective study of 872 renal transplants 2% of grafts were shown to have de novo membranous glomerulopathy with a mean time post-transplant of 62 months [30]. Approximately 60% developed nephrotic syndrome, which was not responsive to steroids. However, overall graft survival was the same as control.

The exact cause of de novo membranous glomerulopathy is unknown but it often coexists with histological features of chronic rejection and therefore may be a manifestation of alloimmune-mediated injury. It is postulated that low-grade chronic vascular and interstitial rejection uncovers unseen epitopes and yields immune complexes. Cases of de novo membranous glomerulopathy associated with the appearance of a donor-specific alloantibody have been described suggesting that it may be an atypical manifestation of acute or chronic humoral rejection. Whether the introduction of more potent immunosuppressive has decreased the incidence of de novo membranous glomerulopathy is unclear. De novo membranous glomerulopathy may be associated with chronic viral infection such as hepatitis B (HBV) or HCV or secondary to drugs. The beneficial effects of steroids, cyclosporine, mycophenolate mofetil, cyclophosphamide, chlorambucil, or other agents have not been validated.

Recurrence of ANCA-Associated Vasculitis

Antineutrophil cytoplasmic antibody (ANCA)-associated vasculitis is the most common cause of rapidly progressive glomerulonephritis and approximately 20% of these patients will develop end-stage renal failure. Nachman et al. performed a pooled analysis of published data consisting of 127 patients with ANCA-associated vasculitis who received a renal transplant [31]. Recurrent ANCA-associated vasculitis occurred in 22 of 127 patients (17%). The average time to relapse was 31 months post-transplantation. Of the 21 with recurrent disease, 12 patients had renal involvement, the remaining patients having recurrence of upper respiratory tract or pulmonary involvement. Neither duration on dialysis prior to transplant, nor type of immunosuppressive therapy (majority received cyclosporine) influenced relapse rate. ANCA status at the time of transplant did not affect outcome. The clinical expression of ANCA-associated disease i.e., Wegener's granulomatosis, microscopic polyangiitis, or necrotizing crescentic glomerulonephritis does not influence risk of relapse. Deegens et al. reported a lower relapse rate in transplanted patients receiving more potent immunosuppression [32]. Mycophenolate mofetil is emerging as an efficacious drug for the treatment of ANCA-associated vasculitis, and it may be the more widespread use of this drug post-transplantation that is leading to lower recurrence rates. Patient and graft survival compare favorable to transplant patients with other forms of primary renal disease.

In general, patients should be in clinical remission and ANCA negative prior to transplantation. However, ANCA levels may remain positive despite disease remission, and a number of groups have reported successful transplantation despite elevated ANCA titers. Nachmann's pooled analysis of trial data concluded that ANCA positivity should not preclude transplant [31]. Clinical recurrence in the renal allograft may manifest as worsening renal function, worsening proteinuria, crescentic glomerulonephritis on biopsy and rising ANCA titers. Rarely, ureteric involvement may lead to transplant hydronephrosis. Extra-renal relapse is more common. When relapse does occur therapy with cyclophosphamide and corticosteroids has been shown to be effective at inducing remission. Rituximab may also be efficacious and allow avoidance of repeated courses of cyclophosphamide [33].

Anti-GBM Disease

Anti-glomerular basement membrane (anti-GBM) disease is characterized by crescentic glomerulonephritis and sometimes lung hemorrhage in the presence of anti-GBM antibodies. This disease usually is mediated by IgG auto-antibodies directed against the noncollagenous domain of the alpha3 chain of Type IV collagen, the Goodpasture autoantigen. There is general consensus that the disease almost never recurs in renal allografts, providing anti-GBM titers are absent prior to transplantation. This is because unlike some other causes of crescentic glomerulonephritis, Goodpasture's disease is a "one-hit" disease that does not relapse. Cameron described successful transplantation of 20 patients with Goodpasture's disease. More recent reports confirm lack of recurrence of anti-GBM disease but warned of an increased rate of malignancy post-transplantation presumably due to the exposure to cyclophosphamide prior to transplantation. Patients should wait for 6–12 months on dialysis until anti-GBM antibodies are absent. Even when antititers are detectable prior to transplantation, most patients develop only mild clinical features despite the detection of liner IgG deposition in the capillary walls.

When recurrence does occur it is usually very soon post-transplantation. However, recurrence has been reported up to 8 years post-transplantation.

De novo anti-GBM disease may occur in allografts transplanted into patients with Alport's disease. Byrne et al. evaluated 52 renal allografts transplanted into 41 patients with Alport's disease [34]. Although 14% of grafts showed linear glomerular basement membrane IgG deposits, only 1 of 52 grafts developed post-transplant anti-GBM disease. Patient and graft survival rates in this population were very good.

Systemic Lupus Erythematosus

Recurrence of SLE-associated renal disease in the transplant is considered rare. In general clinically significant recurrence is seen in less than 5%. Indeed the serological and clinical activity of SLE usually diminishes following the onset of ESKD and relapses are uncommon. Several mechanisms have been proposed for this disease "burn out" following ESKD, including the immunomodulatory effect of uremia, removal of lupus factors by dialysis or loss of renal produced disease mediators. None of these factors satisfactorily explain the lack of recurrence following transplantation; however, maintenance immunosuppression may play an important role in preventing both extra-renal manifestations and recurrent glomerular disease at this stage.

Subclinical histological recurrence may be more common. When protocol biopsies are performed and renal biopsy specimens examined routinely by immunofluorescence and electron microscopy then the reported rate of recurrence may be as high as 30% [35]. However, this high histological recurrence rate was not associated with a poor clinical outcome. All histological variants of lupus-associated glomerular disease have been reported post-transplantation, but mesangial proliferation is the most common histological presentation. It is suggested that a short duration of time on dialysis prior to transplantation and positive lupus serology and hypocomplementemia may be associated with an increased likelihood of recurrence but not all studies demonstrate this. Burgos et al. reported a recurrence rate of 11% in 202 patients [36]. African American race was the strongest risk factor for recurrence. There is no consensus in the literature as to whether recurrence rates differ between living donor and cadaveric kidneys. The use of more potent immunosuppressive agents may further lower the recurrence rate of lupus nephritis. In keeping with the low rate of clinically significant recurrence, patient and graft survival rates in patients with SLE are similar to other transplant populations [36].

Transplantation should be avoided if lupus is clinically active. Early graft loss may be caused by graft thrombosis associated with antiphospholipid antibodies. Long-term anticoagulation should be considered for all SLE patients transplanted with a history of either thrombosis or antiphospholipid antibodies. Antiphospholipid antibodies may also be associated with TMA in renal allograft. Patients with SLE have usually been exposed to corticosteroids and cyclophosphamide. Steroid avoidance protocols may avoid some of the long-term complications of steroids. Due to prior cyclophosphamide exposure, bone marrow suppression and malignancy is more common in patients on maintenance immunosuppression.

Hemolytic Uremic Syndrome

HUS constitutes a triad of acute renal failure, microangiopathic hemolytic anemia, and thrombocytopenia. The pathological finding is a TMA. It represents a common pathophysiological response to a heterogenous group of etiological agents that mediate endothelial injury and/or promote hypercoagulability. These include toxins (shiga toxin), drugs (antineoplastic, antiplatelet, immunosuppressive), viruses (HIV), and autoimmunity (SLE, antiphospholipid antibodies, scleroderma) [37]. In over 50% of cases no triggering condition is recognized. The majority of these patients have a genetic defect in complement regulation that is either inherited or arises de novo in the proband. Both recurrent and de novo HUS can occur in the allograft.

Recurrent HUS

The reported rate of recurrence varies (between 10 and 50%) and is almost certainly related to the etiology of the original disease. When patients develop diarrheal associated HUS from *Escherichia coli* infection (shiga-toxin-induced HUS) leading to ESKD, transplantation is almost never associated with recurrence. Of 118 children transplanted after diarrheal associated HUS only one (0.8%) had recurrence [38]. In contrast atypical or familial HUS, which is not associated with diarrheal prodrome, can result in repeated loss of renal allografts. The genetic defects that result in familial HUS are now well defined. Mutations in three complement regulatory proteins (factor H, factor I, and membrane cofactor protein [MCP]) account for almost all cases. The physiologic function of these proteins is to downregulate the alternative complement pathway. Loss of function or deficiency of one of these proteins leads to excessive complement activation, endothelial injury, and microvascular thrombosis. Complement factor H deficiency appears to carry the worst prognosis in terms of developing ESKD.

Bresin et al. have reported in detail the outcome of renal transplantation in patients with non-shiga-toxin-associated HUS [39]. A total of 78 patients received 100 kidney transplants. Sixty percent had recurrent HUS and 90% of these patients had graft failure. The presence of a factor H mutation or factor I mutation was associated with the highest rate of graft failure (78 vs. 55% in patients without these mutations). The time between renal transplantation and graft loss from recurrence ranged from 3 days to 2 years. Use of CNIs was not associated with an increased risk of recurrence. In contrast, patients with an MCP mutation have a better prognosis.

In this series and others no recurrence was seen. One explanation is that MCP is a transmembrane protein expressed mostly in the kidney. Therefore complement dysregulation related to MCP mutation should be corrected by transplantation of an allograft kidney. It is recommended that genotyping for factor H (CHF), MCP, and factor I (IF) is performed in all patients with ESKD secondary to non-shiga-toxin-associated HUS who are considered for transplantation. The high graft failure rates seen in patients with CHF and IF mutations make transplantation difficult to justify. It is advised not to use live donors because of the rapid failure rate and because of the risk of de novo HUS disease in the donor. Combined liver and kidney transplants may be considered for patients with factor H or factor I mutations. Recent reports suggest graft function can be maintained postrecurrence by prolonged plasmapheresis therapy with fresh frozen plasma replacement. Other groups have adopted calcineurin-free immunosuppression for these patients with some success.

De Novo HUS

De novo HUS in renal allografts is most frequently reported in association with cyclosporine A usage and classically occurs early post-transplantation when the cyclosporin levels are high. However, it is important to note that de novo HUS in renal allografts is also associated with the use of tacrolimus, sirolimus, and induction agents ATG and OKT3 [40]. Other risk factors for the de novo HUS include the use of marginal kidneys, retransplantation, sensitized recipients, infections such as cytomegalovirus (CMV) infection, parvovirus B 19 infection, and BK polyoma virus nephritis, antiphospholipid antibodies, anticardiolipin antibodies in HCV-positive patients, malignancy, and drugs such as clopidogrel. Therefore, de novo HUS is likely multifactorial with immunosuppressive agents playing the most important pathogenetic role.

In the analysis of USRDS data, de novo HUS was reported in only 0.8% of cases [41]. This is likely an underestimate due to failure to diagnose and underreporting. Single-center studies report a greater incidence ranging between 5 and 15%. Usually, de novo HUS occurs in the first few weeks post-transplant, but it may also develop several years after transplantation. The clinical presentation is variable and will range from acute graft dysfunction to mild increase in creatinine. Frequently the hematological changes are only mild. Glomerular thrombi may not be seen on biopsy. Evidence for endothelial injury with thickening and reduplication of the basement membrane is common.

The prognosis is less severe than with recurrent HUS and is reflected by the severity of clinical, hematologic, and histological features. Prognosis is more favorable when HUS occurs later in the post-transplant course. Graft loss is rare. Several studies have examined treatment options in de novo transplant HUS but currently therapeutic guidelines are not well defined. The mainstay of treatment is good blood pressure control, early institution of dialysis, and withdrawal of the offending drug. Plasmapheresis in addition to CNI withdrawal resulted in a graft salvage rate of 80%

in one series [42]. The addition of intravenous immunoglobulins resulted in a stable remission in a patient with plasmapheresis-resistant HUS after a kidney transplant.

Henoch Schonlein Purpura

Although the natural history of Henoch Schonlein purpura (HSP) is usually one of complete resolutions, a small subpopulation of patients usually with crescentic glomerulonephritis progresses to ESKD. In countries where HSP is common, these cases can make up a significant proportion of the ESKD population transplanted; greater than 10% in one Japanese study. HSP can recur in the renal transplant and when it does it is usually isolated and not associated with the extra-renal manifestations of HSP. The histological appearance of recurrent disease is identical to IgA nephropathy. The rate of recurrence of HSP post-transplantation is less well characterized than IgA nephropathy and frequently cases in individual center reports are pooled with patients with IgA nephropathy. Han reported on 20 patients with HSP transplanted and followed up for over 10 years [43]. Recurrence rate was 15% but graft survival was good and similar to controls. In contrast Moroni et al. reported the outcome of 17 patients with HSP who were transplanted with a mean follow-up of approximately 10 years [44]. Recurrence was seen in 42% of patients of whom approximately half ultimately lost their graft from recurrence; there was a trend for increased recurrence with living donation. Patients who have crescentic disease in native kidneys generally present with crescentic involvement in the transplant and have a poorer prognosis. There is little information on the treatment of recurrent HSP in renal transplant patients. In native renal disease in adults there is little evidence to support that either corticosteroids or cyclophosphamide alter renal outcome even with crescentic disease. Plasmapheresis may be effective in aggressive early recurrence of HSP.

Nodular Glomerulopathy: Fibrillary Glomerulonephritis, Light Chain Deposition Disease and Amyloid

Fibrillary glomerulonephritis is a rare but progressive glomerular disease that leads to ESKD within months to a few years. Clinical features include mixed nephritic/nephritic syndrome, hematuria, renal dysfunction, and hypertension. There are only a few studies reporting the outcome of these patients following renal transplantation and in general recurrence rate is approximately 50%. Czarnecki et al. reported the outcome of 12 patients with fibrillary glomerulonephritis who were transplanted. Recurrence occurred in five patients and the distinguishing factor associated with recurrence was the presence of a monoclonal gammopathy. Several of these patients later developed hematologic malignancy [45].

Light chain deposit disease (LCDD) is a monoclonal plasma cell disorder characterized by tissue deposition of non-amyloid immunoglobulin light chains, predominantly kappa light chains, causing proteinuria and renal insufficiency. It is usually associated with myeloma but can also be seen in association with a "benign" paraproteinemia. LCDD reoccurs almost invariably after renal grafting. The characteristic pathology is nodular glomerulosclerosis; however, an MPGN pattern with crescents has also been described which is associated with a poorer prognosis. Leung et al. described the post-transplant course of seven patients with LCDD [46]. All patients had nodular glomerulopathy with kappa light chains. Recurrence post-transplantation occurred in five patients with a median time to recurrence of 33 months. Mortality was high predominantly due to progression of myeloma. The same group have recently reported improved outcome in patients who receive high-dose chemotherapy and autologous stem cell transplantation prior to renal transplantation. There are reports of a good response to rituximab treatment.

Although ESKD is common in patients with systemic amyloidosis, these patients rarely receive a renal transplant because of the poor underlying patient prognosis. Renal transplantation may however improve the survival of these patients. Appreciation of the type of amyloid is important. The amyloid light chain (AL) amyloid has the worst prognosis due to the development of significant cardiac involvement resulting in ventricular arrhythmias. Patients with AL amyloid fare better if they receive treatment in the form of chemotherapy or autologous stem cell transplantation prior to renal transplantation. However, tolerability of this regimen is reduced if patients have ESKD. Renal transplant should be considered in patients who are in remission. Significant cardiac involvement should be excluded prior to renal transplantation. In contrast amyloid associated (AA) amyloid does not affect the heart and providing the underlying cause has remitted, renal transplantation is advised. However, patient and graft survival in these patients may be reduced compared with other patients with renal transplant. Serum amyloid P scintigraphy was performed in patients with 15 AA amyloidosis who had received a renal transplant [47]. Graft amyloidosis was not detected in any patients in whom the amyloidogenic underlying disorder had remitted, but over half of those in whom it had not. Recurrence of amyloid A deposition in the allograft can be seen in patients with secondary amyloidosis due to familial Mediterranean fever (FMF). Keven et al. reported on 17 transplant patients with FMF [48]. Graft outcome was as good as the general transplant population and recurrence seen in only two patients despite colchicines treatment.

Conclusion and General Recommendations

Recurrent and de novo glomerular disease is a significant problem post-transplantation and the detrimental impact glomerular disease has on graft survival will likely increase as grafts survive longer due to improvements in immunosuppression.

There are several salient points, which can be summarized from the literature on recurrent glomerular disease.

- Recurrent and de novo glomerular disease is more common than previously thought. Protocol biopsies and routine immunostaining and electron microscopy have yielded an increase in the diagnosis of glomerular disease post-transplantation. Close attention to urinalysis in the post-transplant clinic is important.
- Advances in immunosuppression including the use of potent induction agents have not reduced the rate of recurrent glomerular disease.
- Recurrent FSGS is a major problem particularly in the pediatric population and in patients where the underlying pathogenesis involves a circulating permeability factor. In general live donor transplantation should not be discouraged in these patients. Early diagnosis of recurrent FSGS is essential for success of treatment. Prophylactic plasmapheresis should be provided for those with a high risk of recurrence. Treatment of proven recurrence should include plasmapheresis; this may be required for a protracted time period.
- Recurrent IgA nephropathy is a very common histological finding. Its impact on graft survival however is dependent on duration of transplant follow-up due to the relative indolence of the disease. Recurrent disease may be increased in live donor transplants (albeit with no detrimental effect on graft survival) and reduced with ATG induction. Patients with crescentic IgA nephropathy have a poorer outcome post-transplantation. There is no specific treatment for recurrence.
- Recurrent DDD is common and significantly impacts on graft survival. Treatment should include prolonged plasmapheresis and rituximab in the presence of C3 nephritic factor or prolonged plasma infusion in the setting of factor H deficiency.
- De novo MPGN type 1 is common post-transplantation in patients with chronic hepatitis C infection. Attempts at eradication of hepatitis C with interferon and ribaviron should be made pre-transplantation. These agents and rituximab have also been safely used successfully post-transplantation without precipitating acute rejection.
- In general recurrence of ANCA-associated vasculitis, HSP, SLE, and anti-GBM disease is not a significant problem particularly if the activity of these diseases is quiescent prior to transplantation.
- Patients who develop ESKD from diarrhea-associated HUS do not exhibit recurrence. Recurrence is also rare in patients with MCP deficiency. In contrast, patients with familial HUS due to factor H or factor I deficiency have high graft failure rates from recurrence. Live related donation should be avoided in this group. Combined kidney liver transplants may be advised in this group.
- There is limited data on optimal treatment of recurrent glomerulonephritis in general. All patients should have excellent blood pressure control and inhibition of the renin angiotensin aldosterone system.

References

1. Briganti EM, Russ GR, McNeil JJ, Atkins RC, Chadban SJ. Risk of renal allograft loss from recurrent glomerulonephritis. N Engl J Med. 2002;347(2):103–9.
2. Hariharan S, Peddi VR, Savin VJ, et al. Recurrent and de novo renal diseases after renal transplantation: a report from the renal allograft disease registry. Am J Kidney Dis. 1998;31(6):928–31.
3. Mulay AV, van Walraven C, Knoll GA. Impact of immunosuppressive medication on the risk of renal allograft failure due to recurrent glomerulonephritis. Am J Transplant. 2009;9(4):804–11.
4. Choy BY, Chan TM, Lai KN. Recurrent glomerulonephritis after kidney transplantation. Am J Transplant. 2006;6(11):2535–42.
5. Golgert WA, Appel GB, Hariharan S. Recurrent glomerulonephritis after renal transplantation: an unsolved problem. Clin J Am Soc Nephrol. 2008;3(3):800–7.
6. Pollak MR. Focal segmental glomerulosclerosis: recent advances. Curr Opin Nephrol Hypertens. 2008;17(2):138–42.
7. D'Agati VD. The spectrum of focal segmental glomerulosclerosis: new insights. Curr Opin Nephrol Hypertens. 2008;17(3):271–81.
8. Ijpelaar DH, Farris AB, Goemaere N, et al. Fidelity and evolution of recurrent FSGS in renal allografts. J Am Soc Nephrol. 2008;19(11):2219–24.
9. Fine RN. Recurrence of nephrotic syndrome/focal segmental glomerulosclerosis following renal transplantation in children. Pediatr Nephrol. 2007;22(4):496–502.
10. Cibrik DM, Kaplan B, Campbell DA, Meier-Kriesche HU. Renal allograft survival in transplant recipients with focal segmental glomerulosclerosis. Am J Transplant. 2003;3(1):64–7.
11. Savin VJ, McCarthy ET, Sharma M. Permeability factors in focal segmental glomerulosclerosis. Semin Nephrol. 2003;23(2):147–60.
12. Weber S, Gribouval O, Esquivel EL, et al. NPHS2 mutation analysis shows genetic heterogeneity of steroid-resistant nephrotic syndrome and low post-transplant recurrence. Kidney Int. 2004;66(2):571–9.
13. Kuusniemi AM, Qvist E, Sun Y, et al. Plasma exchange and retransplantation in recurrent nephrosis of patients with congenital nephrotic syndrome of the Finnish type (NPHS1). Transplantation. 2007;83(10):1316–23.
14. Canaud G, Zuber J, Sberro R, Royale V, Anglicheau D, Snanoudj R, et al. Intensive and prolonged treatment of focal and segmental glomerulosclerosis recurrence in adult kidney transplant recipients: a pilot study. Am J Transplant. 2009;9(5):1081–6.
15. Gohh RY, Yango AF, Morrissey PE, et al. Preemptive plasmapheresis and recurrence of FSGS in high-risk renal transplant recipients. Am J Transplant. 2005;5(12):2907–12.
16. Raafat RH, Kalia A, Travis LB, Diven SC. High-dose oral cyclosporin therapy for recurrent focal segmental glomerulosclerosis in children. Am J Kidney Dis. 2004;44(1):50–6.
17. Dello Strologo L, Guzzo I, Laurenzi C, Vivarelli M, Parodi A, Barbano G, et al. Use of rituximab in focal glomerulosclerosis relapses after renal transplantation. Transplantation. 2009;88(3):417–20.
18. Floege J. Recurrent IgA nephropathy after renal transplantation. Semin Nephrol. 2004;24(3):287–91.
19. Kessler M, Hiesse C, Hestin D, Mayeux D, Boubenider K, Charpentier B. Recurrence of immunoglobulin A nephropathy after renal transplantation in the cyclosporine era. Am J Kidney Dis. 1996;28(1):99–104.
20. Andresdottir MB, Hoitsma AJ, Assmann KJ, Wetzels JF. Favorable outcome of renal transplantation in patients with IgA nephropathy. Clin Nephrol. 2001;56(4):279–88.
21. Berthoux F, El Deeb S, Mariat C, Diconne E, Laurent B, Thibaudin L. Antithymocyte globulin (ATG) induction therapy and disease recurrence in renal transplant recipients with primary IgA nephropathy. Transplantation. 2008;85(10):1505–7.
22. Kennoki T, Ishida H, Yamaguchi Y, Tanabe K. Proteinuria-reducing effects of tonsillectomy alone in IgA nephropathy recurring after kidney transplantation. Transplantation. 2009;88(7): 935–41.

23. Smith KD, Alpers CE. Pathogenic mechanisms in membranoproliferative glomerulonephritis. Curr Opin Nephrol Hypertens. 2005;14(4):396–403.
24. Lorenz EC, Sethi S, Leung N, Dispenzieri A, Fervenza FC, Cosio FG. Recurrent membranoproliferative glomerulonephritis after kidney transplantation. Kidney Int. 2010;77(8):721–8.
25. Braun MC, Stablein DM, Hamiwka LA, Bell L, Bartosh SM, Strife CF. Recurrence of membranoproliferative glomerulonephritis type II in renal allografts: The North American Pediatric Renal Transplant Cooperative Study experience. J Am Soc Nephrol. 2005;16(7):2225–33.
26. Kamar N, Izopet J, Alric L, Guilbeaud-Frugier C, Rostaing L. Hepatitis C virus-related kidney disease: an overview. Clin Nephrol. 2008;69(3):149–60.
27. Roth D, Cirocco R, Zucker K, et al. De novo membranoproliferative glomerulonephritis in hepatitis C virus-infected renal allograft recipients. Transplantation. 1995;59(12):1676–82.
28. Dabade TS, Grande JP, Norby SM, Fervenza FC, Cosio FG. Recurrent idiopathic membranous nephropathy after kidney transplantation: a surveillance biopsy study. Am J Transplant. 2008;8(6):1318–22.
29. El-Zoghby ZM, Grande JP, Fraile MG, Norby SM, Fervenza FC, Cosio FG. Recurrent idiopathic membranous nephropathy: early diagnosis by protocol biopsies and treatment with anti-CD20 monoclonal antibodies. Am J Transplant. 2009;9(12):2800–7.
30. Schwarz A, Krause PH, Offermann G, Keller F. Impact of de novo membranous glomerulonephritis on the clinical course after kidney transplantation. Transplantation. 1994;58(6):650–4.
31. Nachman PH, Segelmark M, Westman K, et al. Recurrent ANCA-associated small vessel vasculitis after transplantation: a pooled analysis. Kidney Int. 1999;56(4):1544–50.
32. Deegens JK, Artz MA, Hoitsma AJ, Wetzels JF. Outcome of renal transplantation in patients with pauci-immune small vessel vasculitis or anti-GBM disease. Clin Nephrol. 2003;59(1):1–9.
33. Hermle T, Goestemeyer AK, Sweny P, Burns A. Successful therapeutic use of rituximab in refractory Wegener's granulomatosis after renal transplantation. Clin Nephrol. 2007;68(5): 322–6.
34. Byrne MC, Budisavljevic MN, Fan Z, Self SE, Ploth DW. Renal transplant in patients with Alport's syndrome. Am J Kidney Dis. 2002;39(4):769–75.
35. Goral S, Ynares C, Shappell SB, et al. Recurrent lupus nephritis in renal transplant recipients revisited: it is not rare. Transplantation. 2003;75(5):651–6.
36. Burgos PI, Perkins EL, Pons-Estel GJ, Kendrick SA, Liu JM, Kendrick WT, et al. Risk factors and impact of recurrent lupus nephritis in patients with systemic lupus erythematosus undergoing renal transplantation: data from a single US institution. Arthritis Rheum. 2009;60(9):2757–66.
37. Zheng XL, Sadler JE. Pathogenesis of thrombotic microangiopathies. Annu Rev Pathol. 2008;3:249–77.
38. Loirat C, Niaudet P. The risk of recurrence of hemolytic uremic syndrome after renal transplantation in children. Pediatr Nephrol. 2003;18(11):1095–101.
39. Bresin E, Daina E, Noris M, et al. Outcome of renal transplantation in patients with non-Shiga toxin-associated hemolytic uremic syndrome: prognostic significance of genetic background. Clin J Am Soc Nephrol. 2006;1(1):88–99.
40. De PC. De novo thrombotic microangiopathy. An underrated complication of renal transplantation. Clin Nephrol. 2007;67(6):335–40.
41. Reynolds JC, Agodoa LY, Yuan CM, Abbott KC. Thrombotic microangiopathy after renal transplantation in the United States. Am J Kidney Dis. 2003;42(5):1058–68.
42. Karthikeyan V, Parasuraman R, Shah V, Vera E, Venkat KK. Outcome of plasma exchange therapy in thrombotic microangiopathy after renal transplantation. Am J Transplant. 2003;3(10):1289–94.
43. Han SS, Sun HK, Lee JP, Ha JW, Kim SJ, Kim YS. Outcome of renal allograft in patients with Henoch-Schönlein nephritis: single-center experience and systematic review. Transplantation. 2010;89(6):721–6.
44. Moroni G, Gallelli B, Diana A, et al. Renal transplantation in adults with Henoch-Schonlein purpura: long-term outcome. Nephrol Dial Transplant. 2008;23(9):3010–6.
45. Czarnecki PG, Lager DJ, Leung N, Dispenzieri A, Cosio FG, Fervenza FC. Long-term outcome of kidney transplantation in patients with fibrillary glomerulonephritis or monoclonal gammopathy with fibrillary deposits. Kidney Int. 2009;75(4):420–7.

46. Leung N, Lager DJ, Gertz MA, Wilson K, Kanakiriya S, Fervenza FC. Long-term outcome of renal transplantation in light-chain deposition disease. Am J Kidney Dis. 2004;43(1):147–53.
47. Gillmore JD, Madhoo S, Pepys MB, Hawkins PN. Renal transplantation for amyloid end-stage renal failure-insights from serial serum amyloid P component scintigraphy. Nucl Med Commun. 2000;21(8):735–40.
48. Keven K, Sengul S, Kutlay S, et al. Long-term outcome of renal transplantation in patients with familial Mediterranean fever amyloidosis: a single-center experience. Transplant Proc. 2004;36(9):2632–4.

About the Editors

Anil Chandraker, MB, FASN, FRCP, is the Medical Director of Kidney and Pancreas Transplantation at Brigham and Women's Hospital and Assistant Director of the Transplantation Research Center and an Associate Professor at Harvard Medical School. He is the author of over 100 original articles, review, and book chapters in the area of transplantation.

Mohamed H. Sayegh, MD, is the Raja N. Khuri Dean of the Faculty of Medicine and Vice President of Medical Affairs at the American University of Beirut. He is currently a Lecturer of Medicine and Pediatrics at Harvard Medical School, and is the Director of the Schuster Family Transplantation Research Center, Brigham and Women's Hospital and Children's Hospital Boston. In 2005, he was named the Warren E. Grupe and John P. Merrill Endowed Chair in Transplantation Medicine at Harvard Medical School.

Dr. Sayegh served as Council Member and President (2000–2001) of the American Society of Transplantation (AST). He served as the chair of the Transplant Advisory Board of the American Society of Nephrology (ASN). He also served as the chair of the AST Program, Education and Development Committees; as the chair of the 2005 ASN Program Committee; and the chair of the Program Committee of the 2006 World Transplant Congress and the 2007 World Congress of Nephrology. He served as cochair of the Steering Committee of the NIH Immune Tolerance Network and member of the Executive Committee. He also served as the chair of the Steering Committee of the NIH consortium, Clinical Trials in Organ Transplantation (CTOT).

He is recipient of many highly distinguished and prestigious awards and honors including the Clinician Scientist Award, National Kidney Foundation, the First Young Scientist Award, Wyeth-Ayerst-American Society of Transplant Physicians, the First Mentoring Award, American Society of Transplantation and the AST Basic Science Established Investigator Award (Professor Level).

Dr. Sayegh also served as Associate Editor for the *Journal of American Society of Nephrology* and Deputy Editor of the *Clinical Journal of the American Society of Nephrology*.

A. Chandraker et al. (eds.), *Core Concepts in Renal Transplantation*,
DOI 10.1007/978-1-4614-0008-0, © Springer Science+Business Media, LLC 2012

Dr. Sayegh is also a strong international leader. He served as the chair of the Scientific Advisory Board and member of the Board of Trustees of the Harvard Dubai Foundation. Most recently, Dr. Sayegh was elected into Arab Business' 2010 Power 500 – World's Most Influential Arabs.

Ajay K. Singh, MB, FRCP (UK), MBA, is an Associate Professor of Medicine at Harvard Medical School and a senior nephrologist and Director of Postgraduate Education in the Department of Medicine at Brigham and Women's Hospital (BWH) in Boston.

After obtaining his medical degree (MBBS) from University College Hospital of the University of London in London, the United Kingdom, Dr. Singh concluded his medical training with a clinical fellowship in nephrology and a research fellowship at Tufts-New England Medical Center in Boston. Dr. Singh has been Clinical Chief in the renal Division at the Brigham and Women's Hospital/Harvard Medical School for the past 10 years. During this time he has obtained an MBA from Boston University.

Dr. Singh's research interests are primarily focused on chronic kidney disease and anemia, and he is currently a principal investigator or coprincipal investigator on several studies funded by industry, various foundations, and the National Institutes of Health. A national and international presenter, Dr. Singh is the author of over 150 papers and 5 books. He serves on the editorial board of *JASN* and *Kidney International.* He is the editor of seven books in nephrology and internal medicine.

Dr. Singh is actively involved in education, particularly graduate and postgraduate medical education, and is the recipient of several awards for his contributions. He leads several Harvard Medical School courses, including in internal medicine, nephrology, and in clinical research training. He is a member of the NKF Scientific Advisory Board and the Member of the Medicare Evidence Development Advisory Committee.

Dr. Singh is a Fellow of the Royal College of Physicians in the United Kingdom, among other professional organizations.

Index

V

MIX
Papier aus verantwortungsvollen Quellen
Paper from responsible sources
FSC® C105338

If you have any concerns about our products,
you can contact us on
ProductSafety@springernature.com

In case Publisher is established outside the EU,
the EU authorized representative is:
Springer Nature Customer Service Center GmbH
Europaplatz 3, 69115 Heidelberg, Germany

Printed by Libri Plureos GmbH
in Hamburg, Germany